Depression and Personality

The Depression and Personality book series presents cutting edge knowledge regarding the causes, treatment, and prevention of depression from a perspective that takes into account the interaction between depression and personality and the influences of multiple dimensions that contribute to the development, maintenance, and exacerbation of depression in different populations. The series is published in collaboration with the Millennium Institute for Research in Depression and Personality (MIDAP), a scientific center of excellence in Chile made up of psychologists, psychiatrists and professionals from various areas of social sciences and health, who seek to generate knowledge based on a multidimensional understanding of depression.

MIDAP's characteristic multidimensional and multidisciplinary approach implies the development of an empirically-based model that takes into account the etiology, prevention, intervention, and rehabilitation of depression. This multidimensional and multidisciplinary model is evidenced in the titles of the series, which cover, individually or in combination, the following topics:

1. Basic bio-psycho-social structures and processes involved in depression and its interaction with the personality.
2. Health promotion and psychosocial intervention strategies that would prevent early conditions associated with the development of depression and personality dysfunction.
3. Psychotherapeutic interventions and mechanisms involved in symptomatic relief and change processes in diverse types of depressive patients.
4. Rehabilitation and reintegration interventions oriented to reduce the chronicity of depression and to maintain gains after treatment, as well as, topics regarding early-life maltreatment and co-morbid personality dysfunction as risk factors of chronic or recurrent courses of depression.

Vania Martínez • Claudia Miranda-Castillo
Editors

Prevention and Early Treatment of Depression Through the Life Course

Springer

Editors
Vania Martínez
Faculty of Medicine
Universidad de Chile
Santiago, Chile

Claudia Miranda-Castillo
Faculty of Nursing
Universidad Andrés Bello
Santiago, Chile

ISSN 2662-3587 ISSN 2662-3595 (electronic)
Depression and Personality
ISBN 978-3-031-13028-1 ISBN 978-3-031-13029-8 (eBook)
https://doi.org/10.1007/978-3-031-13029-8

This Springer imprint is published by the registered company Springer Nature Switzerland AG
The registered company address is: Gewerbestrasse 11, 6330 Cham, Switzerland

Contents

Chapter 1
Introduction

Thamara Tapia-Muñoz, Claudia Miranda-Castillo, and Vania Martínez

Depression is considered a preventable health disease and an important public health problem (The Lancet, 2022). Different public health services are offered in order to tackle depression globally with increasing effectiveness (Herrman et al., 2022; The Lancet, 2022). So far, countries have made advances in building public health capacity, including national plans and policies to provide care for all ages. Yet, especially after the COVID-19 emergency, it is known that depression is far from being a resolved problem (Santomauro et al., 2021). The Mental Health Gap Action Programme (mhGAP) was settled to address the gap between the need and provision of health services, especially among low- and middle-income countries (World Health Organization, 2015). The program included depression as one of the priorities because of its high prevalence and burden. Actions needed to reduce the mental health gap included improving mental health literacy among the community

T. Tapia-Muñoz
Department of Behavioural Science and Health, University College London, London, UK

Millennium Nucleus on Sociomedicine (SocioMed), Santiago, Chile

Millennium Institute for Care Research (MICARE), Santiago, Chile

C. Miranda-Castillo
Millennium Institute for Care Research (MICARE), Santiago, Chile

Facultad de Enfermería, Universidad Andrés Bello, Santiago, Chile

Millennium Institute for Research in Depression and Personality (MIDAP), Santiago, Chile

V. Martínez (✉)
Millennium Institute for Research in Depression and Personality (MIDAP), Santiago, Chile

CEMERA, Facultad de Medicina, Universidad de Chile, Santiago, Chile

Millennium Nucleus to Improve the Mental Health of Adolescents and Youths (Imhay), Santiago, Chile
e-mail: vmartinezn@uchile.cl

V. Martínez, C. Miranda-Castillo (eds.), *Prevention and Early Treatment of Depression Through the Life Course*, Depression and Personality,
https://doi.org/10.1007/978-3-031-13029-8_1

and health professionals, strengthening primary care, providing universal care, providing nonspecialized and specialized health workers, setting up community-based approaches to address mental health issues, and establishing promotion, prevention actions, and also evidence-based treatments (World Health Organization, 2015). In consequence, decreasing the mental health gap includes preventing depression, diagnosing it on time, and providing proper treatment for all ages, genders, races, and contexts around the world, with the involvement of all sectors (Herrman et al., 2022; Votruba & Thornicroft, 2016).

Additionally, mental health was included as part of the United Nations' 17 Sustainable Development Goals. The third goal stated a 30% reduction of the "premature mortality from non-communicable diseases through prevention, treatment and promotion of mental health and well-being by 2030" (General Assembly, 2015). Depression, as one of the leading noncommunicable diseases, is related to Sustainable Development Goals by both directly affecting mental health and indirectly restricting people's access to education, work, nutrition, and housing, among other negative consequences (Herrman et al., 2022).

Depression is a broader term used to designate a group of depressive disorders characterized by a syndrome of depressive mood accompanied by emotional, behavioral, and cognitive manifestations (World Health Organization, 2019). The current diagnostic manuals, DSM-5 (American Psychiatric Association, 2013) and ICD-11 (World Health Organization, 2019) share common symptoms and signs to identify depressive disorders, that is, if at least two conditions are met, the presence of depressive mood (low mood) or the presence of anhedonia (lack of interest or lack of pleasure in regular activities), plus at least 2 weeks of these manifestations (World Health Organization, 2019). The symptoms have to affect functionality significantly and should not be secondary to a disease or a response to substance use (World Health Organization, 2019). Both manuals recognize single episodes with mild, moderate, and severe manifestations, as well as chronic disorders, recurrent episodes, and suicide risk. Also, the criteria apply to diagnosing depression with melancholia or psychotic symptoms (Herrman et al., 2022) and exclude depression associated with bipolar disorders (World Health Organization, 2019).

The average prevalence of major depressive disorder (MDD) is 4.5% (Bromet et al., 2018). MDD is associated with an increased risk of death due to suicide, disability, and harm to the new generations (Herrman et al., 2022; World Health Organization, 2021). It is also associated with difficulties in a full integration into society due to loss of functionality or stigma (Ferrari et al., 2022; The Lancet, 2016). The Global Burden of Diseases, Injuries, and Risk Factors Study (GBD) 2019 (Ferrari et al., 2022) showed that depressive disorders were among the 25 principal causes of burden for women and men across the lifespan (Vos et al., 2020). They accounted for 37.3 million (32.3–43.0) disability-adjusted life-years (DALYs). Depressive disorder's level of impact did not notoriously change in two decades, remaining the second leading cause of years lived with disability (YLDs) (Ferrari et al., 2022; Vos et al., 2020).

Despite the efforts to tackle depression, the COVID-19 pandemic directly or indirectly affected the mental health of the population, including an increase in the incidence of depressive disorders. In 2020, there were additional 53.2 million cases of MDD attributable to COVID-19 (Santomauro et al., 2021). Thus, the estimated prevalence of MDD was 3152.9 cases per 100,000 population, equivalent to 246 million people. Moreover, 10.7 million DALYs for MDD were estimated globally, with a higher burden for women than men (Santomauro et al., 2021).

Depressive disorders affect people of different ages. Depression across the lifespan has similarities but also has its features. Among children and adolescents, the disease manuals recognize symptoms like lack of interest in school, grades problems, and risk for self-harm and suicide attempt as substitutions for depressive mood (Rao & Chen, 2009). Suicide is one of the most important causes of death in adolescents (Vos et al., 2020). Depressive disorders were also the first cause of years lived with disability (YLDs) for people 14 years and older (Ferrari et al., 2022). In the case of older adults, depression might manifest with somatic symptoms and pain, lack of interest in social involvement activities, cognitive decline, and a low energy level without feeling sad. In male older adults, anger is a common feature (Blazer, 2003). Among older adults with late-onset depression (first episode after 60 years old), the prevalence of depression is 28%, while the prevalence of MDD is 13%. This last one increases in people 80 years and older (Abdoli et al., 2022; Hu et al., 2022).

Depressive disorders are underdiagnosed and undertreated in young and older people (Blazer, 2003; Bromet et al., 2018; Stein & Fazel, 2015). Because of the characteristics of adolescence and older adulthood, people can consider depression signs and symptoms as natural, neglecting a proper diagnosis (Herrman et al., 2022). The barriers identified for the existing gap in mental health services for children and adolescents are associated with both individual factors, such as mental health literacy, not verbalizing their need for help, and low adherence to treatment, and social factors like stigma toward mental illness and lack of trust in professionals, especially related to confidentiality. Additionally, structural barriers might be the cost of mental health services and the difficulties of making an appointment with a mental health professional (Werlen et al., 2020). Regarding older adults, the barriers related to mental health services gaps are, for example, the lack of belief in the effectiveness of treatments, the idea that symptoms are normal, fear of medication, the cost of treatments, and transportation difficulties (Wuthrich & Frei, 2015).

Across countries, there are individual differences and social-economic factors that make some groups more at risk of developing depression. Black women, without a partner, with lower educational levels, lower incomes, and living in low-income countries are at higher risk of negative mental health outcomes, including depression (Allen et al., 2014). In addition, women who have just given birth (within the first 4 weeks) are at increased risk of depression even without a previous history of mental health issues. The postpartum depression prevalence was 17% among women (Shorey et al., 2018). Even though men also experience postpartum depression (PPD), they have a lower risk than women (Wang et al., 2021). The physical and mental health of the mother and her children is impacted by postpartum depression (Dadi et al., 2020).

In adulthood, particular circumstances might increase the risk of depression. This is the case of someone who cares for a person with a chronic disease or disability (del-Pino-Casado et al., 2019; Mårtensson et al., 2020; Scherer et al., 2019). Caregivers of people with dementia have been largely described as a risk group for depression and other mental health issues due to their exposure to a high level of emotional, physical, and economic demand (Collins & Kishita, 2020). Addressing caregivers' mental health is considered part of an integral approach to tackling dementia since people living with dementia's mental health and their prognosis are closely related to caregivers' mental health (Livingston et al., 2020).

A life-course perspective on the analysis of depression might enhance the understanding of the mechanisms associated with the onset of depression and identify/develop proper evidence-based treatments for different ages and in different circumstances (Allen et al., 2014; Colman & Ataullahjan, 2010). Collaborative care programs within public health seem to be the most effective strategy for all ages, particularly for older adults (Herrman et al., 2022). Nevertheless, in some groups, like caregivers with people living with dementia, those collaborative care programs should integrate specific adapted non-pharmacological treatments (Livingston et al., 2020). Cognitive behavioral therapies (Gautam et al., 2020) and mindfulness-based therapies have shown good results for people of all ages and across contexts (Hofmann & Gómez, 2017). Moreover, new technologies have been developed in the past decades. Technology-based interventions apply to children, adolescents, and adults. They reduce the cost and distance difficulties of other non-pharmacological interventions (Cukrowicz & Joiner Jr., 2007; Grist et al., 2019; Köhnen et al., 2021).

This book is part of the "Depression and Personality" book series. Through these pages, we present current evidence of new perspectives for the prevention and appropriate management of depression in people across the life cycle. A special focus has been given to facilitating factors for the development of health system capacity and the effectiveness of the different types of interventions. The first part of the book reviews the innovations in global prevention and non-pharmacological treatments for children, adolescents, and youths. Chapter 2, "Innovations in Closing the Global Prevention and Treatment Gap for Depression in Children, Adolescents, and Youths," presents evidence related to building clinical capacity and expanding mental health coverage, testing the interventions' attainability, agreeableness, utility, and adequacy in different settings, including low- and middle-income countries. Chapter 3, "Preventing Depression in Children and Adolescents Through Mindfulness-Based Interventions in Schools," assesses current evidence on mindfulness-based interventions (MBIs) implemented in the school context. Chapter 4, "Digital Technology Interventions for Preventing and Treating Youth Depression," discusses the use of digital technologies as an alternative or complement treatment to conventional mental health services. Chapter 5, "Contemplation of Nature to Promote Mental Health and Prevent Depression in Youth," describes the effectiveness of nature-based interventions and their applicability for young people in different contexts. Finally, Chap. 6, "Internet-Based Interventions for Prevention and Early Treatment of Depression in Higher Education Students," reviews the benefit of Internet-based interventions for young adults focusing on people living in negative environments within schools.

The second part of this book reviews interventions for adults across the lifespan. Chapter 7, "Interventions for Adult Depression in Primary Health-Care Clinics," discusses the feasibility, effectiveness, and cost-effectiveness of psychosocial, psychological, and pharmacological interventions for depression in primary health-care settings. Chapter 8, "The Potential of Internet-Based Psychological Interventions for Perinatal Depression Prevention and Treatment," covers postpartum depression and how Internet-based treatments could help to overcome barriers for health-care providers and patients, holding promising results for cost-effective interventions. Chapter 9, "Preventive and Early Treatment of Depression in Older Adults," reviews the interventions that have shown positive results in preventing or treating timely and effectively this disorder in older adults. Finally, Chap. 10, "Depressive Disorders Among Family Caregivers of People Living with Dementia," analyzes the context of caregiving for a person living with dementia and evidence-based psychosocial approaches to address depressive symptoms in that group.

Acknowledgments This manuscript was supported by ANID – Millennium Science Initiative Program – ICS13_005, ICS2019_024, and NCS2021_081. In addition, TT-M received funding from ANID – Doctorado Internacional/2020-72210393, CM-C from ANID – FONDECYT – 1191726, and VM from ANID – FONDECYT – 1221230.

References

Abdoli, N., Salari, N., Darvishi, N., Jafarpour, S., Solaymani, M., Mohammadi, M., & Shohaimi, S. (2022). The global prevalence of major depressive disorder (MDD) among the elderly: A systematic review and meta-analysis. *Neuroscience & Biobehavioral Reviews, 132*, 1067–1073. https://doi.org/10.1016/j.neubiorev.2021.10.041

Allen, J., Balfour, R., Bell, R., & Marmot, M. (2014). Social determinants of mental health. *International Review of Psychiatry, 26*(4), 392–407.

American Psychiatric Association. (2013). *Diagnostic and statistical manual of mental disorders* (5th ed.). Author.

General Assembly. (2015). *Resolution adopted by the General Assembly on 11 September 2015*. Retrieved from https://www.eea.europa.eu/policy-documents/resolution-adopted-by-the-general

Blazer, D. G. (2003). Depression in late life: Review and commentary. *The Journals of Gerontology: Series A, 58*(3), M249–M265. https://doi.org/10.1093/gerona/58.3.M249

Bromet, E. J., Andrade, L. H., Bruffaerts, R., & Williams, D. R. (2018). Major depressive disorder. In D. J. Stein, K. M. Scott, P. de Jonge, & R. C. Kessler (Eds.), *Mental disorders around the world: Facts and figures from the WHO world mental health surveys* (pp. 41–56). Cambridge University Press.

Collins, R. N., & Kishita, N. (2020). Prevalence of depression and burden among informal caregivers of people with dementia: A meta-analysis. *Ageing and Society, 40*(11), 2355–2392. https://doi.org/10.1017/S0144686X19000527

Colman, I., & Ataullahjan, A. (2010). Life course perspectives on the epidemiology of depression. *The Canadian Journal of Psychiatry, 55*(10), 622–632. https://doi.org/10.1177/070674371005501002

Cukrowicz, K. C., & Joiner, T. E., Jr. (2007). Computer-based intervention for anxious and depressive symptoms in a non-clinical population. *Cognitive Therapy and Research, 31*(5), 677–693. https://doi.org/10.1007/s10608-006-9094-x

Dadi, A. F., Miller, E. R., & Mwanri, L. (2020). Postnatal depression and its association with adverse infant health outcomes in low- and middle-income countries: A systematic review and meta-analysis. *BMC Pregnancy and Childbirth, 20*(1), 416. https://doi.org/10.1186/s12884-020-03092-7

del-Pino-Casado, R., Rodríguez Cardosa, M., López-Martínez, C., & Orgeta, V. (2019). The association between subjective caregiver burden and depressive symptoms in carers of older relatives: A systematic review and meta-analysis. *PLoS One, 14*(5), e0217648. https://doi.org/10.1371/journal.pone.0217648

Ferrari, A., Santomauro, D., Mantilla Herrera, A., Shadid, J., Ashbaugh, C., Erskine, H. E., et al. (2022). Global, regional, and national burden of 12 mental disorders in 204 countries and territories, 1990–2019: A systematic analysis for the Global Burden of Disease Study 2019. *The Lancet Psychiatry, 9*(2), 137–150. https://doi.org/10.1016/S2215-0366(21)00395-3

Gautam, M., Tripathi, A., Deshmukh, D., & Gaur, M. (2020). Cognitive behavioral therapy for depression. *Indian Journal of Psychiatry, 62*(Suppl 2), S223–S229. https://doi.org/10.4103/psychiatry.IndianJPsychiatry_772_19

Grist, R., Croker, A., Denne, M., & Stallard, P. (2019). Technology delivered interventions for depression and anxiety in children and adolescents: A systematic review and meta-analysis. *Clinical Child and Family Psychology Review, 22*(2), 147–171. https://doi.org/10.1007/s10567-018-0271-8

Herrman, H., Patel, V., Kieling, C., Berk, M., Buchweitz, C., Cuijpers, P., et al. (2022). Time for united action on depression: A Lancet–World Psychiatric Association Commission. *The Lancet, 399*(10328), 957–1022. https://doi.org/10.1016/S0140-6736(21)02141-3

Hofmann, S. G., & Gómez, A. F. (2017). Mindfulness-based interventions for anxiety and depression. *The Psychiatric Clinics of North America, 40*(4), 739–749. https://doi.org/10.1016/j.psc.2017.08.008

Hu, T., Zhao, X., Wu, M., Li, Z., Luo, L., Yang, C., & Yang, F. (2022). Prevalence of depression in older adults: A systematic review and meta-analysis. *Psychiatry Research, 311*, 114511. https://doi.org/10.1016/j.psychres.2022.114511

Köhnen, M., Dreier, M., Seeralan, T., Kriston, L., Härter, M., Baumeister, H., & Liebherz, S. (2021). Evidence on technology-based psychological interventions in diagnosed depression: Systematic review. *JMIR Ment Health, 8*(2), e21700. https://doi.org/10.2196/21700

Livingston, G., Huntley, J., Sommerlad, A., Ames, D., Ballard, C., Banerjee, S., et al. (2020). Dementia prevention, intervention, and care: 2020 report of the Lancet Commission. *The Lancet, 396*(10248), 413–446. https://doi.org/10.1016/S0140-6736(20)30367-6

Mårtensson, E., Blomberg, O., Pettman, D., Sörensdotter, R., von Essen, L., & Woodford, J. (2020). Psychological interventions for depression among informal caregivers of older adult populations: Protocol of a systematic review and meta-analysis of randomised controlled trials. *BMJ Open, 10*(9), e036402. https://doi.org/10.1136/bmjopen-2019-036402

Rao, U., & Chen, L.-A. (2009). Characteristics, correlates, and outcomes of childhood and adolescent depressive disorders. *Dialogues in Clinical Neuroscience, 11*(1), 45–62. https://doi.org/10.31887/DCNS.2009.11.1/urao

Santomauro, D. F., Mantilla Herrera, A. M., Shadid, J., Zheng, P., Ashbaugh, C., Pigott, D. M., et al. (2021). Global prevalence and burden of depressive and anxiety disorders in 204 countries and territories in 2020 due to the COVID-19 pandemic. *The Lancet, 398*(10312), 1700–1712. https://doi.org/10.1016/S0140-6736(21)02143-7

Scherer, N., Verhey, I., & Kuper, H. (2019). Depression and anxiety in parents of children with intellectual and developmental disabilities: A systematic review and meta-analysis. *PLoS One, 14*(7), e0219888. https://doi.org/10.1371/journal.pone.0219888

Shorey, S., Chee, C. Y. I., Ng, E. D., Chan, Y. H., Tam, W. W. S., & Chong, Y. S. (2018). Prevalence and incidence of postpartum depression among healthy mothers: A systematic review and meta-analysis. *Journal of Psychiatric Research, 104*, 235–248. https://doi.org/10.1016/j.jpsychires.2018.08.001

Stein, K., & Fazel, M. (2015). Depression in young people often goes undetected. *Practitioner, 259*(1782), 17–22. 12-13.

The Lancet. (2016). The health crisis of mental health stigma. *The Lancet, 387*(10023), 1027. https://doi.org/10.1016/S0140-6736(16)00687-5

The Lancet. (2022). Ensuring care for people with depression. *The Lancet, 399*(10328), 885. https://doi.org/10.1016/S0140-6736(21)01149-1

Vos, T., Lim, S. S., Abbafati, C., Abbas, K. M., Abbasi, M., Abbasifard, M., et al. (2020). Global burden of 369 diseases and injuries in 204 countries and territories, 1990–2019: A systematic analysis for the Global Burden of Disease Study 2019. *The Lancet, 396*(10258), 1204–1222. https://doi.org/10.1016/S0140-6736(20)30925-9

Votruba, N., & Thornicroft, G. (2016). Sustainable development goals and mental health: Learnings from the contribution of the FundaMentalSDG global initiative. *Global Mental Health, 3*, e26. https://doi.org/10.1017/gmh.2016.20

Wang, D., Li, Y. L., Qiu, D., & Xiao, S. Y. (2021). Factors influencing paternal postpartum depression: A systematic review and meta-analysis. *Journal of Affective Disorders, 293*, 51–63. https://doi.org/10.1016/j.jad.2021.05.088

Werlen, L., Puhan, M. A., Landolt, M. A., & Mohler-Kuo, M. (2020). Mind the treatment gap: The prevalence of common mental disorder symptoms, risky substance use and service utilization among young Swiss adults. *BMC Public Health, 20*(1), 1470. https://doi.org/10.1186/s12889-020-09577-6

World Health Organization. (2015). *Update of the Mental Health Gap Action Programme (mhGAP) guidelines for mental, neurological and substance use disorders, 2015*. World Health Organization.

World Health Organization. (2019). *ICD-11: International classification of diseases* (11th revision). Retrieved from https://icd.who.int/

World Health Organization. (2021, 13 September 2021). *Depression: Key facts*. Retrieved from https://www.who.int/news-room/fact-sheets/detail/depression

Wuthrich, V. M., & Frei, J. (2015). Barriers to treatment for older adults seeking psychological therapy. *International Psychogeriatrics, 27*(7), 1227–1236. https://doi.org/10.1017/S1041610215000241

Part I
Children, Adolescents, and Youths

Chapter 2
Innovations in Closing the Global Prevention and Treatment Gap for Depression in Children, Adolescents, and Youths

Matías Irarrázaval

2.1 Improving Mental Health and Well-Being by Transforming Lives and Communities

Depression is a highly prevalent common mental disorder and a major public health problem worldwide. Worldwide, depression affects 13.6 million adolescents aged 10–14 and 3.5 million of those aged 15–19 (WHO, 2017). During the last three decades, the incidence of depression increased 49.86%, from 172 million in 1990 to 258 million in 2017 (Liu et al., 2020). Most recent estimates from the Global Burden of Disease study show that unipolar depressive conditions represent 4.4% of the global disease burden (65 million impairment changed life years [DALYs] lost in total), ranking third among the leading causes of disability in the world, the same range as the total burden attributable to diabetes, diarrheal diseases, or the combined impact of asthma and chronic obstructive pulmonary disease (GBD, 2019).

The COVID-19 pandemic has exacerbated the burden of depression, and the number of people predicted to experience depression rose by much more than 25% in 2020 (Santomauro et al., 2021).

Too often, depression goes undetected or untreated – even when it is at its most distressing and disabling – because services are not available, cannot be accessed, or are unaffordable, or because widespread stigma stops people from seeking help. Different belief systems, language, and idiomatic expressions around mental health across cultures also influence whether people seek help from traditional health providers, formal health services, or both (Mekonen et al., 2021). Access to effective

M. Irarrázaval (✉)
Pan American Health Organization/World Health Organization, Washington, DC, USA

Millennium Institute for Research in Depression and Personality (MIDAP), Santiago, Chile
e-mail: mirarrazavald@uchile.cl

V. Martínez, C. Miranda-Castillo (eds.), *Prevention and Early Treatment of Depression Through the Life Course*, Depression and Personality,
https://doi.org/10.1007/978-3-031-13029-8_2

mental health treatment is disturbingly limited around the world, especially in low- and middle-income countries (LMICs) (Degenhardt et al., 2017). In some countries, the treatment gap for depression is a staggering 90% (Liu et al., 2020). The World Mental Health surveys showed that in high-income countries, only 22% of all individuals with 12-month MDD received minimally adequate treatment (Thornicroft et al., 2017). Furthermore, there is a significant shortage of human resources for mental health, particularly in LMICs (Sarikhani et al., 2021). As a result, universal mental health coverage for depression remains far out of reach.

Innovative strategies involving healthcare systems, mental health professionals, and consumers can be important to close the depression treatment gap and make the best use of available resources. Evidence-based innovative strategies that have the potential to substantially reduce the disease treatment gap of depression are discussed further below.

2.2 Scaling Up Care for Depression

The high prevalence and extensive treatment gap for depression imply that countries need to diversify and scale up options for care. Innovative evidence-based psychological care is available to expand existing health and mental health services that can be implemented in countries that are willing to reduce the depression treatment gap.

2.2.1 Nonspecialist Counseling

Counseling programs that recruit, train, and deploy nonspecialist counselors to deliver group or individual psychological interventions in the country's territories have proven to be highly effective in the treatment of depression.

Nonspecialist counseling can also add substantial value to specialized psychological care. As an example, in a specialized psychological healthcare center in Islamabad, Pakistan, a quick mental intervention, Problem Management Plus (PM+), was incorporated into regular, mostly medicinal treatment. The intervention was delivered by nonspecialist counselors that had finished a bachelor's degree in psychology. The program was found to substantially improve results for people with depression (Hamdani et al., 2021).

Additionally, counseling may be directed and also supported to be implemented in primary healthcare and community setups, scaling up the intervention in the different levels of care. In Uganda and Zambia, the social enterprise StrongMinds have trained lay employees as well as volunteers in a culturally adapted and locally validated interpersonal treatment to treat depression in adolescents. Groups of usually 12 adolescents meet in their neighborhoods and are trained in eight or more sessions, developing skills that can be used for depression treatment and prevention of future relapses (Bolton et al., 2003). Through this form of therapy, the lay therapists assist team individuals to identify their depression causes (extended bereavement, disagreements, isolation or social seclusion, and adjustments in one's life) and also layout strategies to overcome them. As clinical depression can reoccur, the skills acquired with treatment have both a prompt and long-term preventive effect on the persons treated. Over the past eight years, the program has treated more than 100,000 persons with depression, with a recovery rate of 80%, a 30% increase in school attendance, a 28% increase in social connectedness, and a 13% increase in families sharing meal time together (StrongMinds, 2021).

Nonspecialist counseling programs can be implemented at the primary care level of services and also in community-based settings. Research studies show that these programs can increase the ability of frontline psychological health services as well as considerably improve treatment. As an example, one program in the North-West Province of South Africa identified individuals with depression among patients with the persistent condition in a collective care program and refer those with moderate depressive symptoms to lay counselors for structured counseling based on cognitive behavioral therapy. The research study discovered substantial reductions in symptoms at year follow-up. Users reported feeling more equipped and far better outfitted to deal with social issues (Petersen et al., 2016).

Indeed, nonspecialist counseling programs can be and increasingly are implemented within primary care facilities and other community-based settings, including through stand-alone services run by NGOs. Studies show that these programs can boost the capacity of frontline mental health services and greatly improve care. For example, one program in Peru identified people with depression among patients with HIV in a collaborative care program and refered those with mild to moderate depressive symptoms to lay counselors for Psychological First Aid (PFA) intervention (Galea et al., 2021). The study found that the use of a simple care pathway operationalizing depression screening and nonspecialist delivered psychological support allows for the reduction of symptoms and the integrations of depression and HIV care for adolescents (Andrews et al., 2018).

In Zimbabwe, the Friendship Bench (FB) project has been incorporating psychological wellness into other wellness programs for more than 20 years. The project uses analytical treatments delivered by neighborhood volunteers, known as "grannies," to resolve "kufungisisa" (depression). The model has also been adapted to be more relevant for adolescents and the Youth Friendship Bench intervention (YouFB) task-shifts youth lay health workers to offer a culturally contextualized, manual-based, six-session problem-solving therapy to adolescents, 16–19 years of age. Unlike the "grannies" in FB, YouFB has younger lay health workers, mostly psychology and sociology students who perform a 1-year internship at the YouFB before their last year of college. YouFB is delivered not only in clinics but also in public parks and other community settings, with a focus on topics such as drug use, sex, and relationships in vulnerable populations (Broström et al., 2021).

2.2.2 Self-Help

Self-help can be guided (when a worker helps the person in the use of the materials) or unguided (when the person receives no support or even encouragement in using the materials). Both specialists and nonspecialists can have a role in supporting guided self-help interventions for depression. For example, they can facilitate discussions, demonstrate techniques, and support people to work through self-help materials; and they can do this face-to-face or remotely. Self-help interventions can be delivered rapidly to large numbers of people, making them particularly useful for scale-up. A recent meta-analysis indicates that low-intensity psychological interventions show promising results for children and adolescents in efficacy trials (Bennett et al., 2019).

Improving Access to Psychological Therapies (IAPT) is a national program for evidence-based mental treatments for depression in the United Kingdom. IAPT has a stepped care approach in which gradually intensive therapies are provided according to the needs. People are initially provided low-intensity, guided self-help based on principles of cognitive behavioral therapy (CBT). The self-help is psychoeducational and is delivered over the phone, through digital CBT, in big teams, or separately.

Released in 2008 as a solution for adults, the program has expanded to children and young people (CYP). The CYP IAPT program's goal has shifted from workforce development to workforce growth since 2017, with the program training 1700 additional psychologists. Based on the initial CYP IAPT curriculum, the CYP IAPT program currently has three training streams: (a) a low-intensity workforce, (b) a school-based workforce, and (c) a high-intensity workforce (Ludlow et al., 2020). People who do not improve after guided self-help are stepped up to receive high-intensity psychological therapies by qualified therapists. A meta-analysis of 60 studies on IAPT found that the program has generated large pre- to posttreatment effect sizes for depression (Wakefield et al., 2021).

The program has been a model for establishing comparable services in Australia, Canada, Japan, and also Norway. Step-by-Step is a new guided, technology-supported, intervention for depression developed by the World Health Organization (WHO). It provides psychoeducation through a narrated story and uses interactive exercises to support additional therapeutic techniques focusing on behavior activation combined with stress management (slow breathing), strengths identification, positive self-talk, increasing social support, and relapse prevention. Step-by-Step was created for usage in a variety of cultural contexts and resource availability, as well as to be relevant in adversity-affected communities. Step-by-Step has been culturally adapted to address depression among Chinese young adults (Sit et al., 2020).

In Lebanon, the Ministry of Public Health with partners tested an adapted version of Step-by-Step called "Khoutweh-Khoutweh" with Lebanese citizens and displaced Syrians. A guided self-help format was used in which supervised nonspecialist counselors provided no more than 15 minutes of remote guidance (by phone or online) per week to people with symptoms of depression. It was found to be relevant, acceptable, and beneficial by those who completed it. Two randomized controlled trials with more than 1000 participants suggest that the intervention was effective in reducing symptoms of depression and improving functioning and well-being. After completing the research, the intervention is now offered by the government as a routine service (Harper Shehadeh et al., 2020).

Even unguided, self-help books and materials can be useful in scaling up psychological support for common mental health conditions. Research shows that bibliotherapy (the use of books as therapy) effectively reduces depressive symptoms, including in the long term (Yuan et al., 2018). "Computer therapy" that delivers CBT for depression and anxiety through the Internet has similarly been shown to be effective, acceptable, and practical, providing equal benefits to traditional face-to-face CBT (Andrews et al., 2018; Martínez et al., 2021).

2.3 Supporting Child and Adolescent Mental Health Services

Standard mental healthcare is usually provided via two discrete systems, child and adolescent mental health services (CAMHS) and adult mental health services. In most LMICs, child and adolescent mental health services are much less available than the adult ones (Zhou et al., 2020).

In response, there has been a growing movement to develop integrated community-based hubs providing uninterrupted services for adolescents and young adults. In addition to mental health services, these hubs often deliver other health and social services in a single community-based setting. They are sometimes referred to as 'one-stop services'. Headspace started in 2006 in Australia, to address the gap in traditional services in supporting young people aged 12–25 years experiencing mental health problems. While each center is deliberately located near public transport for easy access, local youth help design each center and the services it provides. Mental health professionals at the centers provide evidence-based psychological care, and young people can also access physical and sexual health services, work and study support.

A key feature of Headspace is the 'no wrong door' policy. This means that young people can refer themselves or be referred from any service. All centers routinely report data to a national database that is used to monitor and evaluate service activity and outcomes, and inform continuous improvement (Jensen et al., 2016; Rickwood et al., 2019). There is now more than 100 Headspace in Australia and 28 in Denmark.

2.4 Mental Health Services Beyond the Health Sector

Healthcare alone is often not enough to meet all the needs of people living with mental health conditions, especially those living in poverty or without housing, education, or the means to generate an income. This means that other sectors have a key role in complementing any mental health services provided by the health sector.

Depression treatment alone is frequently insufficient to address all the requirements of children and adolescents living with mental health conditions, particularly those who are poor or lack housing, education, or the means to earn a living. As a result, other sectors play a critical role in enhancing any mental health treatments given by the health sector (WHO, 2019). Taking a multisectoral approach to depression prevention, treatment and recovery include services for persons with mental health conditions into the policies and activities of all relevant sectors, such as livelihood support, housing, education, vocational training, employment, social welfare, and legal assistance. It is necessary to take a whole-of-government strategy.

2.4.1 Mental Healthcare and Depression Prevention in School Settings

Mental health activities in non-health settings are largely focused on mental health promotion and prevention activities.

Early Detection and Intervention in Schools Schools operate where most school-age children are, have access to families, are free at the point of use, and overcome traditional access barriers such as inconvenient location, costly transportation, and stigma. Therefore, schools provide a strong platform for early detection and treatment of depression in children and adolescents.

Social and emotional learning programs in schools have been related to mental health benefits at all socioeconomic levels (Fazel, Hoagwood et al., 2014; Fazel, Patel et al., 2014). They may be offered to students of all ages, but are especially beneficial in supporting teenage mental health, as they have been shown to increase emotional well-being, social functioning, and academic success. They have also been linked to a lower risk of depression, as well as the prevention of suicide, substance use, antisocial conduct, and risky sexual practices (Greenberg et al., 2017).

The potential role of schools in securing student mental health and well-being is well recognized in WHO's Global School Wellness Initiative. The Initiative proposes that mental health should be included in comprehensive school healthcare, according to the latest WHO recommendations for school health services (WHO & UNESCO, 2021). According to the standards, school health services should be able to conduct screening and clinical assessments (using the HEADSSS instrument) for referral and assistance for a variety of mental health disorders, including depression (Smith & McGuinness, 2017). The guidelines also propose that school health services include crisis and substance use counseling, as well as support policies on bullying and health promotion.

School-based counseling can be used as a preventative intervention for children who are showing early indications of depression, as an evaluation tool, as early intervention, or as a support to specialized mental health services. All counseling seeks to give young people a safe place to talk about their problems in a supportive setting and to help them find their solutions. Counseling may include working with a family or a group. Counselors in schools can help connect students and their families with social and specialized services (WHO, 2021). School professionals, social service organizations, and others can be trained on specific mental health conditions intervention techniques (including depression, suicide, and pathological gaming) and on how to support youths with caregivers experiencing mental health issues. Since 2007, the Response, Early Intervention, and Assessment in Community Mental Health (REACH) project in Singapore has established regional multidisciplinary and intersectoral networks of care to give frontline help to students with mental health problems. School counselors are taught to recognize emotional, social, and behavioral problems in children and refer them to a REACH clinicians' mobile case management team for assessment and intervention. REACH teams are made up of a mix of doctors, psychologists, medical social workers, occupational therapists, and psychiatric nurses who are at a regional hospital to provide continuity of care if further expert services are needed. Counselors have referred over 4000 adolescents to REACH teams between 2007 and 2015 (Lim et al., 2017).

Social and Emotional Learning Programs Helping Adolescents Thrive (HAT) is a joint WHO-UNICEF initiative to strengthen programming and policy responses for adolescents, to promote positive mental health, prevent mental health conditions, and prevent self-harm and other risk behaviors. The HAT initiative aims to protect and promote adolescent mental health by routinely implementing and monitoring evidence-informed and human rights-based strategies for improving mental health and preventing and reducing mental health and substance use conditions in adolescents (Berger et al., 2016). The HAT initiative advocates a broad approach to school-based social and emotional learning that uses a mix of interventions to build mental health awareness; strengthen emotional, cognitive, and social skills; and engage in physical activity (WHO & UNICEF, 2021).

Table 2.1 shows psychosocial interventions for social and emotional learning strategies to promote and protect adolescent mental health and reduce self-harm and other risk behaviors.

Universal school-based social and emotional learning programs can be embedded into the usual school curriculum and delivered by teachers. For example, a universal randomized controlled effectiveness trial to increase depression literacy shows that ADAP, a short school-based intervention (3 hours throughout 2- or 3-course periods), significantly increased depression literacy in both boys and girls (Swartz et al., 2017).

According to research, a whole-school approach to social learning programs might be beneficial. A cluster randomized trial of a whole-school health promotion

Table 2.1 Psychosocial interventions for social and emotional learning

Learning goal		Intervention
Emotional	Emotion regulation	Techniques to improve one's ability to manage and respond to emotions effectively
	Stress management	Techniques to control levels of stress, especially chronic stress that interferes with everyday functioning
	Mindfulness	Activities to enhance abilities to pay attention purposefully, in the present, and without judgment
Cognitive	Problem-solving	Techniques to identify and act on a solution to a challenge or difficult problem
	Drug and alcohol knowledge	Education about the use of drugs and alcohol and their effects
Social	Interpersonal skills	Improving skills to develop or improve close, strong, positive relationships with others
	Assertiveness	Improving skills to communicate one's viewpoint, needs, or wishes clearly and respectfully
Physical	Physical activity	Opportunities to engage in sports or physical activity, either individually or in teams

Source: Helping Adolescents Thrive toolkit: strategies to promote and protect adolescent mental health and reduce self-harm and other risk behaviors. Geneva: World Health Organization and United Children's Fund; 2021. License: CC BY-NC-SA 3.0 IGO (https://apps.who.int/iris/handle/10665/341327, accessed 10 March 2022)

intervention in Bihar, India, found that it was more effective than classroom-based treatments at improving school environment at a 1-year follow-up, with substantial positive benefits on depressive symptoms, bullying, and violence (although only when delivered by lay counselors, not teachers) (Shinde et al., 2018). These effects were shown to last over time, with similar effect sizes during the 2-year follow-up. (Shinde et al., 2020). Overall, there is evidence to support psychological preventive interventions, delivered across the school in preventing depression at the universal level. This is combined with existing review evidence to support physical activity interventions for the prevention of depression (Hoare et al., 2021).

Such programs are not only effective but can bring good economic returns (WHO, 2021) (Table 2.2). One investment case for the Philippines calculated that the return on investment (including productivity gains and social value of health) of universal school-based social and emotional learning programs was 14.8 to 1 over 20 years (WHO, 2021).

Anti-bullying Interventions Within any universal school-based promotion and prevention program, anti-bullying interventions are especially important to improve school safety and protect the mental health of both victims and perpetrators, in the short term and throughout the life span.

Bullying can take many forms: physical, verbal, social, and, since the rise of the Internet and social media, cyberbullying. Nearly one in three adolescents is a victim of bullying (Biswas et al., 2020). People who are bullied as a child are more likely to experience emotional distress and mental health conditions and to have problems

Table 2.2 Costs, health impact, and cost-effectiveness of mental health interventions

	Low- and lower middle-income countries (n = 10)			Upper middle- and high-income countries (n = 10)		
	Cost of implementation per year (I$ million per one million population)	Health impact per year (healthy life years gained per one million population)	Average cost-effectiveness ratio (I$/healthy life year gained)	Cost of implementation per year (I$ million per one million population)	Health impact per year (healthy life years gained per one million population)	Average cost-effectiveness ratio (I$/healthy life year gained)
Universal, school-based socio-emotional learning programs to improve mental health and prevent suicide in adolescents	<0.10	50–100	1000–5000	0.10–0.50	50–100	1000–5000
Indicated, school-based socio-emotional learning programs to improve mental health and prevent suicide in adolescents	<0.10	<10	10,000–50,000	0.10–0.50	<10	10,000–50,000

Adapted from WHO menu of cost-effective interventions for mental health. Geneva: World Health Organization, 2021.

adjusting to school (Smokowski & Kopasz, 2005). When relevant confounders were taken into account, there is a correlation between being bullied at the age of 15 or 18 and reporting depression symptoms at the age of 28 (Winding et al., 2020). Bullying can also result in isolation, low self-esteem, and self-harm.

Childhood bullies themselves are more likely to have academic problems in the short term and are more likely to engage in harmful substance use, antisocial behavior, and interpersonal violence later in life (Smokowski & Kopasz, 2005). Anyone involved in bullying – those who bully and/or are bullied– is more likely to have depression and anxiety (Stephens et al., 2018).

School-based anti-bullying programs focus on addressing factors in the school that fosters bullying behavior. They can decrease subsequent aggression and depression in youths, in addition to lowering bullying rates (Williford et al., 2012). Anti-bullying programs may be carried out in a variety of ways, ranging from parental and peer support interventions to staff and student awareness-raising and social and emotional skill development. Overall, school-based anti-bullying initiatives have been proven to be effective in reducing intimidation by around 20% (Good Thinking, n.d.). According to the findings, one of the most effective interventions is a multi-level, whole-school approach that includes enforcing an anti-bullying policy as well as class rules (including use of electronic devices), providing information to parents and students, including peers, and facilitating cooperative teamwork (Gaffney et al., 2019).

2.4.2 Mental Healthcare in the Child Protection and Juvenile Justice System

Child Protection Childhood adversity is a key risk factor for depression, as well as a variety of other health and social problems. To prevent and respond to all types of violence against children, including exploitation, abuse, and neglect, an efficient child protection system is essential.

Effective child protection requires a comprehensive, multistakeholder approach that can tackle the root causes of violence and abuse. The WHO and its partners advocate a seven-pronged strategy (INSPIRE) to simultaneously (WHO, 2016):

- Enact and implement laws prohibiting the use of violence against children, criminalizing sexual abuse and exploitation, limiting juvenile access to guns, and reducing dangerous alcohol consumption
- Strengthen nonviolent, respectful, caring, positive, and gender-equitable connections for all children and challenge restrictive and harmful norms through bystander interventions and community mobilization activities
- Combat the spread of violence in the community and create safe spaces where children and teens may meet and spend time

- Strengthen parent and caregiver support to prevent harsh parenting and foster strong parent-child connections
- Improve family economic security and stability through strengthening incomes, notably through social protection, group saving and loans, and microfinance
- Provide reaction and support services, such as health and social assistance, as well as psychiatric counseling and psychological therapy programs for both victims and offenders
- Increase school enrollment, create a safe school environment, and enhance children's awareness of sexual abuse and how to protect against it, life and social skills training, and teenage intimate partner violence prevention programs

Many of the youth people in the court system who have depression or other mental health conditions require treatment. According to a meta-analysis, as many as 70% of youths had a diagnosable mental health condition at any justice interaction point. This is in line with other research that shows that children with mental/behavioral health issues are overrepresented in the juvenile justice system (Abram et al., 2015). However, the frequency of mental problems varies depending on where teenagers are in the legal system, with the prevalence of mental disorders increasing as juveniles proceed through the system (Wasserman et al., 2010). Despite the significant prevalence of mental disorders –including depression– among justice-involved youths, many do not have adequate treatment (Abram et al., 2013).

There are several evidence-based programs in the juvenile justice system that specifically target youths with mental health needs –including depression– and focus on reducing delinquency and other related behavioral problems by properly addressing risk factors and mental health needs (Matthews et al., 2013).

Liaison and diversion programs, often known as 'street triage', have been created in certain high-income countries to identify persons with suspected mental health problems when they first come into contact with the juvenile justice system. These services are then used to help persons navigate the juvenile justice system in the early stages, send them to appropriate health or social services, or redirect them away from the juvenile justice system to more appropriate settings.

Crisis Intervention Team (CIT) is a model initially developed in 1988 in Memphis, Tennessee, after a police officer fatally shot a man with a history of mental illness and substance abuse. The model is designed to increase the safety of encounters with the police. Police call center dispatchers are trained to identify mental disturbance calls and assign them to CIT-trained officers; these have access to a designated psychiatric emergency drop-off site that operates a no-refusal policy, reducing officer time with an individual. CIT requires police officer training and changes in police procedures as well as collaboration with mental health providers. CIT is the co-responder model of police mental health 'street', triage with the most robust evidence, but is not widely used in the countries (Puntis et al., 2018).

Integration of mental health into general health services provided to all juvenile offenders, such as the mhGAP with supportive monitoring by mental health specialists, is another recommended strategy for enhancing mental health treatment in the juvenile justice system. Mental health training for staff and juvenile offenders at all levels of the juvenile justice system can help raise awareness, challenge stigmatizing attitudes, and support mental health promotion (Gureje & Abdulmalik, 2019).

In practice, child protection and juvenile justice services are spread across many sectors and may be provided by local governments, nonprofit organizations, and community organizations. Key players in child protection include members of community protection networks, police officers, healthcare professionals, and social workers. These stakeholders have a responsibility to protect and promote the mental health and well-being of the children and adolescents in their care, in addition to protecting them from violence.

2.5 Technological Solutions to Increase Depression Treatment Coverage

The way we prevent and treat depression in children and adolescents is changing because of digital technologies. The recent increase in the accessibility and acceptance of digital interventions may promote a fundamental shift in how depression and other common mental disorders are addressed. Technology has the benefit of being easy –yet not free– accessible to young people and nonspecialist health workers. Digital technology breaks barriers and access to stigma-free mental healthcare, and is also made possible by connecting to fitness, health, and wellness applications. Traditional healthcare might be disrupted, and user interactions with the system could shift because of new types of interventions (Meskó et al., 2017). Self-care and assistance for people to look after their mental health are areas where digital technology excels. However, the impact of its usage, particularly on young people, is a significant concern.

Some research has been done on digital programs that support established healthcare systems, such as providing talking therapy via digital platforms (Fairburn & Patel, 2017). For example, MoodGYM is a free online depression intervention that has been utilized by over three-quarters of a million people since 2001 (Christensen et al., 2002). If there is no supporting assistance, one of the major drawbacks of direct-to-user treatments is the low completion rates. The E-COMPARED (European Comparative Effectiveness Research on Internet-Based Depression Treatment) project is investigating the efficacy and cost-effectiveness of blended Internet-based treatments, which are a combination of in-person and Internet-based therapies. According to the findings, patients have a high level of acceptance of blended therapies, indicating that a progressive integration of technology into normal care may be appropriate for their attitudes and requirements. It also takes into consideration the fact that cost-effectiveness is a major incentive for the implementation of digital solutions (Topooco et al., 2017).

Table 2.3 shows examples of digital solutions for depression prevention in children and adolescents.

Table 2.3 Examples of digital solutions for depression prevention in children and adolescents

Helplines for: • People in crisis, looking for information, or who just want someone to talk to. For example, Crisis Text Line for young people in Chile (Fundación Todo Mejora, 2017)
Information about: • Services, anxiety, depression, and other topics related to general well-being. For example, ReachOut in Australia (ReachOut, 2022)
Connecting with: • Services. For example, the ReachOut NextStep online self-assessment tool asks young people a series of questions to help them identify relevant services in their area (ReachOut NextStep, 2022)
Training and supervision for: • Healthcare settings. In Chile, an online e-platform enhanced collaborative care by providing primary care clinicians with virtual access to specialists who backed adolescent depression treatment. At the 12-week follow-up, satisfaction with psychological care was linked to a substantial reduction in depressed symptomatology in both groups. However, at follow-up, the intervention did appear to have equivalent effectiveness to reduce depressive symptoms compared with enhanced usual care (Martínez et al., 2018) • Schools. In Brazil, a web-based educational program was created to educate primary school teachers on the detection and classroom management of children with mental health problems. Through interactive tutorials, instructional films, and an online discussion forum with mental health professionals, teachers gained more understanding of depression, as well as less stigmatized perspectives on mental disorders, than those who received a text- and video-based program or no training (Pereira et al., 2015)
Prevention and intervention using: • E-delivery of talking therapies. For example, This Way Up in Australia (ReachOut, 2022) • Self-assessment tools and self-care platforms to improve well-being. For example, MoodGYM in Australia and Good Thinking in England (Good Thinking, n.d.) • Conversational agents or chatbots. For example, Woebot in the United States (Good Thinking, n.d.). supporting delivery by: • Screening. For example, the mhGAP depression-screening tool used by nonspecialist health workers in primary care in rural Kenya (Musyimi et al., 2018) • Treatment support. For example, monitoring strategies to help ensure medication or therapy compliance (Mohr et al., 2013) • Telepsychiatry. For example, in Chile, a telepsychiatry consultation program for rural PHC clinics was found to be feasible and useful to support clinicians in the management of institutionalized children and adolescents with complex psychosocial care needs living in a poorly resourced setting (Mundt et al., 2021)

2.6 Conclusions

In many countries of the world, there is a significant and widespread mental health-care gap for depression, which is worsened in limited resource settings. However, innovative strategies to close this gap have been studied and proven to be effective. At least four areas have been discussed that countries can develop to close the depression treatment gap: (1) scaling up care for depression, (2) supporting child and adolescent mental health services, (3) mental health services beyond the health sector, and (4) technological solutions to increase depression treatment coverage. The examples in this chapter demonstrate the effectiveness of these strategies. More research is needed on its feasibility, value, acceptability, and efficacy, particularly in LMICs and other resource-constrained situations.

Finally, here is an action plan for policymakers and other stakeholders based on the innovations described above:

- Take the lead and commit to improving depression prevention and treatment.
- Increase investments in low-cost interventions for depression that might significantly enhance depression therapy.
- Keep track and assess depression services outcomes and indicators, ensuring that they are focused on the needs of service users, their families, and caregivers.
- Provide comprehensive, integrated, and responsive mental health and social care services for depression in community-based settings.
- Integrate and coordinate holistic prevention, promotion, rehabilitation, care, and support that aims at meeting both mental and physical healthcare needs and facilitates the recovery of children and adolescents with depression within and across general health and social services.
- Build the knowledge and skills of general and specialized health workers to deliver evidence-based, culturally appropriate, and human rights-oriented mental health and social care services, for children and adolescents.
- Include mental health into undergraduate and graduate curricula.
- Through training and mentoring health workers in the field, particularly in non-specialized settings, identify and offer treatment and support to people with mental disorders as well as to refer people, as appropriate, to other levels of care.

Conflict of Interest The author has no relevant financial or nonfinancial interests to disclose.

Acknowledgments This manuscript was supported by ANID – Millennium Science Initiative Program – ICS13_005.

References

Abram, K. M., Teplin, L. A., King, D. C., Longworth, S. L., Emanuel, K. M., Romero, E. G., & Olson, N. D. (2013). *PTSD, trauma, and comorbid psychiatric disorders in detained youth*. US Department of Justice, Office of Justice Programs, Office of Juvenile Justice and Delinquency Prevention.

Abram, K. M., Zwecker, N. A., Welty, L. J., Hershfield, J. A., Dulcan, M. K., & Teplin, L. A. (2015). Comorbidity and continuity of psychiatric disorders in youth after detention: A prospective longitudinal study. *JAMA Psychiatry, 72*(1), 84–93.

Alozkan Sever, C., Cuijpers, P., Mittendorfer-Rutz, E., Bryant, R. A., Dawson, K. S., Holmes, E. A., et al. (2021). Feasibility and acceptability of problem management plus with emotional processing (PM+ EP) for refugee youth living in the Netherlands: Study protocol. *European Journal of Psychotraumatology, 12*(1), 1947003.

Andrews, G., Basu, A., Cuijpers, P., Craske, M. G., McEvoy, P., English, C. L., et al. (2018). Computer therapy for the anxiety and depression disorders is effective, acceptable and practical health care: An updated meta-analysis. *Journal of Anxiety Disorders, 55*, 70–78. https://doi.org/10.1016/j.janxdis.2018.01.001

Bennett, S. D., Cuijpers, P., Ebert, D. D., McKenzie Smith, M., Coughtrey, A. E., Heyman, I., et al. (2019). Practitioner review: Unguided and guided self-help interventions for common mental health disorders in children and adolescents: A systematic review and meta-analysis. *Journal of Child Psychology and Psychiatry, 60*(8), 828–847.

Berger, R., Gelkopf, M., Heineberg, Y., & Zimbardo, P. (2016). A school-based intervention for reducing posttraumatic symptomatology and intolerance during political violence. *Journal of Educational Psychology, 108*(6), 761. https://doi.org/10.1037/edu0000066. Accessed 14 March 2022.

Biswas, T., Scott, J. G., Munir, K., Thomas, H. J., Huda, M. M., Hasan, M. M., de Vries, T. D., Baxter, J., & Mamun, A. A. (2020). Global variation in the prevalence of bullying victimisation amongst adolescents: Role of peer and parental supports. *eClinicalMedicine, 20*, 100276. https://doi.org/10.1016/j.eclinm.2020.100276

Bolton, P., Bass, J., Neugebauer, R., Verdeli, H., Clougherty, K. F., Wickramaratne, P., Speelman, L. N., & Weissman, M. (2003). Group interpersonal psychotherapy for depression in rural Uganda: A randomized controlled trial. *Journal of the American Medical Association, 289*(23), 3117–3124.

Broström, S., Johansson, B. A., Verhey, R., & Landgren, K. (2021). "Seeing a brighter future"–experiences of adolescents with common mental disorders receiving the problem-solving therapy "youth friendship bench" in Zimbabwe. *Issues in Mental Health Nursing, 42*(11), 1019–1029.

Christensen, H., Griffiths, K. M., & Korten, A. (2002). Web-based cognitive behavior therapy: Analysis of site usage and changes in depression and anxiety scores. *Journal of Medical Internet Research, 4*(1), e857.

Degenhardt, L., Glantz, M., Evans-Lacko, S., Sadikova, E., Sampson, N., Thornicroft, G., et al. (2017). Estimating treatment coverage for people with substance use disorders: An analysis of data from the world mental health surveys. *World Psychiatry, 16*(3), 299–307.

Fairburn, C. G., & Patel, V. (2017). The impact of digital technology on psychological treatments and their dissemination. *Behaviour Research and Therapy, 88*, 19–25.

Fazel, M., Hoagwood, K., Stephan, S., & Ford, T. (2014). Mental health interventions in schools in high-income countries. *The Lancet Psychiatry, 1*(5), 377–387.

Fazel, M., Patel, V., Thomas, S., & Tol, W. (2014). Mental health interventions in schools in low-income and middle-income countries. *The Lancet Psychiatry, 1*(5), 388–398.

Fundación Todo Mejora. (2017). Materiales sobre diversidad sexual, prevención del suicidio y bullying.

Gaffney, H., Ttofi, M. M., & Farrington, D. P. (2019). Evaluating the effectiveness of school-bullying prevention programs: An updated meta-analytical review. *Aggression and Violent Behavior, 45*, 111–133. https://doi.org/10.1016/j.avb.2018.07.002

Galea, J. T., Contreras, C., Wong, M., Ramos, K., Vargas, V., Sánchez, H., Errea, R. A., Lecca, L., & Franke, M. F. (2021). A non-specialist depression care pathway for adolescents living with HIV and transitioning into adult care in Peru: A nested, proof of concept pilot study. *Global Mental Health (Cambridge, England), 8*, e17. https://doi.org/10.1017/gmh.2021.16

GBD 2019 Mental Disorders Collaborators. (2022). Global, regional, and national burden of 12 mental disorders in 204 countries and territories, 1990–2019: A systematic analysis for the Global Burden of Disease Study 2019. *The Lancet Psychiatry, 9*(2), 137–150.

Good Thinking. (n.d.). Available at www.good-thinking.uk. Accessed 9 March 2022.

Greenberg, M. T., Domitrovich, C. E., Weissberg, R. P., & Durlak, J. A. (2017). Social and emotional learning as a public health approach to education. *The Future of Children, 27*, 13–32.

Gureje, O., & Abdulmalik, J. (2019). Severe mental disorders among prisoners in low-income and middle-income countries: Reaching the difficult to reach. *The Lancet Global Health, 7*(4), e392–e393.

Hamdani, S. U., Huma, Z. E., Masood, A., Zhou, K., Ahmed, Z., Nazir, H., et al. (2021). Effect of adding a psychological intervention to routine care of common mental disorders in a specialized mental healthcare facility in Pakistan: A randomized controlled trial. *International Journal of Mental Health Systems, 15*(1), 1–12.

Harper Shehadeh, M. J., Abi Ramia, J., Cuijpers, P., El Chammay, R., Heim, E., Kheir, W., et al. (2020). Step-by-step, an e-mental health intervention for depression: A mixed methods pilot study from Lebanon. *Frontiers in Psychiatry, 10*, 986.

Hoare, E., Collins, S., Marx, W., Callaly, E., Moxham-Smith, R., Cuijpers, P., et al. (2021). Universal depression prevention: An umbrella review of meta-analyses. *Journal of Psychiatric Research, 144*, 483–493.

Jensen, K. B., Morthorst, B. R., Vendsborg, P. B., Hjorthøj, C., & Nordentoft, M. (2016). Effectiveness of mental health first aid training in Denmark: A randomized trial in waitlist design. *Social Psychiatry and Psychiatric Epidemiology, 51*(4), 597–606.

Lim, C. G., Loh, H., Renjan, V., & Tan, J. (2017). Child community mental health services in Asia Pacific and Singapore's REACH model. *Brain Sciences, 7*(10), 126. https://doi.org/10.3390/brainsci7100126

Liu, Q., He, H., Yang, J., Feng, X., Zhao, F., & Lyu, J. (2020). Changes in the global burden of depression from 1990 to 2017: Findings from the Global Burden of Disease study. *Journal of Psychiatric Research, 126*, 134–140.

Ludlow, C., Hurn, R., & Lansdell, S. (2020). A current review of the children and young People's improving access to psychological therapies (CYP IAPT) program: Perspectives on developing an accessible workforce. *Adolescent Health, Medicine and Therapeutics, 11*, 21–28. https://doi.org/10.2147/AHMT.S196492

Martínez, V., Espinosa-Duque, D., Jiménez-Molina, Á., Rojas, G., Vöhringer, P. A., Fernández-Arcila, M., et al. (2021). Feasibility and acceptability of "Cuida tu Ánimo" (take Care of Your Mood): An internet-based program for prevention and early intervention of adolescent depression in Chile and Colombia. *International Journal of Environmental Research and Public Health, 18*(18), 9628.

Martínez, V., Rojas, G., Martínez, P., Zitko, P., Irarrázaval, M., Luttges, C., & Araya, R. (2018). Remote collaborative depression care program for adolescents in Araucanía region, Chile: Randomized controlled trial. *Journal of Medical Internet Research, 20*(1), e38.

Matthews, S. K., Krivelyova, A., Stephens, R. L., & Bilchik, S. (2013). Juvenile justice contact of youth in systems of care: Comparison study results. *Criminal Justice Policy Review, 24*(2), 143–165.

Mekonen, T., Chan, G. C., Connor, J. P., Hides, L., & Leung, J. (2021). Estimating the global treatment rates for depression: A systematic review and meta-analysis. *Journal of Affective Disorders, 295*, 1234–1242.

Meskó, B., Drobni, Z., Bényei, É., Gergely, B., & Győrffy, Z. (2017). Digital health is a cultural transformation of traditional healthcare. *Mhealth, 3*, 38.

Mohr, D. C., Duffecy, J., Ho, J., Kwasny, M., Cai, X., Burns, M. N., & Begale, M. (2013). A randomized controlled trial evaluating a manualized TeleCoaching protocol for improving adherence to a web-based intervention for the treatment of depression. *PLoS One, 8*(8), e70086.

Mundt, A. P., Irarrázaval, M., Martínez, P., Fernández, O., Martínez, V., & Rojas, G. (2021). Telepsychiatry consultation for primary care treatment of children and adolescents receiving child protective Services in Chile: Mixed methods feasibility study. *JMIR Public Health and Surveillance, 7*(7), e25836.

Musyimi, C. W., Mutiso, V. N., Haji, Z. R., Nandoya, E. S., & Ndetei, D. M. (2018). Mobile based mhGAP-IG depression screening in Kenya. *Community Mental Health Journal, 54*(1), 84–91.

Petersen, I., Fairall, L., Bhana, A., Kathree, T., Selohilwe, O., Brooke-Sumner, C., Faris, G., Breuer, E., Sibanyoni, N., Lund, C., & Patel, V. (2016). Integrating mental health into chronic care in South Africa: The development of a district mental healthcare plan. *The British Journal of Psychiatry: The Journal of Mental Science, 208*(Suppl 56), s29–s39. https://doi.org/10.1192/bjp.bp.114.153726

Puntis, S., Perfect, D., Kirubarajan, A., Bolton, S., Davies, F., Hayes, A., et al. (2018). A systematic review of co-responder models of police mental health 'street' triage. *BMC Psychiatry, 18*(1), 1–11.

Pereira, C. A., Wen, C. L., Miguel, E. C., Polanczyk, G. V. (2015). A randomised controlled trial of a web based educational program in child mental health for school teachers. Eur Child Adolesc Psychiatry 24:931–40. https://doi.org/10.1007/s00787-014-0642-8

ReachOut. (2022). Available at au.reachout.com. Accessed 9 March 2022.

Rickwood, D., Paraskakis, M., Quin, D., Hobbs, N., Ryall, V., Trethowan, J., & McGorry, P. (2019). Australia's innovation in youth mental health care: The headspace Centre model. *Early Intervention in Psychiatry, 13*(1), 159–166.

Santomauro, D. F., Herrera, A. M. M., Shadid, J., Zheng, P., Ashbaugh, C., Pigott, D. M., et al. (2021). Global prevalence and burden of depressive and anxiety disorders in 204 countries and territories in 2020 due to the COVID-19 pandemic. *The Lancet, 398*(10312), 1700–1712.

Sarikhani, Y., Bastani, P., Rafiee, M., et al. (2021). Key barriers to the provision and utilization of mental health services in low- and middle-income countries: A scope study. *Community Mental Health Journal, 57*, 836–852. https://doi.org/10.1007/s10597-020-00619-2

Shinde, S., Weiss, H. A., Khandeparkar, P., Pereira, B., Sharma, A., Gupta, R., et al. (2020). A multicomponent secondary school health promotion intervention and adolescent health: An extension of the SEHER cluster randomised controlled trial in Bihar, India. *PLoS Medicine, 17*(2), e1003021.

Shinde, S., Weiss, H. A., Varghese, B., Khandeparkar, P., Pereira, B., Sharma, A., Gupta, R., Ross, D. A., Patton, G., & Patel, V. (2018). Promoting school climate and health outcomes with the SEHER multi-component secondary school intervention in Bihar, India: A cluster-randomised controlled trial. *Lancet, 392*(10163), 2465–2477. https://doi.org/10.1016/S0140-6736(18)31615-5

Sit, H. F., Ling, R., Lam, A. I. F., Chen, W., Latkin, C. A., & Hall, B. J. (2020). The cultural adaptation of step-by-step: An intervention to address depression among Chinese young adults. *Frontiers in Psychiatry, 11*, 650.

Smith, G. L., & McGuinness, T. M. (2017). Adolescent psychosocial assessment: The HEEADSSS. *Journal of Psychosocial Nursing and Mental Health Services, 55*(5), 24–27. https://doi.org/10.3928/02793695-20170420-03

Smokowski, P. R., & Kopasz, K. H. (2005). Bullying in school: An overview of types, effects, family characteristics, and intervention strategies. *Children and Schools, 27*(2), 101–109. https://doi.org/10.1093/cs/27.2.101

Stephens, M. M., Cook-Fasano, H. T., & Sibbaluca, K. (2018). Childhood bullying: Implications for physicians. *American Family Physician, 97*(3), 187–192.

StrongMinds. (2021). Lusaka: StrongMinds. *Our results: Stopping the depression epidemic in Africa*. https://strongminds.org/our-impact/. Accessed 21 March 2022.

Swartz, K., Musci, R. J., Beaudry, M. B., Heley, K., Miller, L., Alfes, C., Townsend, L., Thornicroft, G., & Wilcox, H. C. (2017). School-based curriculum to improve depression literacy among US secondary school students: A randomized effectiveness trial. *American Journal of Public Health, 107*(12), 1970–1976. https://doi.org/10.2105/AJPH.2017.304088

Thornicroft, G., Chatterji, S., Evans-Lacko, S., et al. (2017). Undertreatment of people with major depressive disorder in 21 countries. *The British Journal of Psychiatry, 210*, 119–124.

Topooco, N., Riper, H., Araya, R., Berking, M., Brunn, M., Chevreul, K., et al. (2017). Attitudes towards digital treatment for depression: A European stakeholder survey. *Internet Interventions, 8*, 1–9.

Wakefield, S., Kellett, S., Simmonds-Buckley, M., Stockton, D., Bradbury, A., & Delgadillo, J. (2021). Improving access to psychological therapies (IAPT) in the United Kingdom: A systematic review and meta-analysis of 10-years of practice-based evidence. *British Journal of Clinical Psychology, 60*(1), 1–37.

Wasserman, G. A., McReynolds, L. S., Schwalbe, C. S., Keating, J. M., & Jones, S. A. (2010). Psychiatric disorder, comorbidity, and suicidal behavior in juvenile justice youth. *Criminal Justice and Behavior, 37*(12), 1361–1376.

Williford, A., Boulton, A., Noland, B., et al. (2012). Effects of the KiVa anti-bullying program on adolescents' depression, anxiety, and perception of peers. *Journal of Abnormal Child Psychology, 40*, 289–300. https://doi.org/10.1007/s10802-011-9551-1

Winding, T. N., Skouenborg, L. A., Mortensen, V. L., et al. (2020). Is bullying in adolescence associated with the development of depressive symptoms in adulthood?: A longitudinal cohort study. *BMC Psychol, 8*, 122. https://doi.org/10.1186/s40359-020-00491-5

World Health Organization. (2017). *Depression and other common mental disorders: Global health estimates* (No. WHO/MSD/MER/2017.2). World Health Organization.

World Health Organization. (2021). *Prevention and management of mental health conditions in the Philippines: The case for investment*. World Health Organization Regional Office for the Western Pacific. https://www.ph.undp.org/content/philippines/en/home/library/prevention-and-management-of-mental-health-conditions-in-the-phi.html. Accessed 9 November 2022.

World Health Organization (WHO). (2016). *INSPIRE: Seven strategies for ending violence against children*. World Health Organization. https://apps.who.int/iris/handle/10665/207717. Accessed 18 November 2021.

World Health Organization (WHO) & UNESCO. (2021). *WHO guideline on school health services*. World Health Organization. https://apps.who.int/iris/handle/10665/341910. Accessed 24 March 2022.

World Health Organization (WHO) & United Nations Children's Fund (UNICEF). (2021). *Helping adolescents thrive toolkit: Strategies to promote and protect adolescent mental health and reduce self-harm and other risk behaviours*. World Health Organization. https://apps.who.int/iris/handle/10665/341327. Accessed 21 March 2022.

World Health Organization (WHO). Regional Office for Europe. (2019). *Multisectoral action for mental health: Thematic brief on mental health*. World Health Organization. Regional Office for Europe. https://apps.who.int/iris/handle/10665/346538

Yuan, S., Zhou, X., Zhang, Y., Zhang, H., Pu, J., Yang, L., et al. (2018). Comparative efficacy and acceptability of bibliotherapy for depression and anxiety disorders in children and adolescents: A meta-analysis of randomized clinical trials. *Neuropsychiatric Disease and Treatment, 14*, 353–365.

Zhou, W., Ouyang, F., Nergui, O.-E., Bangura, J. B., Acheampong, K., Massey, I. Y., & Xiao, S. (2020). Child and adolescent mental health policy in low- and middle-income countries: Challenge and lessons for policy development and implementation. *Frontiers in Psychiatry, 11*, 150.

Chapter 3
Preventing Depression in Children and Adolescents Through Mindfulness-Based Interventions in Schools

Carlos García-Rubio and Catherine I. Andreu

3.1 Prevention of Children's and Adolescents' Depression in Schools

The prevalence of child and adolescent mental health problems continues to grow worldwide. Between 12% and 16% of children and adolescents experience a mental health problem of some type (Polanczyk et al., 2015), while the number of young people who consider suicide has increased in the last decade (Kann et al., 2018). The World Health Organization (WHO, 2018) recognizes that child-adolescent mental health problems are the leading cause of disability in Europe, with one-half of emotional problems starting before the age of 14 (Kessler et al., 2007). Furthermore, these conditions tend to be recurrent and chronic if not prevented or treated early (Pine et al., 1998) and are associated with poor functioning and low quality of life in the short and long term (Fombonne et al., 2001; Zisook et al., 2007). Of particular concern is the increase in mental disorders in children and adolescents since the beginning of the COVID-19 crisis, which has tripled (Save the Children, 2021), with health care services being overwhelmed (Golberstein et al., 2020; Novins et al., 2021). Besides, along with the individual suffering of experiencing a mental health problem in childhood, the economic and social costs are enormous (Fatori et al., 2018). For example, a study carried out in the Netherlands

C. García-Rubio (✉)
Faculty of Psychology, Universidad Autónoma de Madrid, Madrid, Spain

Nirakara Lab, Complutense University of Madrid, Madrid, Spain

C. I. Andreu
Millennium Institute for Research in Depression and Personality (MIDAP), Santiago, Chile

Polibienestar Institute, University of Valencia, Valencia, Spain

V. Martínez, C. Miranda-Castillo (eds.), *Prevention and Early Treatment of Depression Through the Life Course*, Depression and Personality,
https://doi.org/10.1007/978-3-031-13029-8_3

on the cost of depression among children and adolescents showed that the investment amounted to 38 million euros (Bodden et al., 2018). Also, the report *The State of the World's Children 2021 – On My Mind: Promoting, Protecting and Caring for Children's Mental Health* (UNICEF, 2021) has shown that the economic impact of not preventing and treating mental health problems in childhood and adolescence is $387.2 billion per year. Despite these alarming data, several reports from government institutions and experts conclude that mental health problems at an early age are under-recognized and that providing urgent solutions is a priority (European Commission, 2016a; Saunders et al., 2020).

Depression is one of the most prevalent mental disorders in childhood and adolescence, with devastating repercussions for positive development (Garber, 2006). The probability of developing a depressive disorder increases over the life cycle (Kostev et al., 2019). Depressive disorders have an estimated annual prevalence of about 2% in children and 4–8% in adolescents (Lynch & Clarke, 2006), with around 20% of American young people experiencing an episode of depression before the age of 18 (Costello et al., 2003). Depression in childhood and adolescence is characterized by feelings of sadness and hopelessness, irritable mood, and loss of interest in activities. Feelings of underestimation and excessive guilt may be present, together with difficulty concentrating and thinking, recurrent thoughts of death and suicide, sleep and eating disorders, frustration and hostility, agitation or inhibition of movement, fatigue or loss of energy, isolation, and high vulnerability to criticism (Fernández-Hermida & Villamarín-Fernández, 2021). Additionally, depressive disorders tend to run a chronic and recurring course, with comorbidity levels with anxiety disorder nearing 50% (Flannery-Schroeder, 2006). The earlier onset of depression in youth is associated with substance abuse, risky sexual behavior, suicide risk, poor social functioning, decreased school performance, and physical health problems (Lynch & Clarke, 2006).

Several risk factors have been reported to contribute to the development of depression in children and adolescents: exposure to negative life events from childhood (e.g., death of a loved one or being exposed to stress or trauma), maladaptive cognitive style (e.g., excessive rumination and worry, involvement in global and stable attributions, inferring negative characteristics of the self and anticipating negative consequences), deficits in emotional self-regulation skills (e.g., cognitive and emotional reactivity), low self-esteem, self-criticism, feelings of helplessness, being a woman, family risk of depression (e.g., having a father with depression), violence and family instability, poor social support, and subclinical levels of depressive or anxiety symptoms, among others (Carballo et al., 2020; Fernández-Hermida & Villamarín-Fernández, 2021; Garber, 2006; Mendelson & Tandon, 2016; Mezulis et al., 2006; Van der Gucht et al., 2018). Protective factors include positive life events, self-regulation skills (emotion regulation skills and psychological flexibility, mindfulness, and self-compassion), personal resources (resilience, self-efficacy, self-concept, self-esteem, optimism), and supportive relationships (family cohesion, parental support, social support, peer competence and acceptance, sense of belonging, positive teacher-student relationship), among others (Klasen et al., 2015; Muris et al., 2017; Otto et al., 2017; Wang et al., 2012). Therefore, interventions to reduce the risk factors and promote the protective factors for depression are necessary to prevent the early appearance of depressive symptoms and depressive disorders throughout child-adolescent development. In this regard, psychological interventions, which typically target one or more of these risk and protective factors, are cost-effective in the prevention and treatment of depression in young people (Cuijpers et al., 2021; Lynch & Clarke, 2006; Mendelson & Tandon, 2016; Merry et al., 2011).

Psychological prevention depression programs for children and adolescents are divided into universal or targeted approaches. Universal prevention is delivered to a whole population regardless of depression risk (e.g., school-based universal interventions). Targeted prevention approaches are directed either toward those who have an increased risk of depression, such as children with family risk (selective prevention), or adolescents with subclinical depressive symptoms (indicated prevention) (Mendelson & Tandon, 2016). The report *Child and Adolescent Mental Health Policies and Plans* (WHO, 2005) points out the importance of involving all sectors of society in the prevention of mental health problems, highlighting the role of the school. Along the same lines, the European Commission (2016b) points out the need to develop an intersectoral cooperation framework to prevent mental health problems and promote child and youth well-being, highlighting the importance of collaboration between school and health centers in this regard. The school context can be particularly advantageous for depression prevention, since it offers an accessible way to reach youth and provide them with strategies that protect against early depression. In addition, interventions in schools can reduce some of the barriers associated with treating child and adolescent depression, such as stigma or the high cost of individual treatment. A recent meta-analysis of the effectiveness of school-based depression and anxiety prevention programs for young people showed that universal and targeted programs effectively improved mental health (Werner-Seidler et al., 2017). The authors conclude that the school environment provides an ideal context for prevention programs, with the potential to offset the trajectory toward disorder. Furthermore, the effectiveness of these interventions can be amplified by involving other school agents, such as teachers and parents, given that improving the mental health of teachers and parents can indirectly improve that of children and adolescents (Carr, 2000; Durlak, 1998; Restifo & Bögels, 2009; Schonert-Reichl, 2017; Schonert-Reichl & Hymel, 2007).

In recent years, mindfulness-based interventions (MBIs) have been added to the set of preventive psychological interventions implemented in schools to improve young people's mental health. MBIs have been shown to be effective in reducing depression in children and adolescents, teachers, and parents. This chapter proposes that the systematic implementation of MBIs at school can be effective to prevent depression throughout child and adolescent development. As our proposal is based on a systemic approach, in the following sections, we will develop the evidence on MBIs for the reduction of depression in children and adolescents, teachers, and parents.

3.2 Mindfulness-Based Interventions

Mindfulness is defined as "the awareness that emerges through paying attention on purpose, in the present moment, and nonjudgmentally to the unfolding experience moment by moment" (Kabat-Zinn, 2003, p. 145). Along the same lines, Bishop et al. (2006) conceptualized mindfulness as "the self-regulation of attention that is maintained in the immediate experience… (2) with a particular orientation towards the experience in the present moment, characterized by curiosity, openness and acceptance" (p. 232). MBIs have been designed to teach individuals how to cultivate mindfulness skills and incorporate them into their daily lives. The primary aims of MBIs are to teach participants (1) to regulate their attention to monitor their experience of the present moment and (2) to bring an attitude of openness, acceptance, and non-reactivity to the monitored experience (Lindsay & Creswell, 2017).

Recently, Crane et al. (2017) proposed a framework that defines the fundamental characteristics of an MBI. These authors assert that all MBIs must include a set of essential factors and a set of specific adaptations for the population and context to which it is aimed. Regarding the essential factors, they point out that MBIs are programs:

1. That are informed by theories and practices that draw from a confluence of contemplative traditions, science, and the disciplines of medicine, psychology, and education.
2. That help participants to understand how stress and discomfort are created and maintained and how mindfulness practice can help to prevent and treat discomfort generators and maintainers by cultivating a new way of relating to experience.
3. That cultivate the ability to approach and be in contact with the experience of the present moment (e.g., thoughts, emotions, sensations) and promote awareness of the consequences and implications of the different ways of approaching experience (rejection vs. acceptance). Specifically, MBIs facilitate insight into how a rejection-based relationship with the unpleasant experience may generate greater reactivity and suffering, while one based on experiential acceptance can decrease reactivity and suffering. Participants learn the ability of decentering – a metacognitive process that promotes a greater psychological distance from internal experiences, such as thoughts and feelings, and allows the person to disidentify with them (Bernstein et al., 2015) – to recognize how the reactions of rejection, avoidance, or suppression of their thoughts, emotions, and sensations tend to generate greater reactivity and suffering, as well as a more inflexible response pattern, while experiential acceptance allows greater stability, flexibility, mindful decision making, and freedom.
4. That support the development of greater attentional, emotional, and behavioral self-regulation, as well as positive qualities such as kindness, compassion, and equanimity.
5. That involve participants in a systematic training in mindfulness meditation practices (e.g., mindful breathing meditation, body scan, thoughts and emotions meditation, informal practices).

6. That apply a methodology and pedagogy that is experiential, interactive, participatory, student centered, and relationship centered, and a learning process based on an inquiry process.
7. And finally, that are led by facilitators who are experienced mindfulness practitioners with the ability to embody the state of mindfulness in the first person when leading and holding the group.

Regarding the set of specific adaptations that MBIs require, several authors have proposed relevant factors to adjust MBIs to educational settings. The design of an MBI in educational contexts must include all essential factors, adapting them to the school structure and objectives. In educational contexts, MBIs are integrated into (a) the framework of socio-emotional learning (SEL) interventions, whose main objective is to promote socio-emotional competence, and (b) the framework of contemplative education, aimed at promoting mental habits and healthy emotional factors for positive development (Lawlor, 2016). Contemplative education engages the educational community in a set of contemplative practices that help the development of self-awareness to recognize mental and behavioral habits and learn new ways to transcend habitual patterns, thus fostering a more conscious lifestyle, learning, and relationships (Jennings, 2008; Roeser & Peck, 2009). The aims of MBIs for children and adolescents in schools include improving mindfulness skills as well as cognitive (attention and executive function), emotional (emotional regulation), and social (prosocial dispositions) functioning. Improvements in these domains lead to improved mental health, peer relationships, classroom behavior, and student academic performance (Andreu & García-Rubio, 2019). Besides, MBIs for teachers seek to improve their mindfulness and self-compassion skills, reduce burnout, and improve their mental health, which in turn indirectly helps to improve classroom outcomes and student outcomes (Roeser et al., 2012). Furthermore, MBIs in school contexts must be adapted to the specific needs of the multiple agents of the educational community; for example, interventions should be tailored to students' stage of development (Roeser & Pinela, 2014), adapted considering teachers' needs (e.g., practices to reduce burnout or increase emotional support in class) (Jennings, 2015), or adjusted depending on school type (e.g., the secularization of the program in public schools; Jennings, 2016).

3.3 School-Based Mindfulness Interventions for Reducing Children's and Adolescents' Depression

Overall, the evidence suggests that MBIs in schools can reduce some risk factors (e.g., subclinical levels of depression or anxiety, emotional and cognitive reactivity, cognitive vulnerability, self-criticism, victimization) and promote some protective factors (e.g., mindfulness skills, emotional and behavioral self-regulation, self-compassion, peer acceptance) that are involved in the onset or maintenance of depression during child and adolescent development.

About protective factors, MBIs in schools have been shown to be effective in increasing mindfulness skills in children and adolescents (Dunning et al., 2019; Klingbeil et al., 2017). Throughout child-adolescent development, mindfulness skills prevent the early appearance of depressive symptoms and depressive disorders. Cross-sectional studies have shown that children's and adolescents' mindfulness skills correlate with reduced behavioral problems and improved mental health, psychological inflexibility, quality of life, social skills, and academic competence (García-Rubio et al., 2020; Greco et al., 2011). Specifically, mindfulness skills in children are related to less depression, anxiety, negative affect, rumination, and behavioral impulsiveness, as well as greater optimism, academic self-concept, self-efficacy, and school competence (García-Rubio et al., 2019; Lawlor et al., 2014). In adolescents, mindfulness skills have been associated with lower levels of depression, anxiety, stress, and negative affect, as well as greater acceptance, life satisfaction, academic self-concept, and self-efficacy (Pallozzi et al., 2017; Yu et al., 2021).

Furthermore, several studies have shown that mindfulness skills predict a decrease in depressive symptoms during adolescence through a reduction in several psychological mechanisms that facilitate the onset and maintenance of depression. Recently, Royuela-Colomer et al. (2021) found that mindfulness skills in adolescents predicted a reduction in depressive symptoms 1 year later. Similarly, Royuela-Colomer and Calvete (2016) showed that the ability to not react to internal experience and act with awareness predicted a reduction in depressive symptoms at 4 months. Along the same lines, Galla et al. (2020) found that positive changes in not reacting to internal experience during the ages of 13 and 14 are associated with reductions in negative affect and perceived stress 2 years later. Moreover, Tumminia et al. (2020) have shown that adolescents' ability not to judge internal experience reduces rumination at 3 months, which in turn reduces negative affect 6 months later. Likewise, the ability to act with awareness protects against the development of self-injurious behavior during adolescence (Calvete et al., 2017), while mindful attention reduces the association between depressogenic schemas and depressive symptoms (Calvete et al., 2019). Therefore, mindfulness skills can decrease cognitive vulnerability to depression in adolescents. However, more longitudinal studies with children are needed to elucidate the effect of mindfulness skills on the development of depression at an earlier age. Given the protective role of mindfulness skills in child and adolescent depression, it may be useful to promote these skills through school-based preventive interventions. As mentioned above, school-based MBIs have been shown to be effective in increasing mindfulness skills in children and adolescents. Besides, a recent meta-analysis showed that MBIs effectively improve mental health (Kallapiran et al., 2015) and reduce depressive symptoms (Dunning et al., 2019).

Regarding risk factors, MBIs have been shown to be helpful for reducing depressive symptoms in school contexts in the community population (universal prevention) (Raes et al., 2014), in the population at risk (selective prevention) (Fung et al., 2019), and in the population with clinical symptoms (indicated prevention) (Wright et al., 2019). Among the MBIs aimed at reducing depression, there stands out the adaptation for children and adolescents of mindfulness-based cognitive therapy

(MBCT) (Ames et al., 2014; Knowles et al., 2015; Semple & Lee, 2011; Semple & Lee, 2014). In adults, MBCT has been recommended by the National Institute for Health and Clinical Excellence (NICE) to prevent relapse in depression (Segal et al., 2002). MBCT seems to reduce the risk of relapse in patients with recurrent depressions even at a 15-month follow-up (Kuyken et al., 2016). MBCT improves self-regulation, decreasing cognitive reactivity, worry, and rumination, and increasing decentering and self-compassion skills (Gu et al., 2015). In children and adolescents, results are promising, although few studies have evaluated the effectiveness of MBCT for children (MBCT-C). MBCT-C programs at school have been shown to be as effective as cognitive behavioral therapy in reducing symptoms of anxiety and depression in children with high levels of internalizing symptoms (Wright et al., 2019). Also, a study that used MBCT-C for adolescents suggests that it may reduce depressive symptoms in those who are at risk of relapse (Ames et al., 2014). Other trials have shown promising results for improving depression and anxiety in children and adolescents (Cotton et al., 2016; Esmaeilian et al., 2018; Lam, 2016; Lee et al., 2008; Semple et al., 2010).

Recent results with children also suggest that the improvement of emotional regulation skills underlies the effectiveness of MBIs in reducing anxiety-depressive symptoms. In this regard, Bauer et al. (2019) found that school mindfulness training with middle school children can alter the neurocognitive mechanisms of stress. Specifically, the authors showed that children who participated in an MBI integrated into the school curriculum, compared to an active control group, reported lower stress associated with reduced right amygdala activation in response to fearful faces and relatively stronger functional connectivity between the right amygdala and the ventromedial prefrontal cortex while viewing fearful facial expressions. Thus, these results indicate that a school MBI may potentially alter brain correlates of emotional regulation during middle childhood positively, expressly, by altering the neural mechanisms associated with emotional reactivity to unpleasant situations. This finding is consistent with the results of a study with children aged 7–12 years that showed that the increase in dispositional mindfulness after an MBI in school led to reductions in children's anxiety and psychological inflexibility and that positive changes in teacher-rated children's emotional regulation led to improvements in emotional symptoms and decreased peer relationship problems (García-Rubio, 2021). Also, a qualitative study found that children with high social vulnerability (i.e., low family socioeconomic status) can benefit from a school-based MBI by learning to reduce reactivity to unpleasant sensations, thoughts, and emotions (e.g., sadness) and adopting an attitude of openness and non-reactivity to internal experience, being able to shift from reactive to self-regulated behavior (Andreu et al., 2021).

Therefore, although further research is needed, preliminary evidence suggests that children and adolescents learn new strategies of emotional regulation based on mindfulness (e.g., mindful emotion regulation) after participating in an MBI at school. Students are able to get in touch with the present moment and bring an attitude of non-judgment, acceptance, and non-reactivity to internal experience (e.g., not reacting quickly to unpleasant bodily sensations and being able to decenter and disidentify from the ruminative pattern to let go of unpleasant thoughts) instead of engaging in avoidance-based strategies to regulate the unpleasant internal experience, which are involved in the onset and maintenance of depression disorders (e.g., thought suppression, rumination and worry, self-criticism; Ehrenreich-May & Chu, 2013; Greco & Hayes, 2008; Kashdan & Rottenberg, 2010; Muris et al., 2017; Oppo et al., 2019; Tan & Martin, 2015). Furthermore, engaging in mindful emotion regulation from an early age seems to help children and adolescents to develop less inflexible behaviors (i.e., less guided by their psychological reactions to unpleasant internal events and more guided by personal values and goals), which can help to prevent the onset of depressive disorders and relapse (García-Rubio, 2021). Chambers et al. (2015) found that mindful emotion regulation is associated with less depression, anxiety, rumination and dysfunctional attitudes, and a higher quality of life compared to well-studied emotional regulation strategies such as cognitive reappraisal and expressive suppression. Moreover, greater mindful emotion regulation predicted greater recovery from depression in young people with major depression (Chambers et al., 2015). It is also important to mention that students with a higher risk of depression (i.e., women and students with higher baseline depressive symptoms) benefit more from school MBIs in the short and long term (Kang et al., 2018; Van der Gucht et al., 2017; Volanen et al., 2020).

Although there is extensive evidence of the effectiveness of school-based MBIs in reducing depression, very little research has been conducted on their mechanisms of action. Cognitive reactivity and self-compassion are two mechanisms that seem to influence the effectiveness of school MBIs for adolescents. Cognitive reactivity refers to the ease with which negative (often ruminative) thinking patterns are (re) activated when in a mild dysphoric state (Scher et al., 2005). Self-compassion refers to the tendency (or vice versa, the lack thereof) to be caring, warm, and understanding toward oneself when faced with personal shortcomings, problems, or failures (Neff, 2003). Van der Gucht et al. (2018) showed that reduced cognitive reactivity and increased self-compassion after an MBI led to a decrease in students' depressive and anxious symptoms. Similarly, a study conducted with 145 adolescents with high depressive symptoms showed that, after an MBI, reductions in rumination and expressive suppression led to a reduction in internalizing symptoms and perceived stress (Fung et al., 2019). These results suggest that improvements in adolescents' emotional regulation skills are involved in the reduction of depressive symptoms.

Future randomized controlled trials with larger sample sizes and follow-up measures are necessary to generalize the results obtained. Likewise, it is essential for future research to deeply examine the mechanisms of action that underlie the reduction of depressive symptoms in children and adolescents after an MBI, taking into account multiple domains (cerebral, cognitive, emotional) and using diverse methodologies (self-reports, behavioral tasks, neurocognitive measures, teachers' and parents' reports, qualitative methods).

3.4 School-Based Mindfulness Interventions for Reducing Teachers' Depression

Lee Shulman, one of the most relevant American educational psychologists of the XX century, noted: "After 30 years of doing such work, I have concluded that classroom teaching... is perhaps the most complex, most challenging, and most demanding, subtle, nuanced, and frightening activity that our species has ever invented... The only time a physician could possibly encounter a situation of comparable complexity would be in the emergency room of a hospital during or after a natural disaster" (Shulman, 2004, p. 504). Currently, the worldwide prevalence of teacher burnout is very high (Aloe et al., 2014). The MetLife Survey of the American Teacher found that nearly 60% of teachers reported feeling under too much stress (Markow et al., 2013). The increase is dramatic, since in 1985 only 35% reported this. Additionally, the survey found that teacher job satisfaction had dropped dramatically, from 62% in 2008 to 39% in 2012. These data are not exclusive to US teachers, as similar data have been reported for the educational systems of other countries. For example, in the Netherlands, more than half of the teachers report feeling high levels of work stress (Lensen et al., 2021). Almost one in five is quitting their work as teachers and choosing a new profession within 5 years of starting as teachers. These data are alarming since it is well known that repeated exposure to stress over time leads to burnout (Bellingrath et al., 2010). Burnout is considered a syndrome that combines three dimensions: emotional exhaustion, depersonalization, and a lack of personal accomplishment (Maslach et al., 2001). Recent studies have shown a substantial overlap between burnout and depression, with some authors even considering burnout a subtype of depression (Bianchi et al., 2015).

Teacher burnout is associated with greater depressive symptoms, low enthusiasm and motivation, and impaired cognitive ability (García-Carmona et al., 2019; Jennings & Greenberg, 2009). Furthermore, teachers who experience burnout are more likely to fail to meet the instructional and emotional demands that classroom dynamics require (Sandilos et al., 2015). Teachers with high depressive symptoms may be emotionally exhausted and may not be able to provide high-quality care, which can directly affect classroom climate and healthy child development (Jeon et al., 2014). Evidence shows that teachers' depressive symptoms impact children's outcomes directly and indirectly via classroom quality (Roberts et al., 2016). Also, in classrooms where teachers suffer elevated depressive symptoms, children show more internalizing problems (Jeon et al., 2014) and worse socio-emotional competency skills (Roberts et al., 2016). Likewise, teachers' depression and emotional exhaustion are associated with adverse reactions of the children in the classroom. However, teachers' positive coping skills (e.g., emotion regulation skills) are associated with positive responses to children's negative emotions (Buettner et al., 2016).

Therefore, since teaching is a very stressful profession that may directly affect teachers' mental health and indirectly impact on children's mental health, preventive interventions to improve teachers' mental health, teacher-student relationships, and classroom learning environments are necessary. MBIs for teachers are an emerging area of practice and research. Mindfulness training with teachers aims to cultivate their mindfulness, self-regulation, and self-care skills to create a healthy teacher mindset, promoting greater occupational health, well-being, and mental health (Roeser et al., 2012). Also, MBIs seek to provide teachers with tools to foster effective classroom management, a positive interpersonal climate, and positive teacher-student relationships in the classroom. Finally, all of these positive outcomes are aimed at generating a beneficial impact on student outcomes, for example, improving students' mental health. A recent meta-analysis of the effects of MBIs for teachers showed positive effects, increasing mindfulness skills and well-being and reducing psychological distress (Klingbeil et al., 2017). This result is relevant since mindfulness skills in teachers are associated with lower depression and anxiety symptoms, job stress, occupational and emotional burnout, and missed workdays, as well as with greater self-efficacy, job satisfaction, job performance, and emotionally supportive classroom interactions with students, even with the more challenging ones (Abenavoli et al., 2013; Braun et al., 2019; Dane & Brummel, 2014; Hülsheger et al., 2013; Jennings, 2015; Taylor & Millear, 2016). Besides, the association between the teacher's greater dispositional mindfulness and higher-quality relationships with students (e.g., fewer conflicts and positive interactions) is mediated by the teacher's lower burnout and depressive symptoms (Becker et al., 2017; Braun et al., 2019). Therefore, these findings suggest that teachers who have higher levels of dispositional mindfulness may suffer fewer depression symptoms and burnout, leading to higher-quality relationships with students in their classrooms.

Along with improving mindfulness skills, MBIs for teachers have been shown to be effective in improving a set of outcomes relevant to mental health. In a cluster-randomized controlled trial design (RCT) involving 36 American urban elementary schools and 224 teachers, the CARE for Teachers program, a mindfulness-based program specifically designed for teachers, showed positive effects on teachers' emotion regulation, mindfulness, psychological distress, time urgency, and emotional support toward students (Jennings et al., 2017). Almost a year later, the teachers' mental health, mindfulness, and emotional regulation skills continued improving (Jennings et al., 2019). Recently, an RCT in the UK with 206 teachers from 43 different schools showed improvements in mindfulness, self-compassion, well-being, depression, anxiety, perceived stress, and burnout (Montero-Marin et al., 2021). Furthermore, the authors examined the mechanisms of action of the intervention, concluding that the improvement in mindfulness and self-compassion skills led to a reduction in depressive-anxiety symptoms and burnout while also increasing well-being. Likewise, other studies with teachers have shown that the improvement in mindfulness and the reduction in rumination mediate the following benefits of MBIs: decreasing depression, low mood, negative affect, and sleep difficulties (Crain et al., 2017; Roeser et al., 2013). At a biological level, Rodrigues de Oliveira et al. (2021) have examined the impact of an MBI for Brazilian professors on pro-inflammatory and antioxidant biomarkers related to depression. The mindfulness group showed significant decreases in pro-inflammatory markers (IL-6 and IL-8) and increased antioxidant activity (glutathione and cystine) compared to controls at immediate post-intervention. Overall, current evidence suggests that MBIs are effective preventative programs that provide teachers with a set of mindfulness-based socio-emotional competencies, thereby reducing the burnout cascade and preventing depression.

Students also indirectly benefit from teachers' mindfulness skills. Specifically, stronger mindfulness skills in teachers have been indirectly associated with better student outcomes through better interpersonal mindfulness skills or mindful teaching in teachers (Jennings & Greenberg, 2009). In the educational field, interpersonal mindfulness has been defined as the ability of teachers to (1) listen with full attention to students, (2) maintain present-centered awareness of emotions experienced by the self and students during interactions, (3) be open, with acceptance and receptivity to students' thoughts and feelings, (4) be able to self-regulate emotion and behavior in challenging situations (i.e., low emotional and behavioral reactivity and low automaticity in response to the everyday behavior of students), and (5) be compassionate toward the self and students (Frank et al., 2016). Also, Hulburt et al. (2020) have proposed that a mindful teacher is one who is calm in body in challenging situations, clear in mind when making decisions in complex classroom environments, and kind in approach to interactions with students. In this regard, it has been shown that students' perceptions of mindful teaching are associated with changes in mindfulness, self-compassion, and compassion for others. A study with 599 high school students found that those who perceived that their teachers' teaching was more mindful at the beginning of the course developed greater satisfaction with themselves in the middle of the course (i.e., the satisfaction of autonomy, relationship, and competence needs) and improved their skills of mindfulness, self-compassion, and compassion for others at the end of the course (Colaianne et al., 2020). The students seemed to internalize the mindful and compassionate attitude throughout the school year due to their teachers' mindful teaching. There is also evidence that this phenomenon can occur in reverse: the effect of "stress contagion" in the classroom. A higher level of teacher burnout has been found to correlate with higher student cortisol, showing that teacher mental health is linked to the regulation of student stress (Oberle & Schonert-Reichl, 2016). However, teachers' interpersonal mindfulness has been found to moderate the relationship between high levels of teacher stress and the quality of the teacher-student relationship. For instance, teachers' interpersonal mindfulness buffers the effects of elevated pressure on emotional supportiveness in the classroom (Molloy Elreda et al., 2019). Therefore, teacher interpersonal mindfulness and mindful teaching are factors that protect both teachers and students from developing the "burnout cascade" and mental health problems. Furthermore, evidence has shown that MBIs for teachers effectively promote interpersonal mindfulness skills. Concretely, a group of teachers, interviewed after participating in an MBI, reported that they felt greater presence in the classroom, greater body awareness and less emotional reactivity, greater capacity to regulate emotionally and reevaluate stressful situations in the classroom, and less feelings of defensiveness in the relationship with students (i.e., greater understanding and compassion) after the program (Sharp & Jennings, 2016).

In summary, current evidence suggests that MBIs for teachers can prevent burnout and depression by increasing their mindfulness and mindful teaching skills. In addition, this learning helps teachers to be more present to address the needs of students in the classroom and engage in emotionally supportive interactions with them, which undoubtedly prevents the development of mental health problems throughout childhood and adolescence.

3.5 Mindfulness-Based Interventions for Reducing Parents' Depression

Parental psychopathology affects children's mental health. There is strong evidence that family factors play a relevant role in the development, maintenance, and course of youth depression (Restifo & Bögels, 2009). Parents' mental health problems predict depressive symptoms in children and adolescents, as well as their development over time. Concretely, children and adolescents of depressed parents are three to four times more likely to develop a depressive disorder and have a greater risk of experiencing a more severe and continuous course of depression (Garber, 2006). Furthermore, the offspring of depressed parents are more likely to develop greater cognitive vulnerability, internalize more maladaptive emotional regulation strategies, and experience fewer positive life events and positive parenting practices (Loechner et al., 2020). However, children with a high family risk of depression tend to show better mental health if the parent-child relationship is characterized by warmth, acceptance, a lack of hostility, and parental control (Thapar et al., 2012). Positive parenting skills and positive family relationships are protective factors for developing child depression (Klasen et al., 2015). Therefore, to reduce child and adolescent depression, preventive interventions must use a family-based approach to reduce risk factors (e.g., reduce parents' depression and negative parental practices) and increase protective factors (positive parenting skills) (Joshi et al., 2019). Preventive interventions to improve parents' mental health have been shown to reduce children's depression (Gladstone & Beardslee, 2009). As mentioned above, the European Commission (2016b) has indicated that preventing child-adolescent mental health problems requires a cooperation framework that includes several sectors, with particular attention to the preventive role that the school can play. In this regard, home-school or family-school collaboration refers to the relationship between families and schools where parents and teachers work together to promote children's and adolescents' socio-emotional, mental, and academic development (Cox, 2005). Family-school interventions have been shown to improve the development of parents and their children while also strengthening their mental and physical health (Zeleke et al., 2020). In addition, parents will agree to participate in these interventions if they are aimed at improving their well-being and that of their children (Parent & DiMarzio, 2021).

Mindfulness-based parenting interventions are a new approach that is yielding positive results (Burgdorf et al., 2019). These interventions aim to promote parent dispositional mindfulness and mindful parenting skills to improve parents' and children's mental health, parent-child relationships, and family climate (Cohen & Semple, 2010). Parent dispositional mindfulness has been linked to mindful parenting, which consists in intentionally bringing present-centered, nonjudgmental awareness to everyday parent-child interactions (Duncan et al., 2009; Kabat-Zinn & Kabat-Zinn, 1997). The model advanced by Duncan et al. (2009) encompasses five dimensions of mindful parenting relevant to the parent-child relationship: (a) listening with full attention to the child, (b) nonjudgmental acceptance of self and child, (c) emotional awareness of self and child, (d) self-regulation in the parenting relationship, and (e) compassion for self and child. Recent evidence shows that mindful parenting can be a protective factor for the early onset of child and adolescent depression.

First, cross-sectional research has found an indirect association between mindful parenting and adolescents' mindfulness and self-compassion through a more secure perception of the relationship with the parents. Adolescents seem to develop higher levels of mindfulness and self-compassion when the parent-child relationship is characterized by affection, self-regulation, and mindful awareness (Moreira et al., 2018). Also, Parent et al. (Parent et al., 2016) found that higher levels of parent dispositional mindfulness are indirectly related to lower levels of youth internalizing and externalizing problems through higher levels of mindful parenting and lower levels of negative parenting practices (e.g., hostility, reactive and intrusive parenting, coercive disciplinary tactics, and ineffective discipline). Second, longitudinal research has found that mindful parenting predicts reduced levels of depressive symptoms, aggression, and victimization in adolescents after 1 year (Calvete et al., 2021) as well as fewer recurrent conflicts after 3 months, leading to fewer internalizing problems in children after 1 year (Park et al., 2020). Similarly, Parent et al. (2021) carried out a relevant study with children and adolescents where they showed that (a) higher levels of parent dispositional mindfulness are related to higher levels of mindful parenting after 4 months, (b) higher levels of mindful parenting are associated with higher levels of positive parenting (parental proactivity, positive reinforcement, warmth, supportiveness) and lower levels of negative parenting practices (hostility, lax control, and physical discipline) after 8 months, and (c) lower levels of negative parenting practices are related to lower levels of youth internalizing (e.g., depression) and externalizing symptoms after 12 months. Some mechanisms that have been proposed to explain the impacts of mindful parenting on parent-child interactions in the context of child and parent mental health problems are (Bögels et al., 2010) (1) the reduction in parental stress and parental reactivity, (2) the reduction in parental concern regarding parental and/or child psychopathology, (3) the improvement of parental executive functioning in impulsive parents, (4) the break of the cycle of intergenerational transmission of dysfunctional parenting schemas and habits, (5) the increase in self-nourishing attention, and (6) the improvement of marital functioning and co-parenting. Therefore, this body of evidence indicating that dispositional parent mindfulness and mindful parenting help to prevent depression in parents and children justifies the importance of implementing interventions that promote mindfulness skills in parents as well as mindful parenting. Mindful parenting interventions seem adequate for this purpose (Bögels & Restifo, 2013).

Mindful parenting interventions targeting only parents, but not children, have shown promising results. A 10-week mindful parenting intervention found improvements in parents' internalizing symptoms and parental stress and children's internalizing and externalizing symptoms (Bögels et al., 2014). Similarly, an 8-week mindful parenting intervention found that increases in parent dispositional mindfulness after the intervention predicted a decrease in parental psychopathology, while increases in mindful parenting skills predicted a reduction in children's psychopathology (Meppelink et al., 2016). For their part, mindful parenting interventions targeting parents and children in parallel are still scarce, but their results are encouraging. A study examining the feasibility of MBCT in parallel for adolescents recovering from a depressive episode and for their parents showed improvements in depression, rumination, decentering, mindfulness, and self-compassion for the adolescents. Moreover, their parents reported that MBCT helped them to better understand their child's depression and improved the family climate. Similarly, the MYMind protocol, which consists of eight weekly 1.5-hour mindfulness-based group sessions for children and parallel ones for parents, has shown positive effects on the mental health of parents of children with autism spectrum disorders, who usually show elevated depressive symptoms, as well as on mindful parenting and parenting style (de Bruin et al., 2015; Haydicky et al., 2017; Ho et al., 2021; Ridderinkhof et al., 2018; Salem-Guirgis et al., 2019). Also, the MYMind program has shown positive effects, such as reducing childhood ADHD (i.e., reducing internalizing and externalizing symptoms while also increasing attention and executive functioning) and improving parental functioning (i.e., reducing parental psychopathology, over-reactivity, and stress while also increasing mindful parenting) (Bögels et al., 2021).

To our knowledge, there are no studies involving parents in mindfulness-based interventions at school aimed at preventing parent and child depression. However, results obtained in clinical settings suggest that including mindful parenting interventions in school contexts may benefit this purpose. Future research on the feasibility and effectiveness of mindful parenting interventions implemented in school contexts is necessary to determine whether the benefits of preventing depression in clinical settings may be generalized to schools.

3.6 Conclusion

The prevalence of depression in children and adolescents is increasing worldwide. The early emergence of a depressive disorder during childhood and adolescence negatively influences socio-emotional and cognitive development and school and family functioning and has a significant associated socioeconomic cost in the short and long term. Therefore, it is necessary to implement interventions that prevent depression in childhood and adolescence across multiple social sectors. In this regard, the school context meets the necessary conditions for implementing interventions that can help to prevent infant-adolescent depression, adopting either a universal approach (for all students) or a selective approach (for children and adolescents at risk of depression). MBIs are among the emerging interventions that can be cost-effective to address this purpose. This chapter has shown that MBIs implemented in school contexts effectively reduce risk factors and increase protective factors involved in child and adolescent depression. MBIs in schools have been shown to have a positive impact on the functioning of multiple agents involved in the early onset of depression, such as children and adolescents themselves, teachers, and parents. In summary, the evidence presented in this chapter (a) shows that MBIs implemented in schools for children and adolescents, teachers, and parents individually and separately effectively reduce child and adolescent depression, and (b) suggests that implementing MBIs in schools from a community and systemic perspective, involving students, teachers, and parents simultaneously in the intervention, may have greater success in preventing child and adolescent depression. Despite all of the above, it is important to mention that there are studies where there have been no results regarding the prevention of depression (Johnson et al., 2016, 2017), so this is a very recent field of research that still requires optimizing key ingredients, dosage, and format of the MBIs applied in schools. Further research must be conducted on the effectiveness of implementing an MBI in parallel for students, teachers, and parents in school contexts to reduce child and adolescent depression.

Conflict of Interest The authors declare that they have no conflict of interest.

Acknowledgments This chapter was supported by a María Zambrano grant from the Ministry of Universities of the Spanish Government to CIA (Reference number: ZA21-056) and by ANID – Millennium Science Initiative Program – ICS13_005.

References

Abenavoli, R. M., Jennings, P. A., Greenberg, M. T., Harris, A. R., & Katz, D. A. (2013). The protective effects of mindfulness against burnout among educators. *Psychology of Education Review, 37*(2), 57–69. https://doi.org/10.1007/s12671-015-0451-2

Aloe, A. M., Amo, L. C., & Shanahan, M. E. (2014). Classroom management self-efficacy and burnout: A multivariate meta-analysis. *Educational Psychology Review, 26*(1), 101–126. https://doi.org/10.1007/s10648-013-9244-0

Ames, C. S., Richardson, J., Payne, S., Smith, P., & Leigh, E. (2014). Mindfulness-based cognitive therapy for depression in adolescents. *Child and Adolescent Mental Health, 19*(1), 74–78. https://doi.org/10.1111/camh.12034

Andreu, C. I., Araya-Véliz, C., & García-Rubio, C. (2021). Benefits of a mindfulness-based intervention at school from the perspective of at-risk children. *Mindfulness, 12*(7), 1611–1623. https://doi.org/10.1007/s12671-021-01624-6

Andreu, C. I., & García-Rubio, C. (2019). How does mindfulness work in schools? An integrative model of the outcomes and the mechanisms of change of mindfulness-based interventions in the classroom. In C. Steinebach & Á. Langer (Eds.), *Enhancing resilience in youth* (pp. 139–157). Springer. https://doi.org/10.1007/978-3-030-25513-8_9

Bauer, C. C. C., Caballero, C., Scherer, E., West, M. R., Mrazek, M. D., Phillips, D. T., Whitfield-Gabrieli, S., & Gabrieli, J. D. E. (2019). Mindfulness training reduces stress and amygdala reactivity to fearful faces in middle-school children. *Behavioral Neuroscience, 133*(6), 569–585. https://doi.org/10.1037/bne0000337

Becker, B. D., Gallagher, K. C., & Whitaker, R. C. (2017). Teachers' dispositional mindfulness and the quality of their relationships with children in head start classrooms. *Journal of School Psychology, 65*, 40–53. https://doi.org/10.1016/j.jsp.2017.06.004

Bellingrath, S., Rohleder, N., & Kudielka, B. M. (2010). Healthy working school teachers with high effort-reward-imbalance and overcommitment show increased pro-inflammatory immune activity and a dampened innate immune defence. *Brain, Behavior, and Immunity, 24*(8), 1332–1339. https://doi.org/10.1016/j.bbi.2010.06.011

Bernstein, A., Hadash, Y., Lichtash, Y., Tanay, G., Shepherd, K., & Fresco, D. M. (2015). Decentering and related constructs: A critical review and metacognitive processes model. *Perspectives on Psychological Science, 10*(5), 599–617. https://doi.org/10.1177/1745691615594577

Bianchi, R., Schonfeld, I. S., & Laurent, E. (2015). Burnout-depression overlap: A review. *Clinical Psychology Review, 36*, 28–41. https://doi.org/10.1016/j.cpr.2015.01.004

Bishop, S. R., Lau, M., Shapiro, S., Carlson, L., Anderson, N. D., Carmody, J., et al. (2006). Mindfulness: A proposed operational definition. *Clinical Psychology: Science and Practice, 11*(3), 230–241. https://doi.org/10.1093/clipsy.bph077

Bodden, D. H. M., Stikkelbroek, Y., & Dirksen, C. D. (2018). Societal burden of adolescent depression, an overview and cost-of-illness study. *Journal of Affective Disorders, 241*, 256–262. https://doi.org/10.1016/j.jad.2018.06.015

Bögels, S. M., Hellemans, J., van Deursen, S., Römer, M., & van der Meulen, R. (2014). Mindful parenting in mental health care: Effects on parental and child psychopathology, parental stress, parenting, coparenting, and marital functioning. *Mindfulness, 5*(5), 536–551. https://doi.org/10.1007/s12671-013-0209-7

Bögels, S. M., Lehtonen, A., & Restifo, K. (2010). Mindful parenting in mental health care. *Mindfulness, 1*(2), 107–120. https://doi.org/10.1007/s12671-010-0014-5

Bögels, S. M., Oort, F. J., Potharst, E., van Roosmalen, R., Williams, J. M. G., & de Bruin, E. I. (2021). Family mindfulness training for childhood ADHD: Short-and long-term effects on children, fathers and mothers. *Mindfulness*, 1–15. https://doi.org/10.1007/s12671-021-01761-y

Bögels, S. M., & Restifo, K. (2013). *Mindful parenting: A guide for mental health practitioners*. Springer Science & Business Media.

Braun, S. S., Roeser, R. W., Mashburn, A. J., & Skinner, E. (2019). Middle school teachers' mindfulness, occupational health and Well-being, and the quality of teacher-student interactions. *Mindfulness, 10*(2), 245–255. https://doi.org/10.1007/s12671-018-0968-2

de Bruin, E. I., Blom, R., Smit, F. M., van Steensel, F. J., & Bögels, S. M. (2015). MYmind: Mindfulness training for youngsters with autism spectrum disorders and their parents. *Autism: The International Journal of Research and Practice, 19*(8), 906–914. https://doi.org/10.1177/1362361314553279

Buettner, C. K., Jeon, L., Hur, E., & Garcia, R. E. (2016). Teachers' social–emotional capacity: Factors associated with teachers' responsiveness and professional commitment. *Early Education and Development, 27*(7), 1018–1039. https://doi.org/10.1080/10409289.2016.1168227

Burgdorf, V., Szabó, M., & Abbott, M. J. (2019). The effect of mindfulness interventions for parents on parenting stress and youth psychological outcomes: A systematic review and meta-analysis. *Frontiers in Psychology, 10*, 1336. https://doi.org/10.3389/fpsyg.2019.01336

Calvete, E., Gómez-Odriozola, J., & Orue, I. (2021). Differential susceptibility to the benefits of mindful parenting depending on child dispositional. *Mindfulness, 12*, 405–418. https://doi.org/10.1007/s12671-020-01467-7

Calvete, E., Morea, A., & Orue, I. (2019). The role of dispositional mindfulness in the longitudinal associations between stressors, maladaptive schemas, and depressive symptoms in adolescents. *Mindfulness, 10*, 547–558. https://doi.org/10.1007/s12671-018-1000-6

Calvete, E., Orue, I., & Sampedro, A. (2017). Does the acting with awareness trait of mindfulness buffer the predictive association between stressors and psychological symptoms in adolescents? *Personality and Individual Differences, 105*, 158–163. https://doi.org/10.1016/j.paid.2016.09.055

Carballo, J. J., Llorente, C., Kehrmann, L., Flamarique, I., Zuddas, A., Purper-Ouakil, D., Hoekstra, P. J., Coghill, D., Schulze, U., Dittmann, R. W., Buitelaar, J. K., Castro-Fornieles, J., Lievesley, K., Santosh, P., Arango, C., & STOP Consortium. (2020). Psychosocial risk factors for suicidality in children and adolescents. *European Child & Adolescent Psychiatry, 29*(6), 759–776. https://doi.org/10.1007/s00787-018-01270-9

Carr, A. (Ed.). (2000). *What works with children and adolescents?: A critical review of psychological interventions with children, adolescents and their families*. Taylor & Frances/Routledge.

Chambers, R., Gullone, E., Hassed, C., Knight, W., Garvin, T., & Allen, N. (2015). Mindful emotion regulation predicts recovery in depressed youth. *Mindfulness, 6*(3), 523–534. https://doi.org/10.1007/s12671-014-0284-4

Cohen, J. A. S., & Semple, R. J. (2010). Mindful parenting: A call for research. *Journal of Child and Family Studies, 19*(2), 145–151. https://doi.org/10.1007/s10826-009-9285-7

Colaianne, B. A., Galla, B. M., & Roeser, R. W. (2020). Perceptions of mindful teaching are associated with longitudinal change in adolescents' mindfulness and compassion. *International Journal of Behavioral Development, 44*(1), 41–50. https://doi.org/10.1177/0165025419870864

Costello, E. J., Mustillo, S., Erkanli, A., Keeler, G., & Angold, A. (2003). Prevalence and development of psychiatric disorders in childhood and adolescence. *Archives of General Psychiatry, 60*(8), 837–844. https://doi.org/10.1001/archpsyc.60.8.837

Cotton, S., Luberto, C. M., Sears, R. W., Strawn, J. R., Stahl, L., Wasson, R. S., Blom, T. J., & Delbello, M. P. (2016). Mindfulness-based cognitive therapy for youth with anxiety disorders at risk for bipolar disorder: A pilot trial. *Early Intervention in Psychiatry, 10*(5), 426–434. https://doi.org/10.1111/eip.12216

Cox, D. D. (2005). Evidence-based interventions using home-school collaboration. *School Psychology Quarterly, 20*(4), 473–497. https://doi.org/10.1521/scpq.2005.20.4.473

Crain, T. L., Schonert-Reichl, K. A., & Roeser, R. W. (2017). Cultivating teacher mindfulness: Effects of a randomized controlled trial on work, home, and sleep outcomes. *Journal of Occupational Health Psychology, 22*(2), 138–152. https://doi.org/10.1037/ocp0000043

Crane, R. S., Brewer, J., Feldman, C., Kabat-Zinn, J., Santorelli, S., Williams, J. M. G., & Kuyken, W. (2017). What defines mindfulness-based programs? The warp and the weft. *Psychological Medicine, 47*(6), 990–999. https://doi.org/10.1017/s0033291716003317

Cuijpers, P., Karyotaki, E., Ciharova, M., Miguel, C., Noma, H., Stikkelbroek, Y., Weisz, J. R., & Furukawa, T. A. (2021). The effects of psychological treatments of depression in children and adolescents on response, reliable change, and deterioration: A systematic review and meta-analysis. *European Child & Adolescent Psychiatry*. https://doi.org/10.1007/s00787-021-01884-6

Dane, E., & Brummel, B. J. (2014). Examining workplace mindfulness and its relations to job performance and turnover intention. *Human Relations, 67*(1), 105–128. https://doi.org/10.1177/0018726713487753

Duncan, L. G., Coatsworth, J. D., & Greenberg, M. T. (2009). A model of mindful parenting: Implications for parent-child relationships and prevention research. *Clinical Child and Family Psychology Review, 12*(3), 255–270. https://doi.org/10.1007/s10567-009-0046-3

Dunning, D. L., Griffiths, K., Kuyken, W., Crane, C., Foulkes, L., Parker, J., & Dalgleish, T. (2019). Research review: The effects of mindfulness-based interventions on cognition and mental health in children and adolescents – A meta-analysis of randomized controlled trials. *Journal of Child Psychology and Psychiatry, 60*(3), 244–258. https://doi.org/10.1111/jcpp.12980

Durlak, J. A. (1998). Common risk and protective factors in successful prevention programs. *American Journal of Orthopsychiatry, 68*(4), 512–520. https://doi.org/10.1037/h0080360

Ehrenreich-May, J., & Chu, B. C. (2013). *Transdiagnostic treatments for children and adolescents: Principles and practice*. Guilford Publications.

Esmaeilian, N., Dehghani, M., Dehghani, Z., & Lee, J. (2018). Mindfulness-based cognitive therapy enhances emotional resiliency in children with divorced parents. *Mindfulness, 9*(4), 1052–1062. https://doi.org/10.1007/s12671-017-0840-9

European Commission. (2016a). *European framework for action on mental health and wellbeing.* http://www.mentalhealthandwellbeing.eu/publications

European Commission. (2016b). Mental health and schools. *Situation analysis and recommendations for action (joint action on mental health and wellbeing).* https://ec.eu-ropa.eu/health/sites/health/files/mental_health/docs/2017_mh_schools_en.pd

Fatori, D., Salum, G., Itria, A., Pan, P., Alvarenga, P., Rohde, L. A., et al. (2018). The economic impact of subthreshold and clinical childhood mental disorders. *Journal of Mental Health, 27*, 588–594. https://doi.org/10.1080/09638237.2018.1466041

Fernández-Hermida, J. R., & Villamarín-Fernández, S. (Eds.) (2021). *Libro Blanco de la Salud Mental Infanto-Juvenil. Volumen 1. Consejo General de la Psicología de España.* https://www.cop.es/pdf/LibroBlanco-Volumen1.pdf

Flannery-Schroeder, E. C. (2006). Reducing anxiety to prevent depression. *American Journal of Preventive Medicine, 31*(6 Suppl 1), 136–S142. https://doi.org/10.1016/j.amepre.2006.07.006

Fombonne, E., Wostear, G., Cooper, V., Harrington, R., & Rutter, M. (2001). The Maudsley long-term follow-up of child and adolescent depression. *British Journal of Psychiatry, 179*(3), 210–217. https://doi.org/10.1192/bjp.179.3.210

Frank, J. L., Jennings, P. A., & Greenberg, M. T. (2016). Validation of the mindfulness in teaching scale. *Mindfulness, 7*(1), 155–163. https://doi.org/10.1007/s12671-015-0461-0

Fung, J., Kim, J. J., Jin, J., Chen, G., Bear, L., & Lau, A. S. (2019). A randomized trial evaluating school-based mindfulness intervention for ethnic minority youth: Exploring mediators and moderators of intervention effects. *Journal of Abnormal Child Psychology, 47*(1), 1–19. https://doi.org/10.1007/s10802-018-0425-7

Galla, B. M., Tsukayama, E., Park, D., Yu, A., & Duckworth, A. L. (2020). The mindful adolescent: Developmental changes in nonreactivity to inner experiences and its association with emotional Well-being. *Developmental Psychology, 56*(2), 350–363. https://doi.org/10.1037/dev0000877

Garber, J. (2006). Depression in children and adolescents: Linking risk research and prevention. *American Journal of Preventive Medicine, 31*(6 Suppl 1), 104–125. https://doi.org/10.1016/j.amepre.2006.07.007

García-Carmona, M., Marín, M. D., & Aguayo, R. (2019). Burnout syndrome in secondary school teachers: A systematic review and meta-analysis. *Social Psychology of Education: An International Journal, 22*(1), 189–208. https://doi.org/10.1007/s11218-018-9471-9

García-Rubio, C. (2021). *Effectiveness and mechanisms of action of the mindfulness-based interventions in the school context* [Doctoral dissertation, Universidad Autónoma de Madrid]. http://hdl.handle.net/10486/696537

García-Rubio, C., Lecuona, O., Blanco Donoso, L. M., Cantero-García, M., Paniagua, D., & Rodríguez-Carvajal, R. (2020). Spanish validation of the short-form of the avoidance and fusion questionnaire (AFQ-Y8) with children and adolescents. *Psychological Assessment, 32*(4), e15–e27. https://doi.org/10.1037/pas0000801

García-Rubio, C., Rodríguez-Carvajal, R., Langer, A. I., Paniagua, D., Steinebach, P., Andreu, C. I., Vara, M. D., & Cebolla, A. (2019). Validation of the Spanish version of the child and adolescent mindfulness measure (CAMM) with samples of Spanish and Chilean children and adolescents. *Mindfulness, 10*(8), 1502–1517. https://doi.org/10.1007/s12671-019-01108-8

Gladstone, T. R. G., & Beardslee, W. R. (2009). The prevention of depression in children and adolescents: A review. *The Canadian Journal of Psychiatry/La Revue Canadienne de Psychiatrie, 54*(4), 212–221.

Golberstein, E., Wen, H., & Miller, B. F. (2020). Coronavirus disease 2019 (COVID-19) and mental health for children and adolescents. *Journal of American Medical Association Pediatrics, 174*(9), 819–820. https://doi.org/10.1001/jamapediatrics.2020.1456

Greco, L. A., Baer, R. A., & Smith, G. T. (2011). Assessing mindfulness in children and adolescents: Development and validation of the child and adolescent mindfulness measure (CAMM). *Psychological Assessment, 23*(3), 606–614. https://doi.org/10.1037/a0022819

Greco, L. A., & Hayes, S. C. (Eds.). (2008). *Acceptance and mindfulness treatments for children and adolescents: A practitioner's guide*. New Harbinger.

Gu, J., Strauss, C., Bond, R., & Cavanagh, K. (2015). How do mindfulness-based cognitive therapy and mindfulness-based stress reduction improve mental health and wellbeing? A systematic review and meta-analysis of mediation studies. *Clinical Psychology Review, 37*, 1–12. https://doi.org/10.1016/j.cpr.2015.01.006

Haydicky, J., Wiener, J., & Shecter, C. (2017). Mechanisms of action in concurrent Parent-child mindfulness training: A qualitative exploration. *Mindfulness, 8*, 1018–1035. https://doi.org/10.1007/s12671-017-0678-1

Ho, R., Zhang, D., Chan, S., Gao, T. T., Lee, E., Lo, H., Au Yeung, P., Lai, K., Bögels, S. M., de Bruin, E. I., & Wong, S. (2021). Brief report: Mindfulness training for Chinese adolescents with autism Spectrum disorder and their parents in Hong Kong. *Journal of Autism and Developmental Disorders, 51*(11), 4147–4159. https://doi.org/10.1007/s10803-020-04729-4

Hulburt, K. J., Coalaiane, B. A., & Roeser, R. W. (2020). The calm, clear, and kind educator: A contemplative educational approach to teacher professional identity development. In O. Ergas & J. K. Ritter (Eds.), *Exploring self toward expanding teaching, teacher education and practitioner research* (pp. 17–35). Emerald Publishing. https://doi.org/10.1108/S1479-368720200000034001

Hülsheger, U. R., Alberts, H. J., Feinholdt, A., & Lang, J. W. (2013). Benefits of mindfulness at work: The role of mindfulness in emotion regulation, emotional exhaustion, and job satisfaction. *The Journal of Applied Psychology, 98*(2), 310–325. https://doi.org/10.1037/a0031313

Jennings, P. A. (2008). Contemplative education and youth development. *New Directions for Youth Development, 2008*(118), 101–105. https://doi.org/10.1002/yd.262

Jennings, P. A. (2015). *Mindfulness for teachers: Simple skills for peace and productivity in the classroom*. W. W. Norton & Company.

Jennings, P. A. (2016). Mindfulness-based programs and the American public school system: Recommendations for best practices to ensure secularity. *Mindfulness, 7*(1), 176–178. https://doi.org/10.1007/s12671-015-0477-5

Jennings, P. A., Brown, J. L., Frank, J. L., Doyle, S., Oh, Y., Davis, R., Rasheed, D., DeWeese, A., DeMauro, A. A., Cham, H., & Greenberg, M. T. (2017). Impacts of the CARE for Teachers program on teachers' social and emotional competence and classroom interactions. *Journal of Educational Psychology, 109*(7), 1010–1028. https://doi.org/10.1037/edu0000187

Jennings, P. A., Doyle, S., Oh, Y., Rasheed, D., Frank, J. L., & Brown, J. L. (2019). Long-term impacts of the CARE program on teachers' self-reported social and emotional competence and Well-being. *Journal of School Psychology, 76*, 186–202. https://doi.org/10.1016/j.jsp.2019.07.009

Jennings, P. A., & Greenberg, M. T. (2009). The prosocial classroom: Teacher social and emotional competence in relation to student and classroom outcomes. *Review of Educational Research, 79*(1), 491–525. https://doi.org/10.3102/0034654308325693

Jeon, L., Buettner, C. K., & Snyder, A. R. (2014). Pathways from teacher depression and child-care quality to child behavioral problems. *Journal of Consulting and Clinical Psychology, 82*(2), 225–235. https://doi.org/10.1037/a0035720

Johnson, C., Burke, C., Brinkman, S., & Wade, T. (2016). Effectiveness of a school-based mindfulness program for transdiagnostic prevention in young adolescents. *Behaviour Research and Therapy, 81*, 1–11. https://doi.org/10.1016/j.brat.2016.03.002

Johnson, C., Burke, C., Brinkman, S., & Wade, T. (2017). A randomized controlled evaluation of a secondary school mindfulness program for early adolescents: Do we have the recipe right yet? *Behaviour Research and Therapy, 99*, 37–46. https://doi.org/10.1016/j.brat.2017.09.001

Joshi, S. V., Jassim, N., & Mani, N. (2019). Youth depression in school settings: Assessment, interventions, and prevention. *Child and Adolescent Psychiatric Clinics of North America, 28*(3), 349–362. https://doi.org/10.1016/j.chc.2019.02.017

Kabat-Zinn, J. (2003). Mindfulness-based interventions in context: Past, present, and future. *Clinical Psychology: Science and Practice, 10*(2), 144–156. https://doi.org/10.1093/clipsy.bpg016

Kabat-Zinn, M., & Kabat-Zinn, J. (1997). *Everyday blessings: The inner work of mindful parenting*. Hachette.

Kallapiran, K., Koo, S., Kirubakaran, R., & Hancock, K. (2015). Review: Effectiveness of mindfulness in improving mental health symptoms of children and adolescents: A meta-analysis. *Child and Adolescent Mental Health, 20*(4), 182–194. https://doi.org/10.1111/camh.12113

Kang, Y., Rahrig, H., Eichel, K., Niles, H. F., Rocha, T., Lepp, N. E., Gold, J., & Britton, W. B. (2018). Gender differences in response to a school-based mindfulness training intervention for early adolescents. *Journal of School Psychology, 68*, 163–176. https://doi.org/10.1016/j.jsp.2018.03.004

Kann, L., McManus, T., Harris, W. A., Shanklin, S. L., Flint, K. H., Queen, B., et al. (2018). Youth risk behavior surveillance — United States, 2017. *MMWR Surveillance Summaries, 67*(8), 1–114. https://doi.org/10.15585/mmwr.ss6708a1

Kashdan, T. B., & Rottenberg, J. (2010). Psychological flexibility as a fundamental aspect of health. *Clinical Psychology Review, 30*(7), 865–878. https://doi.org/10.1016/j.cpr.2010.03.001

Kessler, R. C., Amminger, G. P., Aguilar-Gaxiola, S., Alonso, J., Lee, S., & Ustun, T. B. (2007). Age of onset of mental disorders: A review of recent literature. *Current Opinion in Psychiatry, 20*(4), 359–364. https://doi.org/10.1097/yco.0b013e32816ebc8c

Klasen, F., Otto, C., Kriston, L., Patalay, P., Schlack, R., Ravens-Sieberer, U., & BELLA Study Group. (2015). Risk and protective factors for the development of depressive symptoms in children and adolescents: Results of the longitudinal BELLA study. *European Child & Adolescent Psychiatry, 24*(6), 695–703. https://doi.org/10.1007/s00787-014-0637-5

Klingbeil, D. A., Renshaw, T. L., Willenbrink, J. B., Copek, R. A., Chan, K. T., Haddock, A., et al. (2017). Mindfulness-based interventions with youth: A comprehensive meta-analysis of group-design studies. *Journal of School Psychology, 63*, 77–103. https://doi.org/10.1016/j.jsp.2017.03.006

Knowles, L. M., Goodman, M. S., & Semple, R. J. (2015). Mindfulness with elementary-school-age children. In S. Willard & A. Saltzman (Eds.), *Teaching mindfulness skills to kids and teens* (pp. 19–41). Guilford Publications.

Kostev, K., Teichgräber, F., Konrad, M., & Jacob, L. (2019). Association between chronic somatic conditions and depression in children and adolescents: A retrospective study of 13,326 patients. *Journal of Affective Disorders, 245*, 697–701. https://doi.org/10.1016/j.jad.2018.11.014

Kuyken, W., Warren, F. C., Taylor, R. S., Whalley, B., Crane, C., Bondolfi, G., Hayes, R., Huijbers, M., Ma, H., Schweizer, S., Segal, Z., Speckens, A., Teasdale, J. D., Van Heeringen, K., Williams, M., Byford, S., Byng, R., & Dalgleish, T. (2016). Efficacy of mindfulness-based cognitive therapy in prevention of depressive relapse: An individual patient data meta-analysis from randomized trials. *JAMA Psychiatry, 73*(6), 565–574. https://doi.org/10.1001/jamapsychiatry.2016.0076

Lam, K. (2016). School-based cognitive mindfulness intervention for internalizing problems: Pilot study with Hong Kong elementary students. *Journal of Child and Family Studies, 25*(11), 3293–3308. https://doi.org/10.1007/s10826-016-0483-9

Lawlor, M. S. (2016). Mindfulness and social emotional learning (SEL): A conceptual framework. In K. Schonert-Reichl & R. Roeser (Eds.), *Handbook of mindfulness in education* (pp. 65–80). Springer. https://doi.org/10.1007/978-1-4939-3506-2_5

Lawlor, M. S., Schonert-Reichl, K. A., Gadermann, A. M., & Zumbo, B. D. (2014). A validation study of the mindful attention awareness scale adapted for children. *Mindfulness, 5*(6), 730–741. https://doi.org/10.1007/s12671-013-0228-4

Lee, J., Semple, R. J., Rosa, D., & Miller, L. (2008). Mindfulness-based cognitive therapy for children: Results of a pilot study. *Journal of Cognitive Psychotherapy, 22*(1), 15–28. https://doi.org/10.1891/0889.8391.22.1.15

Lensen, J. H., Stoltz, S. E. M. J., Kleinjan, M., Speckens, A. E. M., Kraiss, J. T., & Scholte, R. H. J. (2021). Mindfulness-based stress reduction intervention for elementary school teachers: A mixed method study. *Trials, 22*(1), 1–10. https://doi.org/10.1186/s13063-021-05804-6

Lindsay, E. K., & Creswell, J. D. (2017). Mechanisms of mindfulness training: Monitor and acceptance theory (MAT). *Clinical Psychology Review, 51*, 48–59. https://doi.org/10.1016/j.cpr.2016.10.011

Loechner, J., Sfärlea, A., Starman, K., Oort, F., Thomsen, L. A., Schulte-Körne, G., & Platt, B. (2020). Risk of depression in the offspring of parents with depression: The role of emotion regulation, cognitive style, parenting and life events. *Child Psychiatry and Human Development, 51*(2), 294–309. https://doi.org/10.1007/s10578-019-00930-4

Lynch, F. L., & Clarke, G. N. (2006). Estimating the economic burden of depression in children and adolescents. *American Journal of Preventive Medicine, 31*(6), 143–151. https://doi.org/10.1016/j.amepre.2006.07.001

Markow, D., Macia, L., & Lee, H. (2013). *The MetLife survey of the American teacher: Challenges for school leadership*. Metropolitan Life Insurance Company. https://www.metlife.com/assets/cao/foundation/MetLife-Teacher-Survey-2012.pdf

Maslach, C., Schaufeli, W. B., & Leiter, M. P. (2001). Job burnout. *Annual Review of Psychology, 52*, 397–422. https://doi.org/10.1146/annurev.psych.52.1.397

Mendelson, T., & Tandon, S. D. (2016). Prevention of depression in childhood and adolescence. *Child and Adolescent Psychiatric Clinics of North America, 25*(2), 201–218. https://doi.org/10.1016/j.chc.2015.11.005

Meppelink, R., de Bruin, E. I., Wanders-Mulder, F. H., Vennik, C. J., & Bögels, S. M. (2016). Mindful parenting training in child psychiatric settings: Heightened parental mindfulness reduces parents' and children's psychopathology. *Mindfulness, 7*, 680–689. https://doi.org/10.1007/s12671-016-0504-1

Merry, S. N., Hetrick, S. E., Cox, G. R., Brudevold-Iversen, T., Bir, J. J., & McDowell, H. (2011). Psychological and educational interventions for preventing depression in children and adolescents. *The Cochrane Database of Systematic Reviews, 12*, CD003380. https://doi.org/10.1002/14651858.CD003380.pub3

Mezulis, A. H., Hyde, J. S., & Abramson, L. Y. (2006). The developmental origins of cognitive vulnerability to depression: Temperament, parenting, and negative life events in childhood as contributors to negative cognitive style. *Developmental Psychology, 42*(6), 1012–1025. https://doi.org/10.1037/0012-1649.42.6.1012

Molloy Elreda, L., Jennings, P. A., DeMauro, A. A., Mischenko, P. P., & Brown, J. L. (2019). Protective effects of interpersonal mindfulness for teachers' emotional supportiveness in the classroom. *Mindfulness, 10*(3), 537–546. https://doi.org/10.1007/s12671-018-0996-y

Montero-Marin, J., Taylor, L., Crane, C., Greenberg, M. T., Ford, T. J., Williams, J. M. G., et al. (2021). Teachers "finding peace in a frantic world": An experimental study of self-taught and instructor-led mindfulness program formats on acceptability, effectiveness, and mechanisms. *Journal of Educational Psychology, 113*(8), 1689–1708. https://doi.org/10.1037/edu0000542

Moreira, H., Gouveia, M. J., & Canavarro, M. C. (2018). Is mindful parenting associated with adolescents' well-being in early and middle/late adolescence? The mediating role of adolescents' attachment representations, self-compassion and mindfulness. *Journal of Youth and Adolescence, 47*(8), 1771–1788. https://doi.org/10.1007/s10964-018-0808-7

Muris, P., Meesters, C., Herings, A., Jansen, M., Vossen, C., & Kersten, P. (2017). Inflexible youngsters: Psychological and psychopathological correlates of the avoidance and fusion questionnaire for youths in nonclinical Dutch adolescents. *Mindfulness, 8*(5), 1381–1392. https://doi.org/10.1007/s12671-017-0714-1

Neff, K. (2003). Self-compassion: An alternative conceptualization of a healthy attitude toward oneself. *Self and Identity, 2*(2), 85–101. https://doi.org/10.1080/15298860309032

Novins, D. K., Stoddard, J., Althoff, R. R., Charach, A., Cortese, S., Cullen, K. R., Frazier, J. A., Glatt, S. J., Henderson, S. W., Herringa, R. J., Hulvershorn, L., Kieling, C., McBride, A. B., McCauley, E., Middeldorp, C. M., Reiersen, A. M., Rockhill, C. M., Sagot, A. J., Scahill, L., et al. (2021). Editors' note and special communication: Research priorities in child and adolescent mental health emerging from the COVID-19 pandemic. *Journal of the American Academy of Child & Adolescent Psychiatry, 60*(5), 544–554. https://doi.org/10.1016/j.jaac.2021.03.005

Oberle, E., & Schonert-Reichl, K. A. (2016). Stress contagion in the classroom? The link between classroom teacher burnout and morning cortisol in elementary school students. *Social Science & Medicine, 159*, 30–37. https://doi.org/10.1016/j.socscimed.2016.04.031

Oppo, A., Schweiger, M., Ristallo, A., Presti, G., Pergolizzi, F., & Moderato, P. (2019). Mindfulness skills and psychological inflexibility: Two useful tools for a clinical assessment for adolescents with internalizing behaviors. *Journal of Child and Family Studies, 28*(12), 3569–3580. https://doi.org/10.1007/s10826-019-01539-w

Otto, C., Haller, A. C., Klasen, F., Hölling, H., Bullinger, M., Ravens-Sieberer, U., & BELLA study group. (2017). Risk and protective factors of health-related quality of life in children and adolescents: Results of the longitudinal BELLA study. *PLoS One, 12*(12), e0190363. https://doi.org/10.1371/journal.pone.0190363

Pallozzi, R., Wertheim, E., Paxton, S., & Ong, B. (2017). Trait mindfulness measures for use with adolescents: A systematic review. *Mindfulness, 8*(1), 110–125. https://doi.org/10.1007/s12671-016-0567-z

Parent, J., Dale, C., McKee, L. G., & Sullivan, A. (2021). The longitudinal influence of caregiver dispositional mindful attention on mindful parenting, parenting practices, and youth psychopathology. *Mindfulness, 12*(2), 357–369. https://doi.org/10.1007/s12671-020-01536-x

Parent, J., & DiMarzio, K. A. (2021). Mindful parenting research: An introduction. *Mindfulness, 12*, 261–265. https://doi.org/10.1007/s12671-020-01572-7

Parent, J., McKee, L. G., Rough, J. N., & Forehand, R. (2016). The association of parent mindfulness with parenting and youth psychopathology across three developmental stages. *Journal of Abnormal Child Psychology, 44*(1), 191–202. https://doi.org/10.1007/s10802-015-9978-x

Park, Y. R., Nix, R. L., Duncan, L. G., Coatsworth, J. D., & Greenberg, M. T. (2020). Unfolding Relations among Mindful Parenting, Recurrent Conflict, and Adolescents' Externalizing and Internalizing Problems. *Family process, 59*(4), 1690–1705. https://doi.org/10.1111/famp.12498

Pine, D. S., Cohen, P., Gurley, D., Brook, J., & Ma, Y. (1998). The risk for early-adulthood anxiety and depressive disorders in adolescents with anxiety and depressive disorders. *Archives of General Psychiatry, 55*(1), 56–64. https://doi.org/10.1001/archpsyc.55.1.56

Polanczyk, G. V., Salum, G. A., Sugaya, L. S., Caye, A., & Rohde, L. A. (2015). Annual research review: A meta-analysis of the worldwide prevalence of mental disorders in children and adolescents. *Journal of Child Psychology and Psychiatry, 56*(3), 345–365. https://doi.org/10.1111/jcpp.12381

Raes, F., Griffith, J. W., Van der Gucht, K., & Williams, J. M. G. (2014). School-based prevention and reduction of depression in adolescents: A cluster-randomized controlled trial of a mindfulness group program. *Mindfulness, 5*(5), 477–486. https://doi.org/10.1007/s12671-013-0202-1

Restifo, K., & Bögels, S. (2009). Family processes in the development of youth depression: Translating the evidence to treatment. *Clinical Psychology Review, 29*(4), 294–316. https://doi.org/10.1016/j.cpr.2009.02.005

Ridderinkhof, A., de Bruin, E. I., Blom, R., & Bögels, S. M. (2018). Mindfulness-based program for children with autism spectrum disorder and their parents: Direct and long-term improvements. *Mindfulness, 9*(3), 773–791. https://doi.org/10.1007/s12671-017-0815-x

Roberts, A., LoCasale-Crouch, J., Hamre, B., & DeCoster, J. (2016). Exploring teachers' depressive symptoms, interaction quality, and children's social-emotional development in head start. *Early Education and Development, 27*(5), 642–654. https://doi.org/10.1080/10409289.2016.1127088

Rodrigues de Oliveira, D., Wilson, D., Palace-Berl, F., de Mello Ponteciano, B., Fungaro Rissatti, L., Sardela de Miranda, F., Piassa Pollizi, V., Fuscella, J. C., Mourão Terzi, A., Lepique, A. P.,

D'Almeida, V., & Demarzo, M. (2021). Mindfulness meditation training effects on quality of life, immune function and glutathione metabolism in service healthy female teachers: A randomized pilot clinical trial. *Brain, Behavior, & Immunity – Health, 18*, 100372. https://doi.org/10.1016/j.bbih.2021.100372

Roeser, R. W., & Peck, S. C. (2009). An education in awareness: Self, motivation, and self-regulated learning in contemplative perspective. *Educational Psychologist, 44*(2), 119–136. https://doi.org/10.1080/00461520902832376

Roeser, R. W., & Pinela, C. (2014). Mindfulness and compassion training in adolescence: A developmental contemplative science perspective. *New Directions for Youth Development, 2014*(142), 9–30. https://doi.org/10.1002/yd.20094

Roeser, R. W., Schonert-Reichl, K. A., Jha, A., Cullen, M., Wallace, L., Wilensky, R., Oberle, E., Thomson, K., Taylor, C., & Harrison, J. (2013). Mindfulness training and reductions in teacher stress and burnout: Results from two randomized, waitlist-control field trials. *Journal of Educational Psychology, 105*(3), 787–804. https://doi.org/10.1037/a0032093

Roeser, R. W., Skinner, E., Beers, J., & Jennings, P. A. (2012). Mindfulness training and teachers' professional development: An emerging area of research and practice. *Child Development Perspectives, 6*(2), 167–173. https://doi.org/10.1111/j.1750-8606.2012.00238.x

Royuela-Colomer, E., & Calvete, E. (2016). Mindfulness facets and depression in adolescents: Rumination as a mediator. *Mindfulness, 7*, 1092–1102. https://doi.org/10.1007/s12671-016-0547-3

Royuela-Colomer, E., Fernández-González, L., & Orue, I. (2021). Longitudinal associations between internalizing symptoms, dispositional mindfulness, rumination and impulsivity in adolescents. *Journal of Youth and Adolescence, 50*(10), 2067–2078. https://doi.org/10.1007/s10964-021-01476-2

Salem-Guirgis, S., Albaum, C., Tablon, P., Riosa, P. B., Nicholas, D. B., Drmic, I. E., & Weiss, J. A. (2019). MYmind: A concurrent group-based mindfulness intervention for youth with autism and their parents. *Mindfulness, 10*(9), 1730–1743. https://doi.org/10.1007/s12671-019-01107-9

Sandilos, L. E., Cycyk, L. M., Hammer, C. S., Sawyer, B. E., López, L., & Blair, C. (2015). Depression, control, and climate: An examination of factors impacting teaching quality in preschool classrooms. *Early Education and Development, 26*(8), 1111–1127. https://doi.org/10.1080/10409289.2015.1027624

Saunders, N. R., Gandhi, S., Chen, S., Vigod, S., Fung, K., De Souza, C., et al. (2020). Health care use and costs of children, adolescents, and young adults with somatic symptom and related disorders. *JAMA Network Open, 3*(7), e2011295. https://doi.org/10.1001/jamanetworkopen.2020.11295

Save the Children. (2021). Crecer Saludable(Mente). *Un análisis sobre la salud mental y el suicidio en la infancia y la adolescencia*. https://www.savethechildren.es/sites/default/files/2021-12/Informe_Crecer_saludablemente_DIC_2021.pdf

Scher, C. D., Ingram, R. E., & Segal, Z. V. (2005). Cognitive reactivity and vulnerability: Empirical evaluation of construct activation and cognitive diatheses in unipolar depression. *Clinical Psychology Review, 25*(4), 487–510. https://doi.org/10.1016/j.cpr.2005.01.005

Schonert-Reichl, K. A. (2017). Social and emotional learning and teachers. *Future of Children, 27*(1), 137–155. [special issue: Social and emotional learning]. https://www.jstor.org/stable/44219025

Schonert-Reichl, K. A., & Hymel, S. (2007). Educating the heart as well as the mind social and emotional learning for school and life success. *Education Canada, 47*, 20–25. https://eric.ed.gov/?id=EJ771005

Segal, Z. V., Williams, J. M. G., & Teasdale, J. D. (2002). *Mindfulness-based cognitive therapy for depression: A new approach to preventing relapse*. Guilford Press.

Semple, R. J., & Lee, J. (2011). *Mindfulness-based cognitive therapy for anxious children: A manual for treating childhood anxiety*. New Harbinger Publications.

Semple, R. J., & Lee, J. (2014). Mindfulness-based cognitive therapy for children. In R. A. Baer (Ed.), *Mindfulness-based treatment approaches: Clinician's guide to evidence base and applications* (pp. 161–188). Elsevier Academic Press. https://doi.org/10.1016/B978-0-12-416031-6.00008-6

Semple, R. J., Lee, J., Rosa, D., & Miller, L. F. (2010). A randomized trial of mindfulness-based cognitive therapy for children: Promoting mindful attention to enhance social-emotional resiliency in children. *Journal of Child and Family Studies, 19*(2), 218–229. https://doi.org/10.1007/s10826-009-9301-y

Sharp, J. E., & Jennings, P. A. (2016). Strengthening teacher presence through mindfulness: What educators say about the cultivating awareness and resilience in education (CARE) program. *Mindfulness, 7*, 209–218. https://doi.org/10.1007/s12671-015-0474-8

Shulman, L. S. (2004). The wisdom of practice: Essays on teaching, learning, and learning to teach. San Francisco, CA: Jossey-Bass

Tan, L., & Martin, G. (2015). Taming the adolescent mind: A randomised controlled trial examining clinical efficacy of an adolescent mindfulness-based group programme. *Child and Adolescent Mental Health, 20*(1), 49–55. https://doi.org/10.1111/camh.12057

Taylor, N. Z., & Millear, P. M. R. (2016). The contribution of mindfulness to predicting burnout in the workplace. *Personality and Individual Differences, 89*, 123–128. https://doi.org/10.1016/j.paid.2015.10.005

Thapar, A., Collishaw, S., Pine, D. S., & Thapar, A. K. (2012). Depression in adolescence. *Lancet, 379*(9820), 1056–1067. https://doi.org/10.1016/S0140-6736(11)60871-4

Tumminia, M. J., Colaianne, B. A., Roeser, R. W., & Galla, B. M. (2020). How is mindfulness linked to negative and positive affect? Rumination as an explanatory process in a prospective longitudinal study of adolescents. *Journal of Youth and Adolescence, 49*(10), 2136–2148. https://doi.org/10.1007/s10964-020-01238-6

UNICEF. (2021). *The state of the world's children 2021: On my mind – Promoting, protecting and caring for children's mental health*. https://www.unicef.org/reports/state-worlds-children-2021

Van der Gucht, K., Takano, K., Kuppens, P., & Raes, F. (2017). Potential moderators of the effects of a school-based mindfulness program on symptoms of depression in adolescents. *Mindfulness, 8*(3), 797–806. https://doi.org/10.1007/s12671-016-0658-x

Van der Gucht, K., Takano, K., Raes, F., & Kuppens, P. (2018). Processes of change in a school-based mindfulness programme: Cognitive reactivity and self-coldness as mediators. *Cognition and Emotion, 32*(3), 658–665. https://doi.org/10.1080/02699931.2017.1310716

Volanen, S.-M., Lassander, M., Hankonen, N., Santalahti, P., Hintsanen, M., Simonsen, N., et al. (2020). Healthy learning mind – Effectiveness of a mindfulness program on mental health compared to a relaxation program and teaching as usual in schools: A cluster-randomised controlled trial. *Journal of Affective Disorders, 260*, 660–669. https://doi.org/10.1016/j.jad.2019.08.087

Wang, B., Li, X., Barnett, D., Zhao, G., Zhao, J., & Stanton, B. (2012). Risk and protective factors for depression symptoms among children affected by HIV/AIDS in rural China: A structural equation modeling analysis. *Social Science & Medicine (1982), 74*(9), 1435–1443. https://doi.org/10.1016/j.socscimed.2012.01.007

Werner-Seidler, A., Perry, Y., Calear, A. L., Newby, J. M., & Christensen, H. (2017). School-based depression and anxiety prevention programs for young people: A systematic review and meta-analysis. *Clinical Psychology Review, 51*, 30–47. https://doi.org/10.1016/j.cpr.2016.10.005

WHO. (2005). *Child and adolescent mental health policies and plans. WHO mental health policy and service guidance package – Module 11*. World Health Organization. https://www.who.int/mental_health/policy/services/9_child%20ado_WEB_07.pdf?ua=1

WHO. (2018). *Situation of child and adolescent health in Europe (9289053488)*. https://www.euro.who.int/__data/assets/pdf_file/0007/381139/situation-child-adolescent-health-eng.pdf

Wright, K. M., Roberts, R., & Proeve, M. J. (2019). Mindfulness-based cognitive therapy for children (MBCT-C) for prevention of internalizing difficulties: A small randomized controlled trial with Australian primary school children. *Mindfulness, 10*, 2277–2293. https://doi.org/10.1007/s12671-019-01193-9

Yu, M., Zhou, H., Xu, H., & Zhou, H. (2021). Chinese adolescents' mindfulness and internalizing symptoms: The mediating role of rumination and acceptance. *Journal of Affective Disorders, 280*(Pt A), 97–104. https://doi.org/10.1016/j.jad.2020.11.021

Zeleke, W. A., Hughes, T. L., & Drozda, N. (2020). Home–school collaboration to promote mind–body health. In C. Maykel & M. A. Bray (Eds.), *Promoting mind–body health in schools: Interventions for mental health professionals* (pp. 11–26). American Psychological Association. https://doi.org/10.1037/0000157-002

Zisook, S., Lesser, I., Stewart, J. W., Wisniewski, S. R., Balasubramani, G. K., Fava, M., et al. (2007). Effect of age at onset on the course of major depressive disorder. *American Journal of Psychiatry, 164*(10), 1539–1546. https://doi.org/10.1176/appi.ajp.2007.06101757

Chapter 4
Digital Technology Interventions for Preventing and Treating Youth Depression

Daniela Lira and Vania Martínez

4.1 Current Evidence Regarding Mental Health in Young People

Good mental health is essential for positive development in children and adolescents, including optimal psychological development, establishing and maintaining good interpersonal relationships, effective learning, and good physical health (Clarke et al., 2015). Thus, the presence of mental health problems in childhood and adolescence is of great relevance given their prevalence, early onset, and impact on multiple areas of young people's lives (Liverpool et al., 2020).

In recent years, a significant increase in mental health problems has been reported in youth (Scholten & Granic, 2019). Estimated prevalence ranges between 10% and 20% worldwide (Liverpool et al., 2020), with depression being one of the most frequent problems in adolescents (Christ et al., 2020).

D. Lira
Doctoral Program in Psychotherapy, Pontificia Universidad Católica de Chile & Universidad de Chile, Santiago, Chile

Millennium Institute for Research in Depression and Personality (MIDAP), Santiago, Chile

Millennium Nucleus to Improve the Mental Health of Adolescents and Youths (Imhay), Santiago, Chile

V. Martínez (✉)
Millennium Institute for Research in Depression and Personality (MIDAP), Santiago, Chile

Millennium Nucleus to Improve the Mental Health of Adolescents and Youths (Imhay), Santiago, Chile

CEMERA, Facultad de Medicina, Universidad de Chile, Santiago, Chile
e-mail: vmartinezn@uchile.cl

V. Martínez, C. Miranda-Castillo (eds.), *Prevention and Early Treatment of Depression Through the Life Course*, Depression and Personality,
https://doi.org/10.1007/978-3-031-13029-8_4

Unipolar depressive disorders are one of the leading causes of disability among adolescents (Topooco et al., 2018). Studies estimate that around one in nine adolescents will meet the criteria for major depressive disorder (MDD), with similar percentages of adolescents experiencing subthreshold symptoms (Wozney et al., 2017). Thus, studies indicate that by the age of 18, 20% of young people will have experienced at least one clinically significant depressive episode, with 75% of these experiencing a subsequent episode within 5 years (Grist et al., 2019).

Depression affects youth development, reduces commitment to education, and can lead to lifelong disabilities (Garrido et al., 2019). Furthermore, depression can have persistent impacts on daily functioning and a negative impact on social, family, and peer relationships (Wozney et al., 2017). Early depressive symptoms have been linked to various mental health problems in adulthood, including anxiety, depressive, and substance use disorders (Christ et al., 2020). Increased risk of suicide is among the most alarming consequences of depression in youth, as those who suffer from MDD are seven times more likely to commit suicide than people without MDD. This is one of the main causes of death in this population (Das et al., 2016).

In turn, pandemic-related measures and consequences (e.g., lockdowns and social distancing) may have had negative impacts, including increased depressive symptoms and feelings of loneliness (Rauschenberg et al., 2021). Although young people are less susceptible to severe COVID-19 infections, they are more at risk regarding the negative psychosocial effects of the pandemic (Power et al., 2020). Moreover, according to the research that has emerged in this context, more negative mental health consequences are expected in the future (Rauschenberg et al., 2021).

However, studies indicate that 64–87% of mental health problems are not detected or treated (Scholten & Granic, 2019). Thus, only a small percentage of youth with depressive symptoms receive treatment, and those who are treated generally receive only a few sessions (Stiles-Shields et al., 2016). Therefore, several deficits and disparities currently exist in health systems, which are often affected by problems of coverage, accessibility, efficiency, and cost (Stiles-Shields et al., 2016).

In addition, several studies have reported ethnic, racial, and economic disparities, with lack of access to effective services and the financial burden of treatment being established as some of the barriers to accessing treatment (Stiles-Shields et al., 2016). Nevertheless, the low percentage of treatment is associated not only with a lack of availability but also with low rates of help-seeking behavior resulting from the perceived stigma of mental health problems (Ebert et al., 2015; Grist et al., 2019).

4.2 Digital Technologies as an Opportunity for Mental Health in Young People

Digital mental health interventions are those that are delivered or supported through mobile technology (Clough & Casey, 2015). Given the existing barriers and disparities, the mental healthcare needs of youth cannot be addressed using traditional interventions alone (Stiles-Shields et al., 2016). Thus, coupled with the high presence of digital devices, interest in digital mental health interventions for this population has increased notably (Schleider et al., 2020). The accelerated development of technological innovations has been identified as an opportunity to address the gap in mental health services in various settings (Scholten & Granic, 2019).

Although access to these technologies varies between countries with different levels of economic development, studies show that one in three Internet users in the world is under 18 years of age (Odgers & Jensen, 2020). Thus, digital interventions are a highly viable choice for delivering youth depression treatment, given young people's access to this type of technology and their familiarity with it (O'Dea et al., 2015).

In recent years, the use of digital technologies to deliver interventions tailored to the needs and preferences of the youth population has been promoted (Liverpool et al., 2020). These interventions present several advantages such as greater availability and privacy (O'Dea et al., 2015).

The COVID-19 pandemic has become a catalyst to rethink service delivery in order to make it more accessible, equitable, and efficient (Power et al., 2020). Thus, digital interventions provide unique opportunities for the delivery of mental health services, even under the restrictive conditions associated with the COVID-19 pandemic (Rauschenberg et al., 2021; Taylor et al., 2020).

There is currently a great diversity of types of digital interventions, which have different levels of development and diffusion (Andersson, 2018). These interventions, which have different objectives, can be therapeutic and preventive (Buntrock et al., 2014) or be based on a stepped care approach (Ebert et al., 2017). Thus, it has been proposed that these interventions can be implemented in a way that is tailored to the individual needs of people (Mohr et al., 2019).

4.2.1 General Definitions of Digital Technologies in Mental Health

TeleMental Health One of the best-known terms for digital intervention in mental health is TeleMental Health. The American Telemedicine Association (ATA) (2009) has stated that TeleMental Health is the practice of mental health specialties at distance, a broad definition that points to the delivery of health information and services by electronic means. Thus, the prefix "tele" primarily refers to the communication tools used for these remote services (Craig & Petterson, 2005). However, the terminology used to refer to this type of intervention has not been consistent in the literature, with authors employing other terms such as e-health, cybertherapy, or teletherapy (Andersson, 2018).

This type of intervention consists in the exchange of mental health information between people who are not in the same physical space, utilizing devices (e.g., computers, smartphones) connected to the Internet (Orsolini et al., 2021). This exchange, aimed at improving the patient's health status, can be established between mental health professionals (e.g., psychiatrist, psychologist) or between a professional and a patient (ATA, 2009). Thus, this type of intervention can be regarded as equivalent to one conducted in a clinician's office, but with remote contact over the Internet (Bernardy et al., 2019).

Web- and Computer-Based Interventions After nearly two decades of development, web- and computer-based interventions are one of the most developed types of digital interventions today (Andersson et al., 2019). Interventions of this type are backed by controlled trials of self-help interventions and the first computer-based interventions conducted via CD-ROM or email in the late 1990s (Andersson, 2018).

Throughout their history, web- and computer-based interventions have used – among others – psychodynamic and interpersonal therapeutic approaches (Moshe et al., 2020), with most interventions being based on the principles of cognitive behavioral therapy (CBT) (Andersson et al., 2019). Thus, web- and computer-based CBT laid the groundwork for this type of interventions, which were initially developed as programs designed to replicate traditional face-to-face treatments in terms of content and duration (Carlbring et al., 2018). Currently, regarding features and components, they typically include screening or diagnostic stages, psychoeducational information, and exercise modules (Andersson, 2018; Carlbring et al., 2018).

Mental Health Apps Mental health apps consist of discrete, stand-alone software that works on mobile devices such as smartphones, tablets, and personal digital assistants (Lui et al., 2017). Their features include visual appeal, extensive multimedia capabilities, self-paced use, content sharing, customizability, and the ability to track user progress anytime, anywhere (Bricker et al., 2014).

Currently, as the acquisition of mobile devices continues to increase worldwide, it has been proposed that apps, due to their connectivity, mobility, and availability, can become an important vector for mental health interventions (Lecomte et al., 2020). Thus, apps with mental health-related objectives have rapidly proliferated in recent years, with more than 10,000 apps currently available (Torous et al., 2019). These apps encompass various intervention types and generally feature elements such as symptom monitoring, delivery of various therapeutic tools (e.g., relaxation exercises), psychoeducation, recruitment of social support, and positive reinforcement (Lui et al., 2017). Thus, these applications seek to provide mental health benefits in a variety of ways, making it possible to measure, monitor, and actively manage problems, among other functions (Yardley et al., 2016).

Virtual Reality and Augmented Reality Accelerated advances in the creation of artificial or altered environments in recent years have also impacted on mental health interventions through technologies such as virtual reality (VR) and augmented reality (AR) (Vinci et al., 2020). VR is a digital technology that artificially creates sensory experiences while allowing the user to manipulate objects within the virtual environment (Zeng et al., 2018). Thus, VR combines 3D graphics, motion trackers, vibration platforms, and audio to create immersive and interactive environments (Vinci et al., 2020). This technology makes it possible to produce therapeutic situations that are difficult to recreate in real life, providing repeated and immediately available treatment (Freeman et al., 2017). In general, VR interventions incorporate exposure and social skills training, strategies that are well suited to naturalistic virtual environments, allowing greater control of the stimuli presented in therapeutic strategies and lower risk compared to strategies such as in vivo exposure (Vinci et al., 2020). In addition, simulations can be designed to be presented repeatedly and graded in terms of difficulty until the desired change occurs (Freeman et al., 2017). For its part, AR "affects the perception of the real-world environment by 'augmenting' it with computer-generated digital objects" (Vinci et al., 2020). Therefore, AR can be considered an extension of VR: while VR integrates the person into the virtual environment, AR integrates virtual data or objects into the real environment (Bin et al., 2020). Thus, AR combines real and virtual objects in the real world, aligning them with each other and operating in response to the user in real time (Vinci et al., 2020).

Video Games Among mediated virtual experiences, video games have recently attracted attention given the potentialities of their use to promote positive functioning (Villani et al., 2018). Thus, in recent years, game-based digital interventions have been developed to address mental health problems (Fleming et al., 2017). The literature in this field has mainly focused on two approaches: the so-called "serious games," which are designed to educate, alleviate symptoms, train, or change behaviors while entertaining players (Lau et al., 2017), and "gamification," which consists in the inclusion of game elements (e.g., scoring and rewards) in nongame contexts (Fleming et al., 2017). Importantly, research has shown the potential of video games in the development of various cognitive, emotional, and social skills (Villani et al., 2018). In addition, video games have been observed to be useful both as a psychoeducational tool (Shah et al., 2018) and for assessment and rapport building in psychotherapy (Colder Carras et al., 2018). Depending on the developmental capacity of their target audience, video games can vary greatly in their level of complexity, interactivity, social interaction, immersion, and story development (Shah et al., 2018).

Chatbots Chatbots (conversational agents, conversational bots, or chatterbots) are computer programs that can interact with human users through spoken, written, and visual language (Abd-Alrazaq et al., 2019). Recently, the use of this technology has increased significantly in the field of mental health (Abd-Alrazaq et al., 2020). For example, chatbots have been used to assess self-esteem and anxiety, promote user engagement, and increase symptom awareness in those who are reluctant to seek treatment (Cameron et al., 2017), as well as to complement evidence-based therapies by targeting symptoms of depression (Abd-Alrazaq et al., 2019).

Websites Finally, the increased use of web technologies and resources has influenced the way people seek help, as their accessibility has created opportunities to make available more sources of care and information (Pretorius, Chambers, & Coyle, 2019). Thus, individuals can access various websites and web-based materials to support the self-management of mental health problems (Stawarz et al., 2019). In this domain, formal and informal resources such as social media and discussion forums exist to promote help-seeking (Pretorius, Chambers, Cowan, & Coyle, 2019). Therefore, the growing role of alternative sources of help such as YouTube, blogs, self-help websites, and discussion forums needs to be studied to determine how they are used and how they can be positively enhanced (Pretorius, Chambers, & Coyle, 2019). In addition, these tools are used as a source of peer support, with evidence suggesting that they promote a sense of community, help raise awareness and combat stigma, and provide spaces for expression and coping (Stawarz et al., 2019).

4.2.2 Uses of Digital Technologies in Mental Health

Just as there is diversity in the types of digital mental health interventions, these interventions can also be administered in diverse ways. For instance, interventions can be delivered synchronously, that is, in real time (Bernardy et al., 2019). Most of the literature on synchronous digital interventions focuses on services delivered via video calls, as they are the most similar to face-to-face treatments (Berryhill et al., 2019). Interventions can also be asynchronous, with communication occurring at different times and being delivered through means such as email, voicemail, or text messages (Orsolini et al., 2021). Asynchronous interventions include protocolized self-help programs, which may involve contact with healthcare professionals or staff (i.e., guided interventions) or be used without therapeutic support (i.e., unguided interventions) (Bernardy et al., 2019).

Another mode of administration consists in using digital interventions as a tool attached to traditional face-to-face formats (i.e., blended treatment). This approach is aimed at strengthening the effectiveness and efficacy of said interventions (Neary & Schueller, 2018; Schuster et al., 2020).

Lastly, collaborative programs (Martínez et al. 2018b) and distance consultancies or teleconsultations (Mundt et al., 2021) represent another way of implementing digital technologies. In this case, technologies are used to allow teams of mental health specialists to collaborate with primary healthcare teams in centers where there are no specialists (Orsolini et al., 2021). Thus, the objective is to enhance the resolution capacity of primary care, improve the referral of patients across all levels of care, and safeguard the continuity of care for the population with mental health problems (Martínez et al. 2018b).

4.3 Digital Interventions for Youth Depression

4.3.1 Digital Interventions for Preventing Youth Depression

Evidence indicates that mental health problems can be prevented and that interventions during childhood and adolescence enhance the benefits of prevention efforts (Baños et al., 2017). Prevention focuses on reducing the incidence, prevalence, or severity of mental health problems (Clarke et al., 2015), involving various actions that seek to reduce risk factors, interrupt the progress of problems, and reduce their negative consequences (Baños et al., 2017).

Prevention includes interventions termed universal (i.e., for the entire population), selective (i.e., for people with risk factors), and indicated (i.e., for people who show early signs of mental health problems) (Ebert et al., 2017). Also, since reaching as many people as possible is another fundamental element of prevention, the accessibility of digital interventions makes them especially suitable for young people (Baños et al., 2017).

Preventive digital interventions for young people have attracted less scholarly attention than those aimed at the adult population (Ebert et al., 2017). However, several authors have sought to synthesize the current evidence for preventive digital interventions for young people in reviews and meta-analyses. For example, in their systematic review of preventive interventions for young people, Clarke, Kuosmanen, and Barry (Clarke et al., 2015) identified a total of 20 studies of digital interventions, most of which are computer-based CBT programs designed to prevent depression and/or anxiety. The authors found that the studies varied in quality, classing them as weak, moderate, or strong in this regard. Those deemed to be "strong" showed significant positive effects in reducing depressive symptoms, with these improvements being maintained in those studies that included follow-up assessments at 6–12 months. However, the authors note that these results should be viewed with caution because of the generally small sample sizes used (Clarke et al., 2015). In addition to the above, the studies indicated high acceptability, especially in those interventions that included support from therapists over the Internet. Regarding support, the authors point out that, given the diversity of the studies in terms of design and quality, it is difficult to establish what type of support is necessary – and how intense it must be – to promote the participation of young people in interventions of this type. Finally, dropout was a significant issue for digital preventive interventions, as participants completed an average of 50% of the modules included in the programs (Clarke et al., 2015). This problem is consistent with the evidence for digital interventions in other populations (Batterham & Calear, 2017).

Another study, which consisted in a systematic review and meta-review by Hollis et al. (2017), analyzed the results of 30 randomized controlled trials (RCTs), of which 7 were preventive interventions for young people. These preventive interventions included a total of 1345 participants aged 12–25 years. The interventions were both universal and indicated, featuring components such as behavioral activation, CBT, psychoeducation, interpersonal psychotherapy, and modification of attention bias. Overall, the analyses revealed that the most effective digital interventions used the CBT approach, attaining small to moderate effects, whereas the rest of the interventions yielded poorer results. However, it is worth noting that the strongest effects were found in interventions with non-active comparators (e.g., waiting list control). Furthermore, the interventions varied in terms of the level of human and technical support offered, leading to particularly deficient acceptance and adherence results for unguided interventions. Finally, the authors note that none of the studies presented cost-effectiveness data.

Garrido et al. (2019) examined, quantitatively and qualitatively, the effectiveness and engagement results of research on digital interventions published between 2007 and 2017. The interventions were diverse (e.g., web- and computer-based, applications, games, text messages) and were implemented in various contexts (schools, hospitals, and community settings). Most of the interventions were based on CBT strategies or a combination of CBT with other models. Analyses indicated that digital interventions had small effects compared to non-active control groups, and no differences were found compared to active controls. Regarding support, most of the interventions were guided, and these were found to be more effective than the unguided ones. Regarding adherence and commitment, qualitative data from the studies were categorized as characteristics that participants liked or disliked and as characteristics that predicted adherence. One of the characteristics that the participants liked was the social support associated with the interventions, as they perceived that contact with professionals and/or the possibility of connecting with peers with similar difficulties was useful to them. Another of the main attractions of the interventions was their digital nature, with the participants highlighting aspects such as privacy, anonymity, and the possibility of adapting the interventions to their routines and interests, added to the possibility of accessing them in various locations. Another aspect evaluated positively was the content of the interventions, as the participants indicated that the topics covered helped them to learn more about mental health and become familiar with specific techniques for their difficulties (e.g., questioning negative thoughts). With respect to the negatively evaluated characteristics, one of the aspects pointed out by the participants was the so-called educational content, which they criticized when the modules were seen as too long, exhausting and/or tedious, and not adjusted to their needs (e.g., possibility of skipping modules). The participants also evaluated interventions negatively when they found them too youth-oriented or condescending. They also mentioned the negative impact of technical failures or navigation difficulties, which were among the reasons cited for low adherence and commitment. Finally, few studies reported factors predictive of adherence, which included the context of the intervention (greater adherence in school settings), gender (greater adherence of female participants), and mental health (higher initial symptomatology scores and previous history of mood disorders predicting greater adherence) (Garrido et al., 2019).

Recently, Bergin et al. (2020) published the results of a scoping review of digital interventions aimed at examining factors related to implementation. This review included 30 studies of preventive interventions (universal, selective, and indicated) for depressive and/or anxiety symptoms. Most were web- and computer-based interventions targeting adolescents between 15 and 16 years of age (Bergin et al., 2020). The results showed diversity in terms of the reporting and measurement methods used to collect information about the usability, participation, and implementation features of the interventions, as well as with respect to how the sociodemographic characteristics of the samples were reported. Regarding the barriers and facilitators related to implementation, the results showed that these varied according to the contexts in which the programs were implemented. For example, in school-based programs, completeness was affected by absenteeism (Bergin et al., 2020). However, aspects such as technical difficulties affected all implementation settings and were overcome with the support of the research teams. In general, the authors state that, since few studies consistently report the factors related to the implementation of digital interventions, they still cannot reach their full potential, given that there is a lack of understanding of the optimal implementation choices (Bergin et al., 2020).

4.3.2 Digital Interventions for Treating Youth Depression

Although digital interventions for the treatment of youth depression are a rapidly developing field, it remains limited compared to research in the adult population. However, various efforts are being made to examine the current evidence for this type of intervention. For example, in a systematic review and meta-analysis, Grist et al. (2019) examined the results of 34 RCTs of digital interventions for the treatment of depression and/or anxiety in children and adolescents. The studies analyzed included a total of 3113 participants aged 6–22 years, with an average of less than 18 years. Most of the interventions consisted in web- and computer-based CBT (50%), while the rest included attention bias modification training, cognitive bias modification training, problem solving therapy, acceptance and commitment therapy, biofeedback, and emotion regulation training. Regarding effectiveness, analyses revealed that CBT-based digital intervention produced moderate effect sizes ($g = 0.66$) compared to non-active control groups (e.g., waiting list). However, the quality of the studies was varied, with most studies showing low risk of bias in aspects such as participant randomization, but showing high risk of bias in the reports and in the blinding of participants and personnel involved in the trials. Regarding program completion, the studies varied widely regarding whether and how it was reported, with an average of 64%. The authors also presented subgroup analyses, for example, of therapeutic support. These analyses pointed to a significant effect of the guided interventions, which produced larger effect sizes compared to the unguided ones. However, both the guided and unguided interventions were significantly better than the control groups. Therapeutic support was also identified as a moderating factor of commitment and therapeutic outcomes. Other analyses showed that interventions with parental support significantly differed from and had larger effect sizes than those without support. Furthermore, it was also observed that interventions that featured participants with a confirmed diagnosis of depression produced significantly larger effect sizes than those that targeted participants with severe symptoms. Finally, there were no significant differences between studies with children, adolescents, and mixed ages, with all the age subgroups of the intervention groups exhibiting a significant benefit over the control groups.

Another recent systematic review and meta-analysis by Christ et al. (2020) evaluated the results of 24 RCTs of computer- and web-based CBT for adolescents, emerging adults, and mixed samples with depression and/or anxiety. In more than half of the studies, interventions were guided by a therapist or researcher who monitored progress and provided personalized support, encouragement, clarification, or feedback. Regarding adherence, the results indicated an average of 57.12% in the 19 studies in which it was reported. Regarding control groups, most studies compared interventions with a non-active control group (e.g., waiting list), while the remaining studies used placebo controls (e.g., information control) or treatment as usual (TAU). The pooled effect sizes of the interventions with respect to depressive symptoms were moderate compared to the control groups (active and non-active), with moderate to high heterogeneity. Regarding effectiveness at short-term follow-up (i.e., up to 5 months), only three studies reported these results, with no significant differences being found between the interventions and their control groups. However, in the three studies in which the results of long-term follow-up effects (i.e., 6–12 months) were reported, the interventions were noted to be effective in reducing depressive symptoms compared to non-active control groups. Regarding the quality of the studies, most of their results were found to be poor overall. Thus, the high risk of bias observed was mainly due to bias in outcome measurement and missing outcome data. Christ et al. (2020) also performed subgroup analysis, which revealed no evidence that aspects such as diagnosis, age, level of support offered, adherence, recruitment type, or number of modules completed were associated with differential effect sizes.

Liverpool et al. (2020) recently published the results of a systematic review focused on modes of delivery, facilitators, and barriers in digital interventions for children and young people (up to 25 years). The review indicated that six types of digital intervention exist: websites, computer-based games and programs, apps, robots and digital devices, VR, and text messaging. The factors presented as barriers and facilitators of digital interventions were categorized into two broad themes, which included intervention and person-specific influences. Regarding intervention-related factors, the authors identified suitability (accessibility and convenience), usability (ease of use and/or understanding), and acceptability of the characteristics of the intervention. In this area, one of the main factors was acceptability, where elements such as images, language, and interfaces could constitute a barrier to engagement if they were unappealing to the participants. In contrast, the participants highlighted features such as the inclusion of videos, personalization or creation of profiles, and the possibility of connecting with others as features that promoted the use of the interventions. Regarding usability, those interventions that were described as self-paced, user-friendly, age-appropriate, simple, and straightforward were favored by the participants (Liverpool et al., 2020). On the contrary, those interventions in which participants encountered problems understanding the task or did not receive enough instructions decreased the probability of continuing to use them. The possibility of including interventions according to their lifestyle was another facilitating factor, as it enabled participants to access them anytime and anywhere. With respect to person-specific factors, motivation (usefulness) and opportunity (trust and anonymity) were deemed fundamental. Regarding motivation, curiosity and perceived need stood out, as less interest was shown in interventions considered not very useful or too general. Regarding opportunity, the participants indicated that social connection (peer interaction or therapist support) promoted the use of the interventions. Furthermore, participants also identified trust as a critical issue, with interventions that raised concerns regarding privacy, anonymity, or uncertainty of their validity being less accepted and used (Liverpool et al., 2020).

4.4 Advantages and Challenges of Digital Interventions

The advantages of digital mental health interventions have been widely covered in the literature, with authors proposing several benefits that include better uptake and accessibility, efficiency, clinical effectiveness, and customization (Hollis et al., 2017). Digital interventions offer greater availability and accessibility, with participants being able to use them at a time and place of their choice (O'Dea et al., 2015). This has been pointed out as an important benefit for disadvantaged populations and/or people living in isolated geographic areas (Clarke et al., 2015). In addition, digital interventions offer greater privacy and anonymity, which increases access among people who are not willing to seek face-to-face help due to the stigma associated with mental health problems (Grist et al., 2019). Other widely discussed advantages of digital interventions include their potential to reduce health system costs, rapid scalability, and dissemination (O'Dea et al., 2015) as well as low-cost delivery (Grist et al., 2019). Thus, digital interventions promise cost-effective evidence-based interventions at scale, reducing disparities and removing barriers in access to mental healthcare (Odgers & Jensen, 2020). In addition, these types of interventions also offer flexibility in self-direction and self-pacing, high fidelity due to automated delivery, ease of use, quick feedback, and the appeal of interactivity and visual features (Ebert et al., 2015; Liverpool et al., 2020; O'Dea et al., 2015).

It has been proposed that the advantages of digital interventions could be especially relevant for young people (Ebert et al., 2015), given their greater digital literacy, access to and use of technology (Liverpool et al., 2020), and ownership of digital devices (Garrido et al., 2019). Thus, young people, considered to be digital natives, exhibit high acceptance of technology and digital formats, which are suited to their activities, habits, culture, communications, relationships, and social connection (Baños et al., 2017). In addition, several studies show that young people use the Internet as an important source of information on mental health, preferring it and feeling more comfortable when addressing personal problems in the relative anonymity of an online context (Garrido et al., 2019).

Despite the numerous advantages that digital interventions can offer, their potential benefits are hindered by various difficulties and limitations (Bergin et al., 2020).

Therefore, although current evidence from youth depression prevention and treatment programs is promising, challenges are observed in several areas (Topooco et al., 2018). The most commonly mentioned issues include limitations in program acceptance, commitment, and adherence (Bergin et al., 2020). Thus, the evidence indicates that, despite the great accessibility offered by digital interventions, these limitations make it difficult to use, disseminate, and research them (O'Dea et al., 2015). It has been proposed that these difficulties are linked to methodological and design aspects (e.g., how human support is incorporated) and that they can be overcome by attaining a deep understanding of the intended behavior of users and their environments (Orlowski et al., 2015).

Other challenges stem from the clinical limitations of digital interventions, including restricted adaptation to the needs of the patient, difficulties in addressing comorbidity, and problems dealing with acute crises (Liverpool et al., 2020). In addition, several concerns have been raised regarding digital interventions: their impact on the therapeutic relationship, their efficacy in treating more serious problems, their high attrition rates, and concerns about technology failure during therapeutic processes and quality control (Grist et al., 2019). Other challenges arise from the cautious or negative attitudes of professionals towards digital interventions; among other issues, they mention the inability to address important aspects of the disease, data security, and accessibility (Liverpool et al., 2020).

Furthermore, several research gaps have been identified, for example, with respect to the wide diversity and methodological and reporting quality of RCTs, which results in difficulties for combining and comparing research in systematic reviews and meta-analyses (Hollis et al., 2017). In addition, current evidence points to the presence of highly heterogeneous studies and a clear scarcity of longitudinal results that might allow us to determine whether the benefits of the interventions hold in the long term (Baños et al., 2017). The scarcity of economic evaluations and implementation studies constitutes another relevant limitation, as there is very little evidence showing that digital interventions for young people can be successfully implemented (Bergin et al., 2020). Given these limitations, and since the field of digital interventions advances at such an accelerated rate, it has been suggested that the capacity of traditional research designs (such as RCTs) to generate evidence has been overwhelmed (Hollis et al., 2017). Finally, although research on the young population has increased in recent years, it is still limited compared to research in adults (Christ et al., 2020).

4.5 Ethical and Legal Considerations of the Use of Digital Interventions

There are important aspects that must be considered for an ethical use of digital interventions, the first of which is selecting evidence-based interventions to ensure their quality and rigorousness (Baños et al., 2017). This is relevant because the rapid development of digital interventions (such as apps) has led to an explosive increase in their availability, causing many of them to remain unevaluated (Torous et al., 2019).

Security, privacy, and confidentiality are other fundamental aspects of digital interventions (Grist et al., 2019). To meet these requirements, the literature suggests using safe and proven platforms such as Skype for Business, Updox, VSee, Zoom for Healthcare, Doxy.me, and thera-LINK (Chiauzzi et al., 2020). In addition, it is relevant to consider that aspects such as the use of other people's devices or the recording of sessions (which require explicit consent) can increase the risk of breaches of confidentiality (McSwain et al., 2017; Myers et al., 2017). Thus, it is essential that professionals take reasonable measures to preserve confidentiality, considering aspects such as the context in which the person will be treated and their preferences to agree on how, where, and through what means the intervention will be carried out (Chiauzzi et al., 2020). Finally, with respect to safety, professionals must consider the possibility of emergencies and/or acute crises and prepare accordingly (McSwain et al., 2017; Myers et al., 2017).

Regarding the young population, it must be considered that the implementation of digital interventions for minors requires parental consent. However, since reliably obtaining consent online can be difficult, this can be a barrier to reaching these groups (Ebert et al., 2017). In consequence, it has been suggested that these procedures should include information on why the interventions are justified, their benefits, risks, limitations, duration, costs and conditions, and connections with their implementation settings, among other issues (Myers et al., 2017).

Finally, given the rapid adoption and development of digital interventions, equitable and inclusive research, policies, and interventions are required to prevent their use from amplifying inequalities in youth mental health and benefiting only those who are best positioned to take advantage of the possibilities that they provide (Odgers & Jensen, 2020). Thus, this field requires laws, regulatory frameworks and policies, political will, and financing conducive to the proper use, development, and implementation of digital interventions (Titov et al., 2019).

4.6 Implementation Recommendations for the Use of Digital Interventions

Despite the promising results, advantages, and benefits of digital interventions for the prevention and treatment of mental health problems in young people, current evidence indicates that more research and development are required (Bergin et al., 2020). For example, users' and health professionals' expectations and preferences regarding digital interventions are among the most frequently mentioned barriers to scalability (Vis et al., 2018). Thus, researchers have suggested that, for an effective implementation and sustained use, interventions must be adequately designed in terms of both their purpose and practical implementation (Liverpool et al., 2020).

Thus, the importance of involving young people, communities, and stakeholders in the multiple stages of development and implementation has been pointed out in order to strengthen the adoption, adherence, acceptability, and effectiveness of digital interventions (Orlowski et al., 2015). Thus, evidence suggests that participatory research strategies and the co-design of interventions can ensure that these are developed according to the needs, stage of development, lifestyle, and preferences of young people (Liverpool et al., 2020). The authors have also proposed moving away from traditional computer-based interventions and using the most up-to-date technology (such as apps, games, VR, and AR) in interventions aimed at this modern technology-oriented population to increase their attractiveness and usability (Ebert et al., 2017). In addition, researchers have suggested including elements such as rewards and reminders (which are part of persuasive design methods) to promote user engagement and adherence (Liverpool et al., 2020).

Additionally, to improve acceptance by mental health professionals, it is important that they also get involved in the strategy design and decision-making processes of digital mental health interventions (Vis et al., 2018). Likewise, researchers have suggested that interventions should be developed and implemented by interdisciplinary teams that combine knowledge and experiences from various areas (not only mental health), including professionals from fields such as communication and computer science (Odgers & Jensen, 2020). In addition, to ensure the proper implementation of digital interventions, it is necessary to design training programs for health professionals and offer them continuous guidance (Titov et al., 2019).

4.7 Future Directions for Digital Interventions

If digital interventions are the way to overcome current deficits and disparities in health systems, more research is required, especially in young people, since less evidence is available for this age group than for the adult population (O'Dea et al., 2015). This entails improving the quality of research to collect more solid evidence of the effectiveness of these interventions as well as considering other methodologies in addition to traditional RCTs (Hollis et al., 2017). Given the fast pace of technological advances, new methodological frameworks and research designs are required (e.g., micro-randomized trials) that are adapted to emerging needs in this area and allow a timely response to them (Liverpool et al., 2020).

In addition, it is necessary to accumulate a larger and deeper body of evidence in relation to elements such as long-term outcomes and cost-effectiveness data (Das et al., 2016). This can help to corroborate the expectation that digital interventions can reduce the health and economic burden of mental health problems in young people (O'Dea et al., 2015). Furthermore, it is necessary to deepen our understanding of the differences between guided and unguided interventions in order to determine what type of support can generate the greatest benefits (and under what conditions) (Ebert et al., 2017).

Likewise, differential reports are required with respect to characteristics such as gender, ethnicity, socioeconomic status, and geographic and social contexts, since the impact of digital interventions may vary depending on these factors (Das et al., 2016). The scarce evidence in this area makes it difficult to generalize current findings to populations with the greatest need for digital interventions and that might benefit the most from them (e.g., minorities; Bergin et al., 2020). Along the same lines, given that most studies have been conducted in high-income countries, it is necessary to obtain rigorous and high-quality evidence of effective interventions for the prevention and treatment of young people's mental health problems in low- and middle-income countries (Jiménez-Molina et al., 2019; Martínez et al., 2018a; Naslund et al., 2017; Rojas et al., 2019).

Furthermore, future research should incorporate other types of digital interventions in addition to traditional web- and computer-based interventions (Ebert et al., 2017). This can improve engagement and intervention outcomes through technologies that are better matched to the characteristics and lifestyles of the young population (Liverpool et al., 2020). In addition, current technological developments offer a wide variety of opportunities and new functionalities, such as greater interactivity and the possibility of connecting with other types of devices (e.g., sensors), which could enhance the benefits and use of digital interventions (Stiles-Shields et al., 2016).

Finally, future research should address those aspects of implementation that have yet to be fully addressed, such as workforce issues, training of professionals, and the transfer of evidence for real-world adoption (Bergin et al., 2020). It is also important to take into account the contexts in which the interventions will be delivered (Baños et al., 2017). Since digital interventions offer flexibility regarding when, how, and where they are used, specific application contexts (e.g., school and primary care) can offer unique challenges and opportunities (Bergin et al., 2020). Furthermore, current evidence highlights the importance of participatory research and co-design (Orlowski et al., 2015): it has been proposed that the inclusion of young people, their parents, various groups of specialists, and stakeholders in the design and development of these types of interventions is necessary to enhance their benefits and overcome obstacles such as low adherence (Bergin et al., 2020).

4.8 Conclusions

There is some promising evidence for the effectiveness of digital interventions in preventing and treating youth depression. This is relevant given its high prevalence, its negative consequences, and the current deficits of health systems when it comes to addressing this problem. In this context, digital interventions offer various advantages and opportunities, such as accessibility, flexibility, and interactivity. In addition, these types of interventions can be especially useful for the young population, since they match their preferences and lifestyles while also offering more privacy, thus reducing the stigma associated with mental health problems. However, for this type of intervention to achieve its full potential, it is necessary to address various challenges and obstacles. For instance, research and implementation processes need to be improved, which requires new methodological frameworks that are capable of adjusting to a constantly changing and developing field while also making it possible to respond to the current knowledge gaps. Thus, participatory research and design involving all agents (young people, researchers, professionals, communities, and stakeholders) are key to developing effective interventions that are tailored to the needs and preferences of this population and that can be adopted and used sustainably. In addition, cost-effectiveness data are essential to fulfill the promise that digital interventions can be effective, low cost, and rapidly scalable. This is highly relevant considering that these interventions could be especially beneficial to vulnerable populations. However, current evidence does not allow clear conclusions to be drawn in this regard, which might cause gaps and disparities in youth mental health to remain unchanged. Finally, it is necessary to generate regulatory legal frameworks that allow digital interventions to be developed, researched, and ethically implemented.

Conflict of Interest The authors declare that they have no conflict of interest.

Acknowledgments This manuscript was supported by ANID – Millennium Science Initiative Program – ICS13_005 and NCS2021_081, and by ANID – FONDECYT N°1221230. DL received funding from ANID/BECA DOCTORADO NACIONAL/21200952.

References

Abd-Alrazaq, A. A., Alajlani, M., Alalwan, A. A., Bewick, B. M., Gardner, P., & Househ, M. (2019). An overview of the features of chatbots in mental health: A scoping review. *International Journal of Medical Informatics, 132*, 103978. https://doi.org/10.1016/j.ijmedinf.2019.103978

Abd-Alrazaq, A. A., Rababeh, A., Alajlani, M., Bewick, B. M., & Househ, M. (2020). Effectiveness and safety of using chatbots to improve mental health: Systematic review and meta-analysis. *Journal of Medical Internet Research, 22*(7), e16021. https://doi.org/10.2196/16021

American Telemedicine Association. (2009). *Telemental health standards and guidelines working group.*

Andersson, G. (2018). Internet interventions: Past, present and future. *Internet Interventions, 12*, 181–188. https://doi.org/10.1016/j.invent.2018.03.008

Andersson, G., Carlbring, P., Titov, N., & Lindefors, N. (2019). Internet interventions for adults with anxiety and mood disorders: A narrative umbrella review of recent meta-analyses. *The Canadian Journal of Psychiatry, 64*(7), 465–470. https://doi.org/10.1177/0706743719839381

Baños, R. M., Etchemendy, E., Mira, A., Riva, G., Gaggioli, A., & Botella, C. (2017). Online positive interventions to promote Well-being and resilience in the adolescent population: A narrative review. *Frontiers in Psychiatry, 8*, 10. https://doi.org/10.3389/fpsyt.2017.00010

Batterham, P. J., & Calear, A. L. (2017). Preferences for internet-based mental health interventions in an adult online sample: Findings from an online community survey. *JMIR Mental Health, 4*(2), e26. https://doi.org/10.2196/mental.7722

Bergin, A. D., Vallejos, E. P., Davies, E. B., Daley, D., Ford, T., Harold, G., et al. (2020). Preventive digital mental health interventions for children and young people: A review of the design and reporting of research. *NPJ Digital Medicine, 3*(1), 1–9. https://doi.org/10.1038/s41746-020-00339-7

Bernardy, K., Klose, P., Welsch, P., & Häuser, W. (2019). Efficacy, acceptability and safety of internet-delivered psychological therapies for fibromyalgia syndrome: A systematic review and meta-analysis of randomized controlled trials. *European Journal of Pain, 23*(1), 3–14. https://doi.org/10.1002/ejp.1284

Berryhill, M. B., Culmer, N., Williams, N., Halli-Tierney, A., Betancourt, A., Roberts, H., & King, M. (2019). Videoconferencing psychotherapy and depression: A systematic review. *Telemedicine and e-Health, 25*(6), 435–446. https://doi.org/10.1089/tmj.2018.0058

Bin, S., Masood, S., & Jung, Y. (2020). Virtual and augmented reality in medicine. In *Biomedical information technology* (pp. 673–686). Academic Press. https://doi.org/10.1016/B978-0-12-816034-3.00020-1

Bricker, J. B., Mull, K. E., Kientz, J. A., Vilardaga, R., Mercer, L. D., Akioka, K. J., & Heffner, J. L. (2014). Randomized, controlled pilot trial of a smartphone app for smoking cessation using acceptance and commitment therapy. *Drug and Alcohol Dependence, 143*, 87–94. https://doi.org/10.1016/j.drugalcdep.2014.07.006

Buntrock, C., Ebert, D. D., Lehr, D., Cuijpers, P., Riper, H., Smit, F., & Berking, M. (2014). Evaluating the efficacy and cost-effectiveness of web-based indicated prevention of major depression: Design of a randomised controlled trial. *BMC Psychiatry, 14*(1). https://doi.org/10.1186/1471-244X-14-25

Cameron, G., Cameron, D., Megaw, G., Bond, R., Mulvenna, M., O'Neill, S., et al. (2017). Towards a chatbot for digital counselling. In *Proceedings of the 31st international BCS human computer interaction conference (HCI 2017) 31* (pp. 1–7). https://doi.org/10.14236/ewic/HCI2017.24

Carlbring, P., Andersson, G., Cuijpers, P., Riper, H., & Hedman-Lagerlöf, E. (2018). Internet-based vs. face-to-face cognitive behavior therapy for psychiatric and somatic disorders: An updated systematic review and meta-analysis. *Cognitive Behaviour Therapy, 47*(1), 1–18. https://doi.org/10.1080/16506073.2017.1401115

Chiauzzi, E., Clayton, A., & Huh-Yoo, J. (2020). Videoconferencing-based Telemental health: Important questions for the COVID-19 era from clinical and patient-centered perspectives. *JMIR Mental Health, 7*(12), e24021. https://doi.org/10.2196/24021

Christ, C., Schouten, M. J., Blankers, M., van Schaik, D. J., Beekman, A. T., Wisman, M. A., Stikkelbroek, Y. A., & Dekker, J. J. (2020). Internet and computer-based cognitive behavioral therapy for anxiety and depression in adolescents and young adults: Systematic review and meta-analysis. *Journal of Medical Internet Research, 22*(9), e17831. https://doi.org/10.2196/17831

Clarke, A. M., Kuosmanen, T., & Barry, M. M. (2015). A systematic review of online youth mental health promotion and prevention interventions. *Journal of Youth and Adolescence, 44*(1), 90–113. https://doi.org/10.1007/s10964-014-0165-0

Clough, B., & Casey, L. (2015). The smart therapist: A look to the future of smartphones and mHealth technologies in psychotherapy. *Professional Psychology: Research and Practice, 46*(3), 147–153. https://doi.org/10.1037/pro0000011

Colder Carras, M., Van Rooij, A. J., Spruijt-Metz, D., Kvedar, J., Griffiths, M. D., Carabas, Y., & Labrique, A. (2018). Commercial video games as therapy: A new research agenda to unlock the potential of a global pastime. *Frontiers in Psychiatry, 8*, 300. https://doi.org/10.3389/fpsyt.2017.00300

Craig, J., & Petterson, V. (2005). Introduction to the practice of telemedicine. *Journal of Telemedicine and Telecare, 11*(1), 3–9. https://doi.org/10.1177/1357633X0501100102

Das, J. K., Salam, R. A., Lassi, Z. S., Khan, M. N., Mahmood, W., Patel, V., & Bhutta, Z. A. (2016). Interventions for adolescent mental health: An overview of systematic reviews. *Journal of Adolescent Health, 59*(4), S49–S60. https://doi.org/10.1016/j.jadohealth.2016.06.020

Ebert, D. D., Cuijpers, P., Muñoz, R. F., & Baumeister, H. (2017). Prevention of mental health disorders using internet- and Mobile-based interventions: A narrative review and recommendations for future research. *Frontiers in Psychiatry, 8*(116), 1–16. https://doi.org/10.3389/fpsyt.2017.00116

Ebert, D. D., Zarski, A.-C., Christensen, H., Stikkelbroek, Y., Cuijpers, P., Berking, M., et al. (2015). Internet and computer-based cognitive behavioral therapy for anxiety and depression in youth: A meta-analysis of randomized controlled outcome trials. *PLoS One, 10*(3), e0119895. https://doi.org/10.1371/journal.pone.0119895

Fleming, T. M., Bavin, L., Stasiak, K., Hermansson-Webb, E., Merry, S. N., Cheek, C., Lucassen, M., Lau, H. M., Pollmuller, B., & Hetrick, S. (2017). Serious games and gamification for mental health: Current status and promising directions. *Frontiers in Psychiatry, 7*, 215. https://doi.org/10.3389/fpsyt.2016.00215

Freeman, D., Reeve, S., Robinson, A., Ehlers, A., Clark, D., Spanlang, B., & Slater, M. (2017). Virtual reality in the assessment, understanding, and treatment of mental health disorders. *Psychological Medicine, 47*(14), 2393–2400. https://doi.org/10.1017/S003329171700040X

Garrido, S., Millington, C., Cheers, D., Boydell, K., Schubert, E., Meade, T., & Nguyen, Q. V. (2019). What works and what doesn't work? A systematic review of digital mental health interventions for depression and anxiety in young people. *Frontiers in Psychiatry, 10*, 759. https://doi.org/10.3389/fpsyt.2019.00759

Grist, R., Croker, A., Denne, M., & Stallard, P. (2019). Technology delivered interventions for depression and anxiety in children and adolescents: A systematic review and meta-analysis. *Clinical Child and Family Psychology Review, 22*(2), 147–171. https://doi.org/10.1007/s10567-018-0271-8

Hollis, C., Falconer, C. J., Martin, J. L., Whittington, C., Stockton, S., Glazebrook, C., & Davies, E. B. (2017). Annual research review: Digital health interventions for children and young people with mental health problems–a systematic and meta-review. *Journal of Child Psychology and Psychiatry, 58*(4), 474–503. https://doi.org/10.1111/jcpp.12663

Jiménez-Molina, A., Franco, P., Martínez, V., Martínez, P., Rojas, G., & Araya, R. (2019). Internet-based interventions for the prevention and treatment of mental disorders in Latin America: A scoping review. *Frontiers in Psychiatry, 10*, 664. https://doi.org/10.3389/fpsyt.2019.00664

Lau, H. M., Smit, J. H., Fleming, T. M., & Riper, H. (2017). Serious games for mental health: Are they accessible, feasible, and effective? A systematic review and meta-analysis. *Frontiers in Psychiatry, 7*, 209. https://doi.org/10.3389/fpsyt.2016.00209

Lecomte, T., Potvin, S., Corbière, M., Guay, S., Samson, C., Cloutier, B., Francoeur, A., Pennou, A., & Khazaal, Y. (2020). Mobile apps for mental health issues: Meta-review of meta-analyses. *JMIR mHealth and uHealth, 8*(5), e17458. https://doi.org/10.2196/17458

Liverpool, S., Mota, C. P., Sales, C., Čuš, A., Carletto, S., Hancheva, C., Sousa, S., Cerón, S. C., Moreno-Peral, P., Pietrabissa, G., Moltrecht, B., Ulberg, R., Ferreira, N., & Edbrooke-Childs, J. (2020). Engaging children and young people in digital mental health interventions: Systematic review of modes of delivery, facilitators, and barriers. *Journal of Medical Internet Research, 22*(6), e16317. https://doi.org/10.2196/16317

Lui, J. H., Marcus, D. K., & Barry, C. T. (2017). Professional psychology: Research and practice evidence-based apps? A review of mental health mobile applications in a psychotherapy context evidence-based apps? A review of mental health Mobile applications in a psychotherapy context. *Professional Psychology: Research and Practice, 48*(3), 199–210. https://doi.org/10.1037/pro0000122

Martínez, P., Rojas, G., Martínez, V., Lara, M. A., & Pérez, J. C. (2018a). Internet-based interventions for the prevention and treatment of depression in people living in developing countries: A systematic review. *Journal of Affective Disorders, 234*, 193–200. https://doi.org/10.1016/j.jad.2018.02.079

Martínez, V., Rojas, G., Martínez, P., Zitko, P., Irarrázaval, M., Luttges, C., & Araya, R. (2018b). Remote collaborative depression care program for adolescents in Araucanía region, Chile: Randomized controlled trial. *Journal of Medical Internet Research, 20*(1), e38. https://doi.org/10.2196/jmir.8021

McSwain, S. D., Bernard, J., Burke, B. L., Jr., Cole, S. L., Dharmar, M., Hall-Barrow, J., Herendeen, N., Herendeen, P., Krupinski, E. A., Martin, A., McCafferty, D., Mulligan, D. A., North, S., Ruschman, J., Waller, M., Webster, K., Williams, S., Yamamoto, S., & Yeager, B. (2017). American telemedicine association operating procedures for pediatric telehealth. *Telemedicine Journal and e-Health: The Official Journal of the American Telemedicine Association, 23*(9), 699–706. https://doi.org/10.1089/tmj.2017.0176

Mohr, D. C., Lattie, E. G., Tomasino, K. N., Kwasny, M. J., Kaiser, S. M., Gray, E. L., Alam, N., Jordan, N., & Schueller, S. M. (2019). A randomized noninferiority trial evaluating remotely-delivered stepped care for depression using internet cognitive behavioral therapy (CBT) and telephone CBT. *Behaviour Research and Therapy, 123*, 103485. https://doi.org/10.1016/j.brat.2019.103485

Moshe, I., Terhorst, Y., Cuijpers, P., Cristea, I., Pulkki-Råback, L., & Sander, L. (2020). Three decades of internet- and computer-based interventions for the treatment of depression: Protocol for a systematic review and meta-analysis. *JMIR Research Protocols, 9*(3), e14860. https://doi.org/10.2196/14860

Mundt, A. P., Irarrázaval, M., Martínez, P., Fernández, O., Martínez, V., & Rojas, G. (2021). Telepsychiatry consultation for primary care treatment of children and adolescents receiving child protective Services in Chile: Mixed methods feasibility study. *JMIR Public Health and Surveillance, 7*(7), e25836. https://doi.org/10.2196/25836

Myers, K., Nelson, E. L., Rabinowitz, T., Hilty, D., Baker, D., Barnwell, S. S., et al. (2017). American telemedicine association practice guidelines for telemental health with children and adolescents. *Telemedicine and e-Health, 23*(10), 779–804. https://doi.org/10.1089/tmj.2017.0177

Naslund, J. A., Aschbrenner, K. A., Araya, R., Marsch, L. A., Unützer, J., Patel, V., & Bartels, S. J. (2017). Digital technology for treating and preventing mental disorders in low-income and middle-income countries: A narrative review of the literature. *The Lancet Psychiatry, 4*(6), 486–500. https://doi.org/10.1016/S2215-0366(17)30096-2

Neary, M., & Schueller, S. (2018). State of the field of mental health apps. *Cognitive and Behavioral Practice, 25*(4), 531–537. https://doi.org/10.1016/j.cbpra.2018.01.002

O'Dea, B., Calear, A. L., & Perry, Y. (2015). Is e-health the answer to gaps in adolescent mental health service provision? *Current Opinion in Psychiatry, 28*(4), 336–342. https://doi.org/10.1097/YCO.0000000000000170

Odgers, C. L., & Jensen, M. R. (2020). Annual research review: Adolescent mental health in the digital age: Facts, fears, and future directions. *Journal of Child Psychology and Psychiatry, 61*(3), 336–348. https://doi.org/10.1111/jcpp.13190

Orlowski, S. K., Lawn, S., Venning, A., Winsall, M., Jones, G. M., Wyld, K., et al. (2015). Participatory research as one piece of the puzzle: A systematic review of consumer involvement in design of technology-based youth mental health and well-being interventions. *JMIR Human Factors, 2*(2), e4361. https://doi.org/10.2196/humanfactors.4361

Orsolini, L., Pompili, S., Salvi, V., & Volpe, U. (2021). A systematic review on TeleMental health in youth mental health: Focus on anxiety, depression and obsessive-compulsive disorder. *Medicina, 57*(8), 793. https://doi.org/10.3390/medicina57080793

Power, E., Hughes, S., Cotter, D., & Cannon, M. (2020). Youth mental health in the time of COVID-19. *Irish Journal of Psychological Medicine, 37*(4), 301–305. https://doi.org/10.1017/ipm.2020.84

Pretorius, C., Chambers, D., Cowan, B., & Coyle, D. (2019). Young people seeking help online for mental health: Cross-sectional survey study. *JMIR Mental Health, 6*(8), e13524. https://doi.org/10.2196/13524

Pretorius, C., Chambers, D., & Coyle, D. (2019). Young people's online help-seeking and mental health difficulties: Systematic narrative review. *Journal of Medical Internet Research, 21*(11), e13873. https://doi.org/10.2196/13873

Rauschenberg, C., Schick, A., Hirjak, D., Seidler, A., Paetzold, I., Apfelbacher, C., et al. (2021). Evidence synthesis of digital interventions to mitigate the negative impact of the COVID-19 pandemic on public mental health: Rapid meta-review. *Journal of Medical Internet Research, 23*(3), e23365. https://doi.org/10.2196/23365

Rojas, G., Martínez, V., Martínez, P., Franco, P., & Jiménez-Molina, A. (2019). Improving mental health care in developing countries through digital technologies: A mini narrative review of the Chilean case. *Frontiers in Public Health, 7*, 391. https://doi.org/10.3389/fpubh.2019.00391

Schleider, J. L., Dobias, M., Sung, J., Mumper, E., & Mullarkey, M. C. (2020). Acceptability and utility of an open-access, online single-session intervention platform for adolescent mental health. *JMIR Mental Health, 7*(6), e20513. https://doi.org/10.2196/20513

Scholten, H., & Granic, I. (2019). Use of the principles of design thinking to address limitations of digital mental health interventions for youth. *Journal of Medical Internet Research, 21*(1), e11528. https://doi.org/10.2196/11528

Schuster, R., Topooco, N., Keller, A., Radvogin, E., & Laireiter, A. (2020). Advantages and disadvantages of online and blended therapy: Replication and extension of findings on psychotherapists' appraisals. *Internet Interventions, 21*, 100326. https://doi.org/10.1016/j.invent.2020.100326

Shah, A., Kraemer, K. R., Won, C. R., Black, S., & Hasenbein, W. (2018). Developing digital intervention games for mental disorders: A review. *Games for Health Journal, 7*(4), 213–224. https://doi.org/10.1089/g4h.2017.0150

Stawarz, K., Preist, C., & Coyle, D. (2019). Use of smartphone apps, social media, and web-based resources to support mental health and well-being: Online survey. *JMIR Mental Health, 6*(7), e12546. https://doi.org/10.2196/12546

Stiles-Shields, C., Ho, J., & Mohr, D. C. (2016). A review of design characteristics of cognitive behavioral therapy-informed behavioral intervention technologies for youth with depression and anxiety. *Digital Health, 2*. https://doi.org/10.1177/2055207616675706

Taylor, C. B., Fitzsimmons-Craft, E. E., & Graham, A. K. (2020). Digital technology can revolutionize mental health services delivery: The COVID-19 crisis as a catalyst for change. *International Journal of Eating Disorders, 53*(7), 1155–1157. https://doi.org/10.1002/eat.23300

Titov, N., Hadjistavropoulos, H. D., Nielssen, O., Mohr, D. C., Andersson, G., & Dear, B. F. (2019). From research to practice: Ten lessons in delivering digital mental health services. *Journal of Clinical Medicine, 8*(8), 1239. https://doi.org/10.3390/jcm8081239

Topooco, N., Berg, M., Johansson, S., Liljethörn, L., Radvogin, E., Vlaescu, G., et al. (2018). Chat-and internet-based cognitive–behavioural therapy in treatment of adolescent depression: Randomised controlled trial. *BJPsych Open, 4*(4), 199–207. https://doi.org/10.1192/bjo.2018.18

Torous, J., Wisniewski, H., Bird, B., Carpenter, E., David, G., Elejalde, E., et al. (2019). Creating a digital health smartphone app and digital phenotyping platform for mental health and diverse healthcare needs: An interdisciplinary and collaborative approach. *Journal of Technology in Behavioral Science, 4*(2), 73–85. https://doi.org/10.1007/s41347-019-00095-w

Villani, D., Carissoli, C., Triberti, S., Marchetti, A., Gilli, G., & Riva, G. (2018). Videogames for emotion regulation: A systematic review. *Games for Health Journal, 7*(2), 85–99. https://doi.org/10.1089/g4h.2017.0108

Vinci, C., Brandon, K. O., Kleinjan, M., & Brandon, T. H. (2020). The clinical potential of augmented reality. *Clinical Psychology: Science and Practice, 27*(3), e12357. https://doi.org/10.1111/cpsp.12357

Vis, C., Mol, M., Kleiboer, A., Bührmann, L., Finch, T., Smit, J., & Riper, H. (2018). Improving implementation of emental health for mood disorders in routine practice: Systematic review of barriers and facilitating factors. *JMIR Mental Health, 5*(1), e9769. https://doi.org/10.2196/mental.9769

Wozney, L., Huguet, A., Bennett, K., Radomski, A. D., Hartling, L., Dyson, M., McGrath, P. J., & Newton, A. S. (2017). How do eHealth programs for adolescents with depression work? A realist review of persuasive system design components in internet-based psychological therapies. *Journal of Medical Internet Research, 19*(8), e266. https://doi.org/10.2196/jmir.7573

Yardley, L., Choudhury, T., Patrick, K., & Michie, S. (2016). Current issues and future directions for research into digital behavior change interventions. *American Journal of Preventive Medicine, 51*(5), 814–815. https://doi.org/10.1016/j.amepre.2016.07.019

Zeng, N., Pope, Z., Lee, J. E., & Gao, Z. (2018). Virtual reality exercise for anxiety and depression: A preliminary review of current research in an emerging field. *Journal of Clinical Medicine, 7*(3), 42. https://doi.org/10.3390/jcm7030042

Chapter 5
Contemplation of Nature to Promote Mental Health and Prevent Depression in Youth

Sebastián Medeiros, Álvaro I. Langer, and Sandra Stolzenbach

5.1 Losing Contact with Nature in Current Times

For millions of years, *Homo sapiens* have evolved and developed in natural habitats dominated by plants, animals, rivers, mountains, lakes, hills, and grasslands. Now, an estimated 55% of the world's population lives in urban areas, as urbanization continues to increase worldwide, and is estimated to reach 68% by 2050 (United Nations, 2018). The highly urbanized and artificial environment is a contributing cause of the "state of stress" in modern people (Song et al., 2016). The triggers of urban life, such as intense noise, traffic, and frenetic pace, as well as overload at work, university, and school, in addition to the pressure of social expectations, tend

S. Medeiros (✉)
Millennium Institute for Research in Depression and Personality (MIDAP), Santiago, Chile

Department of Psychiatry, Facultad de Medicina, Pontificia Universidad Católica de Chile, Santiago, Chile

Centro Mindfulness y Medicina, Santiago, Chile

Fundación Floresta, Santiago, Chile
e-mail: smedeiro@uc.cl

Á. I. Langer
Millennium Institute for Research in Depression and Personality (MIDAP), Santiago, Chile

Mind-Body Lab, Instituto de Estudios Psicológicos, Facultad de Medicina, Universidad Austral de Chile, Valdivia, Chile

Millennium Nucleus to Improve the Mental Health of Adolescents and Youths (Imhay), Santiago, Chile

S. Stolzenbach
Fundación Floresta, Santiago, Chile

V. Martínez, C. Miranda-Castillo (eds.), *Prevention and Early Treatment of Depression Through the Life Course*, Depression and Personality,
https://doi.org/10.1007/978-3-031-13029-8_5

to prolong stress, generating chronic stress (Arvay, 2015). Living in urban environments has been documented to have a negative impact on emotional health, and it is especially related to an increased risk of depressive disorders (Kovess-Masféty et al., 2005; Wang, 2004). It appears that the loss of contact with the healing and restorative properties of nature contributes to the generation and perpetuation of stress.

Increasing urbanization and less access to green spaces are affecting the physical and mental health in children and adolescents. A strong relationship has been observed between living environments with less green space and anxiety disorder and depression, especially in children and people with lower socioeconomic status (Maas et al., 2009). Socioeconomically deprived children and adolescents, especially in urban areas, are also at an increased risk of behavioral disorders (Trivedi et al., 2008). Urbanization has been associated with increased rates of substance use and technology addiction among youth, as well as high rates of self-harm in adolescent females (Chandra et al., 2018).

In addition, the current pandemic times pose an exponential burden and threat to the mental health of children and young people (Ford et al., 2021). Physical restraints and social distancing measures are affecting the development of self and interpersonal regulatory systems at critical periods of personal development, contributing to vulnerability to stress. For example, Meherali et al. (2021) conducted a systematic review, selecting 18 articles, and reported that children and adolescents are more likely to experience anxiety, depression, sleep and appetite disorders, and impaired social interactions during and after a pandemic. They highlight the impact of mitigation measures and describe common affective symptoms such as stress, worry, helplessness, and social and risk behavior problems.

5.2 Contemplation of Nature as a Practice of Connection

Contemplative practices (e.g., sitting meditation, breath awareness, walking meditation, yoga) are activities or actions that allow us to slow down and deepen awareness and connection as ways to promote well-being and alleviate human suffering. Awareness refers to seeing clearly the phenomena of experience, including thoughts, emotions, and sensory information as they occur: “What am I noticing now?” Connection refers to an intimate attunement to the experience: “What is my relationship/attitude to the present moment like?” Over the past several decades, contemplative interventions have been incorporated at a secular level among diverse populations, age ranges, and within clinical and educational perspectives, with the goal of achieving well-being and resilience (MLERN, 2012). The most studied interventions include mindfulness-based interventions, compassion training programs, and other mind-body practices, showing benefits across a wide array of conditions in physical, mental, and emotional domains including changes at neurological and immunological levels (Goldberg et al., 2018; Guendelman et al., 2017; Khoury et al., 2015; Rosenkranz et al., 2013). Specifically in youth, contemplative practices can foster the development of self-regulatory, mentalizing, and empathic capacities contributing to the building of internal resources for resilience (Medeiros & Guendelman, 2019).

Nature contemplation can be understood as a contemplative practice that can help us recover our embodied, embedded, and interconnected experience. Different nature-based interventions (NBIs) have emerged and are being incorporated in different contexts and age ranges. Some examples are horticulture therapy, community gardening, nature meditation, and forest therapy, among others (Chaudhury & Banerjee, 2020). Franco et al. (2017) recall how interest in nature as a therapeutic resource has ancient foundations, including Hippocrates, who extolled the benefits of air, water, and natural environments for physical and mental well-being. Shamans and healers from all traditions have always recognized the healing power of nature.

We have all experienced the peace of mind and tranquility that arise when we are in contact with nature: being in a forest, by the sea, on a lake or a mountain, listening to the sound of the wind, the waves, the current of a stream, the singing of birds, the smells of a forest or flowers, the light reflecting off a lake or coming through the leaves of a forest. Connecting with and exploring nature allows a sense of comfort, security, and belonging and offers promising benefits for promoting mental health.

5.2.1 Coming Back to Our Senses Through the Forest: "Shinrin-Yoku"

One of the most scientifically explored examples of NBIs is "shinrin-yoku," a term proposed in Japan in 1982. Its literal meaning corresponds to "forest bathing" (also referred to as forest therapy) and consists of immersing oneself in nature by mindfully using all the senses (Hansen et al., 2017). The duration of each session can vary, for example, a single session from 2 to 4 hours, short 15-min sessions twice a day for 3 consecutive days, 12-week forest-based programs, and others. Some activities are conducted with the guidance of a therapist, while others are realized individually (following instructions and behavioral recommendations) or in a group. According to Clifford (2018), "forest bathing is not the same as hiking." "The destination in forest bathing is here, not there. The pace is slow." "We walk slowly so we can focus our senses on the myriad ways the living forest surrounds and touches us. Feeling the breeze on our skin, hearing the gurgle of the stream and the calls of the birds, seeing the movement of the trees in the wind… When the forest is allowed to take its place within you, it supports your body's natural capacity for wellness and healing" (p. 2).

5.2.2 Key Factors of Nature Contemplation to Enhance Mental Health Promotion and Depression Prevention

We consider NBIs to be contemplative practices in themselves. However, when formal meditative practices or instructions to train attention (such as mindfulness practices) are incorporated, there appears to be an enhancing effect. In fact, a recent study demonstrated that mindfulness instructions improve mood during exposure to nature in an urban setting (Nisbet et al., 2019). Specifically, 100 participants were randomly assigned to 20-min guided walks under the following conditions: outdoors, outdoors with mindfulness, or indoors. The results indicated that walking outdoors presented more relationship with nature and better mood than those who walked indoors. However, the group with mindfulness practice, compared to the group walking outdoors, reported greater awareness of their environment, greater connection with nature, and lower negative affect. In a similar perspective, mindfulness practice in NBIs has been argued to be a key component to acquire the potential health benefits of exposure to nature (Djernis et al., 2019; Huynh & Torquati, 2019). Based on existing mindfulness research and theory, we highlight two attentional and attitudinal contemplative skills that may underlie benefits and should be further explored, particularly in youth at risk for depression. These are (1) sensory awareness of present moment experience in nature and (2) feeling gratitude and the perception of beauty.

Sensory Awareness of Present Moment Experience in Nature Our brains, including the limbic system, have evolved to inform us of whether we can relax and connect in a certain place or situation or, on the contrary, if we are in alarm mode and should activate fight or flight reactions. According to De De Wit (2008), from a contemplative perspective, suffering arises when we resist the changing and sometimes difficult nature of experience. This resistance can include hyperactivity and overthinking, as well as disconnection or avoidance of emotional and physical difficulties. The stressed mind constantly wanders or clings to things being different; the stressed body is in a state of hyperarousal and unease. Chronic stress can lead to a dysregulated neurocircuitry that underlies mental illnesses such as depression, schizophrenia, and anxiety disorders. Dysfunctional modes of thinking, in particular repetitive negative self-referential thinking (rumination), and experiential avoidance of emotions appear at the base of depression (Cribb et al., 2006; Mellick et al., 2019).

Contemplative practices cultivate focused attention as a means of stabilizing the mind in the present moment and counteracting dysfunctional thinking and disembodied patterns (Guendelman et al., 2017). Among these, nature-based practices that deliberately increase awareness and connection to the sensory experience of the present moment may offer profound healing properties, as greater inner calm and safety are experienced. A contemplative approach while in nature can facilitate a shift from self-referential narratives to direct, present-centered contact with the body and senses, i.e., touch, sight, hearing, smell, and taste. The senses help us to situate ourselves in the present moment and thus absorb all that nature offers us, to welcome it and let it settle in us. As Clifford (2018) suggests, "By giving attention to your senses, you turn down the volume on the cacophony of inner thoughts. Your senses bring you into the present moment, where you can take in all the forest has to offer" (p. 2).

Franco et al. (2017) reveal the importance of multisensory pathways through which the benefits of nature are provided. Beyond visual components, for example, sounds such as wind, rushing water, birdsong, and chatter can counteract anthropogenic sounds such as traffic, recreational, and industrial sounds that contribute to stress. Similarly, many natural smells such as flowers, freshly cut grass, and damp earth evoke pleasant and calming sensations and mood. Furthermore, these authors differentiate a passive reception of the benefits with a more active engagement with the environment, in line with the idea of deliberately cultivating sensory awareness of present moment experience in nature.

Feeling Gratitude and the Perception of Beauty In the modern world, we tend to forget something very important: that we depend on the earth and that the sun, the climate, and the plants are fundamental for our existence. In his book, *A Song of Love to the Earth*, mindfulness teacher Nhất Hạnh suggests that we tend to think of ourselves as the center of the universe and our interest is focused almost exclusively on our survival. Much of our fear, hatred, anger, and our feelings of loneliness may stem from a sense of separation. We are so caught up in our work and our problems that we have forgotten that we are more than just our minds. A contemplative attitude toward nature that perceives beauty and cultivates a sense of gratitude can counteract that illusion of separateness, helping to recognize interdependence and foster care and belonging. According to Nhất Hạnh (2013), if one looks deeply and reflects on all the virtues of nature, one can experience the connection that binds one to the earth and realize that nature is not just the environment around us, arising in us great respect and admiration for the miracle of life.

To perceive beauty, we must train our attention capacity, something that mindfulness does (Langer et al., 2017). In other words, focusing on sensory awareness is training attention. Once the mind and the body are in a state of "attentive calm," we are more "available" to perceive what is around us. A central point of interest is that contact with nature could be a catalyst for perceiving beauty in a bidirectional way, i.e., that nature contemplation can reveal both a new point of view on what is perceived and, potentially, an insight of the self through what is observed (Langer et al., 2017).

A new view or appreciation of ourselves or the environment can trigger the feeling of gratitude. It has been often defined as "a generalized tendency to recognize and respond with gratefulness to the role of other people's benevolence in the positive experiences and outcomes that one obtains" (McCullough et al., 2002). According to Sansone and Sansone (2010), gratitude refers to "what is valuable and meaningful to oneself." It has been claimed that gratitude is a key element of psychological well-being (Wood et al., 2010) and that mindfulness meditation enhances gratitude (Sawyer et al., 2021). Thus, we propose that nature contemplation is a specific way to cultivate gratitude and thus promote mental health. Specifically, contemplative practices include a caring and responsible relationship with nature, recognizing the interdependence between nature and our health. In fact, the relationship between these concepts has been noted: “Simply by experiencing nature and practicing gratitude, personal well-being and quality of life can be vastly improved. Experiencing the beauty of nature and giving gratitude towards its beauty is quite an experience” (Kachru & Taylor, 2017, p. 17).

5.3 Studies on Nature, Well-Being, and Mental Health

In recent decades, there has been a growing research interest in the impact of nature on health. Exposure to nature can improve physiological and biological markers of well-being including autonomic nervous system regulation and neuroimmunological dynamics, which are often impaired by chronic stress. White et al. (2019) examined associations between recreational contact with nature and self-reported health and well-being in 19,806 participants, estimating that spending at least 120 min per week in a natural environment may promote well-being when compared with spending less time in green spaces. Also in well-being research, a meta-analysis showed that people who were more connected to nature (i.e., not just contact) tended to experience more positive affect, vitality, and life satisfaction compared to those less connected to nature (Capaldi et al., 2014). Similarly, Pritchard et al. (2020) demonstrated that connection with nature was associated with dimensions of flourishing personal resources such as personal growth (i.e., the studies pointed out the increase of positive emotions).

On a more interventionist level, Kotera et al. (2020) conducted a systematic review and meta-analysis examining 20 studies on adults conducted in Asia and Europe indicating effectiveness of forest bathing in reducing mental health symptoms in the short term, particularly anxiety. Similarly, Stier-Jarmer et al. (2021) look at the effectiveness of forest-based interventions on the cardiovascular system, immune system, and mental health. According to Antonelli et al. (2021), there is a strong evidence to recommend the use of forest bathing as a complementary practice for the improvement of mental well-being in cases of stress, anxiety, emotional imbalance, and mild mood impairments. Regarding depression in adults, research shows that forest therapy is effective in preventing and improving symptoms. For example, using the Profile of Mood States (POMS) test, Li et al. (2007) demonstrated that forest bathing (three-day/two-night trip to forest fields) significantly increases vitality and decreases anxiety, depression, anger, and fatigue in healthy female subjects. Extensive research on disease and health problems (including cancer, chronic pain, and chronic stroke) has shown the effect of forest therapy in reducing associated symptoms of depression and anxiety (Chun et al., 2016; Han et al., 2016; Lee et al., 2017; Oh et al., 2017).

In children and adolescents, exposure to nature shows mental, physical, and social health benefits. Recent systematic reviews and meta-analyses (including randomized controlled trials and cross-sectional studies) have found reductions in emotional and behavioral problems including stress, depression, and attention-deficit/hyperactivity disorder and promotion of emotional well-being, cognitive development, self-esteem, resilience, and health-related quality of life (Mygind et al., 2019; Tillmann et al., 2018). In youth with affective and behavioral disorders and heterogeneous mental health disorders, a recent pretest-posttest non-randomized controlled study in 50 adolescent probationers explored the psychological and physiological effects of forest therapy programs. The forest therapy program, which consisted in 2 days and 1 night (vs. lecture room), offered beneficial effects on psychological and physiological measures of well-being (Jeon et al., 2021). Similarly, Macháčková et al. (2021) found a significant effect on psychopathology, irritability, restlessness, emotional instability, egocentrism, relativity, and negativism in 68 institutionalized adolescents with affective and behavioral disorders. Interestingly, this nature-based intervention included observation of patterns of prosocial behavior in forest animals. More research is needed to understand the role of nature in this population while recognizing their specific psychological needs and socio-emotional development.

To our knowledge, there are no studies designed to directly evaluate the effect of NBIs on young people presenting clinical depression. Most studies have assessed depressive symptoms among other psychological variables. For example, Chang (2015) observed a significant reduction in the Children's Depression Inventory (CDI) scores in 47 adolescents living in Seoul who participated in a forest experience program. Interestingly, they also found positive changes in Self-Confidence and Idealism Scales in the Offer Self-Image Questionnaire-Revised (OSIQ-R). Also, in Korea, the effects of a combined health promotion program using urban forests and mentoring on the perceived and psychological health of vulnerable elementary school students (from low-income families) were assessed. The results of this study showed that self-esteem and depression were significantly improved in the experimental group compared to the control group (Bang et al., 2018). Also, in university students who participated in forestry activities, a decrease in depressive symptoms was found compared to the control group (Mao et al., 2012). In addition, Furuyashiki et al. (2019) studied a sample of working-age people (including youth) with and without depressive symptoms that participated in day-long sessions of forest bathing. The results indicated that those with depressive symptoms demonstrated significantly greater improvement on many of the POMS items compared to those without depressive symptoms.

5.4 Connection with Nature and Arousal: A Regulated Mind and a Regulated Body

Going back to our physiology, when we perceive that a situation threatens our life, the body mobilizes a large amount of energy to prepare to fight or flee and to repair in case of injury. Our body knows how to cope with acute stress situations by counteracting them through neurobiological and hormonal control systems that lead to allostasis. The autonomic nervous system (ANS) plays a fundamental role in orchestrating mind-body interactions, and its optimal functioning indicates adaptive self-regulation. Chronic stress involves dysregulation of the ANS and arousal, as excessive demands are felt as a threat and the whole organism is in survival mode. The neurobiological and systemic effects of chronic stress are well established (see McEwen, 2017). In the brain, chronic stress can cause alterations in regions such as the hippocampus, prefrontal cortex, and amygdala (McEwen, 2008) which are involved in memory, executive functions, and emotional regulation, among other functions.

At the physiological research level, heart rate variability (HRV) is a measure of autonomic nervous activity (primarily assessing parasympathetic-vagal tone) used as an index of health (Shaffer et al., 2014). An altered ANS regulation of the heart has been observed in various psychiatric disorders (Kemp et al., 2010; Quintana et al., 2016). Although the underlying mechanisms are still unclear, it seems that HRV-indexed arousal dysregulation is associated with depression (Hartmann et al., 2019). Studies in children and adolescents also point to a correlation between HRV and depressive symptoms (Blood et al., 2015). In adults, HRV has been introduced in the contemplative field to assess the effects of attentional and attitudinal practices on ANS modulation (Christodoulou et al., 2020; Medeiros et al., 2021). Regarding nature-embedded practice, the measurement of HRV has gained attention to understand its beneficial effects. For instance, Kobayashi et al. (2018) observed higher HRV in young male participants walking for ~15 min in forest environments compared to walking in urban environments. Forest bathing has been shown to reduce blood pressure (Ochiai et al., 2015; Park et al., 2009), probably accounting for reduced sympathetic activity and increased vagal-relaxed tone in blood vessels. Farrow and Washburn (2019) describe a positive relationship between parasympathetic nervous system activation and reduced anxiety. At younger ages, Jeon et al. (2021) have recently found improvement in HRV dynamics in the adolescents tested, along with beneficial effects on psychological well-being.

5.5 Nature, Inflammation, and Immune System in Mental Health

Acute stress is a potent trigger of inflammation as an adaptive response that prepares the body for eventual tissue repair and defense against pathogens. The hypothalamic-pituitary-adrenal (HPA) axis coordinates a hormonal response system to regulate stress. Through glucocorticoids, mainly cortisol, stress hormones increase to terminate the inflammatory response. Chronic stress induces endocrine and immune dysregulation and is associated with low-grade systemic inflammation that has serious long-term health consequences (Gouin, 2011; Rohleder, 2019). Such is the case in depression, where chronic exposure to stress can lead to dysregulation of physiological and neurochemical processes including elevation of proinflammatory markers (leading to neuroinflammation) and alterations in the neurotransmitters' function (Davis et al., 2017; Howren et al., 2009). In addition, childhood adversity and early stress are associated with immune dysregulation at the epigenetic level, which results in the production of proinflammatory cytokines, leading to disease and susceptibility to infection (Chen et al., 2021). Indeed, Miller and Cole (2012) found that in adolescents at risk of depression, higher levels of childhood adversity were associated with greater increases in inflammation (measured by C-reactive protein and interleukin-6), suggesting that childhood adversity affects neuroimmune functioning, amplifying inflammatory signaling between the brain and the periphery.

Several studies in healthy adult and clinical populations exposed to nature have reported increased health and upregulation of cortisol levels and dynamics, as well as other markers of dysregulated immunology (Mao et al., 2012; Sung et al., 2012; for a review, see Antonelli et al., 2019). The case of natural killer (NK) cells is interesting as they are important contributors to cell-mediated immune response. NK cells release proteins and lymphokines such as perforin, GNR (granulysin), and GrA/B (granzyme A/B-expressing cells) that play a key role in the innate response to infections and tumors (Li et al., 2007, 2010). It is noted that NK cells may play a key role in the development of several diseases, including cancer risk, susceptibility to infections, and occurrence of autoimmune and allergic disorders (Antonelli et al., 2021). Similarly, findings of immune alterations in the pathogenesis of depression show decreased numbers and functions of NK cells (and other T cells) (Grosse et al., 2016). Chae et al. (2021) recommend the use of the number or activity of NK cells and cytotoxic molecules as effective outcome measures of the immunological effects of forest therapy. They conducted a systematic review in healthy and unhealthy participants and found that most studies reported improvement in these measures after the intervention. For college students, a recent study by Lyu et al. (2019) in 60 men observed that a "bamboo" forest therapy significantly increased well-being along with NK cells' number and activity and decreased cortisol level after a 3-day immersion. Further studies are needed to evaluate the impact of nature on inflammatory and immune functions in young people.

5.6 Psychological and Environmental Mechanisms

Experiences in nature, as we have named, provide multiple benefits for health and well-being; however, the mechanisms of how they work are not yet fully understood or are at an early stage. The underlying mechanisms are complex, as they appear to be multifactorial and intertwine internal-psychological and sensory aspects with external-environmental non-sensory factors, including chemicals and therapeutic aromatic compounds. In terms of mental health and the impact of forest therapy, studies of psychological therapies in which nature itself is not integrated are excluded, even though they may be developed in nature-based settings.

5.6.1 Psychological Mechanisms

Attention restoration theory (ART) (Kaplan & Kaplan, 1989; Kaplan & Talbot, 1983) and stress reduction theory (SRT) (Ulrich, 1983) are some of the psychological avenues that have been argued to substantiate the above results and the primarily restorative effect that occurs in contact with nature. ART suggests that mental fatigue and concentration can be improved by spending time in or looking at nature. As summarized by Wolf et al. (2014), Rachel and Stephen Kaplan proposed ART to explain responses to the effects of natural environments noting that environments need the following conditions to be restorative: (a) being away, (b) extension, (c) compatibility, and (d) fascination. Specifically, fascination would be essential for cognitive recovery since when an environment has fascinating qualities, it attracts involuntary attention, which in turn would require less mental effort. Recent empirical findings have demonstrated the plausibility of ART for understanding the role of intentional attention in the benefits of being in nature. For example, being in nature with a portable electronic device would not be as beneficial in restoring attention in students who do not have these devices in the same natural environment (Jiang et al., 2018).

On the other hand, SRT states that natural settings would promote psychophysiological positive affective response (Ulrich et al., 1991). In short, nature environments are perceived as involving little threat, which allows generating a calm response, thus decreasing stress reactions. These effects would imply a reduction of several stress markers as mentioned above by translating the regulation of the ANS and the immune-endocrine systems. From a psychological and evolutionary perspective of emotion regulation (Gilbert, 2010), nature would promote the calm and appeasement system in counterpart to the threat detection (sympathetic activity, adrenaline) and goal-oriented systems (dopamine), typical autopilot and survival mode.

5.6.2 Environmental Mechanisms

Of particular interest is the study of therapeutic aromatic compounds known as phytoncides, which are volatile and essential oils produced by plants and trees. Most of these compounds are known as terpenes or terpenoids and represent one of the major components of forest aerosols (Cho et al., 2017). Terpenes in the air originate from leaves and tree needles. They also emanate from tree trunks, their bark, weeds, herbs, shrubs, fungi, mosses, ferns, and decaying humus. These molecules fulfill a great number of functions; for example, they confer protection to plants by avoiding solar radiation, they have antimicrobial and antiparasitic properties, and they help to attract or avoid other species to collaborate or defend themselves.

When we walk through the forest, we come into contact with plant terpenes in gaseous form. Some of these are absorbed through the skin, but mostly through the lungs. Studies on terpenes show beneficial effects on inflammatory diseases, tumorigenesis, and neurodegeneration. For example, most of the anti-inflammatory functions of terpenes and terpenoids occur due to the decreased levels of proinflammatory mediators such as nitric oxide (NO), interleukins, tumor necrosis factor-alpha (TNF-α), and prostaglandin E2 (PGE2) (Kim et al., 2020). Terpenes produced by conifers have shown beneficial effects on human health (Cho et al., 2017). Terpenes also have several immunostimulatory properties. For example, breathing near trees for a single day in a wooded area causes a 40% increase in NK cells. Even more, spending two consecutive days in a forest can increase NK cells by more than 50% (Arvay, 2015).

5.7 Fostering an Embodied Relation with Nature and Current Times

Modern urbanization, current lifestyles, hyper-technologization, global health, and climate uncertainty, along with individual vulnerabilities and contexts, are outstripping our coping resources. A study by Killingsworth and Gilbert (2010), which ecologically assessed people's mental states as they engaged in various daily activities, found that regardless of the activity people engage in, they are happiest when their thoughts do not wander. Their research shows that a wandering mind has negative emotional consequences and feelings of unhappiness. Young people are especially vulnerable at this moment in history. Hyperactivity, digital addiction, overthinking, and other forms of autopilot functioning serve to disconnect from the present moment, especially when it is difficult, and appear as maladaptive strategies for coping with life today. Perhaps, urbanization and associated stress contribute to an autopilot mode of cognitive and emotional processing, in which disconnection leads to dysregulation. Under stress, we experience less awareness of what we are experiencing, of our emotions, thoughts, and sensations. In addition, survival mode limits resources for deepening connection and the possibility of healing. Chronic stress and loss of contact with nature translate into disorders that explain the difficulties in taking care of ourselves and self-regulating. When our physical body is sick, we need to stop, rest, and pay attention to it. Also, when we suffer, we need love and understanding. It seems natural to turn to nature, as it possesses all the virtues we seek, such as strength, stability, patience, and compassion. Being in conscious contact with nature brings feelings of relief and helps to restore mood and vitality.

Along with other therapeutic interventions and lifestyle measures such as rest, exercise, nutrition, relationships, and avoidance of toxic substances (Kushner & Mechanick, 2015), getting back to nature appears as a natural necessity in promotion and prevention. Being in nature allows us to return to a safe sensory self-experience, as the five senses are easily stimulated, it does not speed us up as is usually the case with the frenetic pace of everyday life, and it usually takes us into relaxation mode. Its practice can be part of lifestyle changes to cultivate attentional and attitudinal qualities to be in relation with life. Despite observed benefits, a recent systematic review of observational studies found some limited evidence suggesting a beneficial association between exposure to urban green space (distance to nearest green space and average greenness) and mental well-being in children and depressive symptoms in adolescents and young adults (Vanaken & Danckaerts, 2018). Thus, the contemplative dimension of being in nature and how nature can teach contemplative abilities needs to be studied further to understand its benefits and its application in youth at risk for depression.

From a cognitive perspective, maladaptive patterns of information processing in adolescents with depression include difficulties in the voluntary deployment of attention to and from emotional stimuli, negative interpretation biases, and overgeneralized autobiographical memories (Oliver et al., 2019). At the brain level, depressed adolescents show increased functional connectivity in the default mode network (DMN) (Zhang et al., 2016). DMN includes the medial prefrontal, posterior cingulate, and precuneus, and its increased functional connectivity with the subgenual prefrontal cortex (sgPFC) is associated with depressive rumination (Hamilton et al., 2015). Multisensory stimuli present in nature can serve as available anchors to focus attention helping to decrease mental rumination in young. Interestingly, Bratman et al. (2015) reported decreased rumination, as well as decreased neural activity in the sgPFC, following a 90-min walk in a natural (vs. urban) environment in healthy adults.

From an emotional perspective, experiential avoidance refers to an "unwillingness to remain in contact with uncomfortable private events by escaping or avoiding these experiences" (Hayes et al., 1996). In adolescence, experiential avoidance has also been studied in depression and its symptom intensity and persistence (Kring, 2008; Mellick et al., 2019). Nature can foster stability and teaches us to relate it to ourselves in a more caring attitude. As difficult inner experience can be softened "naturally" by multisensory stimulation, repetitive exposure to nature can create safety, allowing for a more embodied sense of self. Contemplation of nature can temper experiential avoidance of bodily and emotional difficulties, as awareness of sensory stimuli helps to calm and regulate arousal. New ways of being present, along with recognition of the impermanent dimension of nature (i.e., cycles, weather, seasons, plant growth processes, death, and decay), can foster acceptance of life's changes and losses. These qualities carry over to other times in life and act as valuable resources for coping with difficulties.

Considering that positive correlations have been described between nature, mindfulness traits, and measures of psychological well-being (Sadowski et al., 2020; Timko Olson et al., 2020), we suggest that intentionally developing contemplative skills while in nature may enhance their effects, especially in depression where mere exposure to nature may be insufficient. This is in line with research suggesting mindfulness practice as a key component of NBIs to maximize its benefits (Nisbet et al., 2019).

5.8 The Need to Implement Nature Therapy in Today's Youth

According to Antonelli et al. (2021), the positive impact of forest bathing on the quality of life of individuals, together with its favorable cost-effectiveness profile, may justify its possible adoption for public health strategies to promote well-being in different contexts. Nature therapy as promotion and prevention should begin at early childhood and continue throughout all ages, recognizing critical periods of development of self- and interpersonal regulatory systems. Promoting nature contemplation from an early age can teach young people to relate more healthily to life's difficulties and changes. Special interest has been placed on bringing NBIs into the educational settings, including schools and universities. Through simple interventions in nature, it is possible to pause, return to the senses, and cultivate appreciation and gratitude.

In university students, NBIs have started to be used as a preventive model for mental health problems (Bang et al., 2017). Thus, one of the interesting topics in universities is the possibility of using the campus itself as part of the recreational activities in which students may participate. These activities could reduce stress and anxiety and improve well-being in a relatively short period of time (Lee et al., 2014; Rajoo et al., 2019). For example, a recent study by Kim et al. (2021) with university students who participated in forest activities in a Korean university campus, using the Concise Measure of Subjective Well-Being (COMOSWB), found positive increases in subjective well-being compared with those participants who did not participate in any forest activities. A Chilean example of a university campus of forest therapy intervention was conducted in a Valdivian Forest hotspot (southern Chile) with 21 students who were randomly assigned to perform a walk and contemplation in a forest or city space in a single, 1-hour session. This pilot study evaluated its effect on mental health, well-being, and mindfulness. The results indicate that the overall protocol can be feasibly administered and that anxiety as a state was the only variable that decreased significantly in the forest therapy group compared to the city group (Langer et al., under review).

Future research is needed to explore the mechanisms of action of nature therapy in promoting effective responses to stress and preventing mental health disorders, especially depression. We suggest that studies should cover the NBIs at all stages of development, recognizing specific and critical needs. By understanding specific depressive psychopathology and the potential of contemplative resources in nature, more specific interventions can be designed for both universal and targeted prevention. This is in line with Owens and Bunce (2022) proposal of candidate mechanisms involved in both nature exposure and depression pathogenesis (i.e., stress, rumination, mindfulness, sleep, and exercise) that should be analyzed in more rigorous studies.

Neurologically, studies could further assess the change in activity of self-referential processing regions (e.g., DMN), characteristics of depressive cognitions, and enhancement of somatosensory areas and interoceptive pathways. Autonomic nervous system and immunological markers could provide further insight into the positive correlates of nature exposure in youth. Mixed methodological studies can articulate quantitative and subjective data to explore underlying mechanisms of action. Particularly in youth, qualitative methods should assess how specific contemplative skills (sensory awareness and appreciation/gratitude) may contribute to daily life coping and mental health. Future studies can deepen the understanding of the influence of the social and relational aspects of NBIs, thus recognizing the needs of youth as well as the environmental variables of local natural environment.

5.9 Conclusion

Given the deteriorating mental health of young people in recent years and the threat of rapid global urbanization, regaining contact with nature represents a great opportunity for well-being. There is capacity for healing and personal growth in the interaction with nature, as it provides us with a protective atmosphere in which, in a very concrete and tangible way, we feel sustained, and allows us to settle down. From a brief contemplation of a green space to a walk in the forest, whether from an individual motivation or as a public health measure or educational activity, contact with nature emerges as necessary to prevent and counteract the effects of stress and the underlying mechanisms of depression. More research is needed to understand the specific contribution of contemplative skills in nature in promoting mental health. Attentional and attitudinal qualities in nature and in everyday life appear to be especially relevant in the prevention of depression, as a less ruminative and more embodied sense of self serves as a prerequisite for perceiving beauty and, in turn, flourishing the sense of gratitude, key aspects of well-being.

Conflict of Interest The authors declare that they have no conflict of interest.

Acknowledgements This manuscript was supported by ANID – Millennium Science Initiative Program – ICS13_005 and NCS2021_081 and ANID – FONDECYT Program – 1221034.

References

Antonelli, M., Barbieri, G., & Donelli, D. (2019). Effects of forest bathing (shinrin-yoku) on levels of cortisol as a stress biomarker: A systematic review and meta-analysis. *International Journal of Biometeorology, 63*(8), 1117–1134. https://doi.org/10.1007/s00484-019-01717-x

Antonelli, M., Donelli, D., Carlone, L., Maggini, V., Firenzuoli, F., & Bedeschi, E. (2021). Effects of forest bathing (shinrin-yoku) on individual well-being: An umbrella review. *International Journal of Environmental Health Research, 1–26.* https://doi.org/10.1080/09603123.2021.1919293

Arvay, C. G. (2015). *Der Biophilia Effekt – Heilung aus dem Wald*. Edition a.

Bang, K.-S., Kim, S., Song, M., Kang, K., & Jeong, Y. (2018). The effects of a health promotion program using urban forests and nursing student mentors on the perceived and psychological health of elementary school children in vulnerable populations. *International Journal of Environmental Research and Public Health, 15*(9), 1977. https://doi.org/10.3390/ijerph15091977

Bang, K.-S., Lee, I., Kim, S., Lim, C. S., Joh, H.-K., Park, B.-J., & Song, M. K. (2017). The effects of a campus forest-walking program on undergraduate and graduate students' physical and psychological health. *International Journal of Environmental Research and Public Health, 14*(7). https://doi.org/10.3390/ijerph14070728

Blood, J. D., Wu, J., Chaplin, T. M., Hommer, R., Vazquez, L., Rutherford, H. J. V., Mayes, L. C., & Crowley, M. J. (2015). The variable heart: High frequency and very low frequency correlates of depressive symptoms in children and adolescents. *Journal of Affective Disorders, 186*, 119–126. https://doi.org/10.1016/j.jad.2015.06.057

Bratman, G. N., Hamilton, J. P., Hahn, K. S., Daily, G. C., & Gross, J. J. (2015). Nature experience reduces rumination and subgenual prefrontal cortex activation. *Proceedings of the National Academy of Sciences, 112*(28), 8567–8572. https://doi.org/10.1073/pnas.1510459112

Capaldi, C. A., Dopko, R. L., & Zelenski, J. M. (2014). The relationship between nature connectedness and happiness: A meta-analysis. *Frontiers in Psychology, 5*(976). https://doi.org/10.3389/fpsyg.2014.00976

Chae, Y., Lee, S., Jo, Y., Kang, S., Park, S., & Kang, H. (2021). The effects of forest therapy on immune function. *International Journal of Environmental Research and Public Health, 18*(16), 8440. https://doi.org/10.3390/ijerph18168440

Chandra, P. S., Shiva, L., & Nanjundaswamy, M. H. (2018). The impact of urbanization on mental health in India. *Current Opinion in Psychiatry, 31*(3), 276–281. https://doi.org/10.1097/YCO.0000000000000408

Chang, J. (2015). The forest experience program and improvement of depression, anxiety, and self-concept in adolescents. *Journal of Korean Forest Society, 104*(1), 127–132. https://doi.org/10.14578/jkfs.2015.104.1.127

Chaudhury, P., & Banerjee, D. (2020). "Recovering with nature": A review of ecotherapy and implications for the COVID-19 pandemic. *Frontiers in Public Health, 8*. https://doi.org/10.3389/fpubh.2020.604440

Chen, M. A., LeRoy, A. S., Majd, M., Chen, J. Y., Brown, R. L., Christian, L. M., & Fagundes, C. P. (2021). Immune and epigenetic pathways linking childhood adversity and health across the lifespan. *Frontiers in Psychology, 12*. https://doi.org/10.3389/fpsyg.2021.788351

Cho, K. S., Lim, Y., Lee, K., Lee, J., Lee, J. H., & Lee, I.-S. (2017). Terpenes from forests and human health. *Toxicological Research, 33*(2), 97–106. https://doi.org/10.5487/tr.2017.33.2.097

Chun, M., Chang, M., & Lee, S. (2016). The effects of forest therapy on depression and anxiety in patients with chronic stroke. *International Journal of Neuroscience, 127*(3), 199–203. https://doi.org/10.3109/00207454.2016.1170015

Christodoulou, G., Salami, N., & Black, D. S. (2020). The utility of heart rate variability in mindfulness research. *Mindfulness, 11*(3), 554–570.

Clifford, M. A. (2018). *Your guide to forest bathing: Experience the healing power of nature*. Conari Press.

Cribb, G., Moulds, M. L., & Carter, S. (2006). Rumination and experiential avoidance in depression. *Behaviour Change, 23*(03), 165–176. https://doi.org/10.1375/bech.23.3.165

Davis, M. T., Holmes, S. E., Pietrzak, R. H., & Esterlis, I. (2017). Neurobiology of chronic stress-related psychiatric disorders: Evidence from molecular imaging studies. *Chronic Stress, 1*, 2470547017710916. https://doi.org/10.1177/2470547017710916

De Wit, H. (2008). Working with existential and neurotic suffering. In F. J. Kaklauskas, S. Nimanheminda, L. Hoffman, & M. S. Jack (Eds.), *Brilliant sanity: Buddhist approaches to psychotherapy*. University Of The Rockies Press.

Djernis, D., Lerstrup, I., Poulsen, D., Stigsdotter, U., Dahlgaard, J., & O'Toole, M. (2019). A Systematic Review and Meta-Analysis of Nature-Based Mindfulness: Effects of Moving Mindfulness Training into an Outdoor Natural Setting. *International journal of environmental research and public health, 16*(17), 3202. https://doi.org/10.3390/ijerph16173202

Farrow, M. R., & Washburn, K. (2019). A review of field experiments on the effect of forest bathing on anxiety and heart rate variability. *Global Advances in Health and Medicine, 8*, 2164956119848654. https://doi.org/10.1177/2164956119848654

Ford, T., John, A., & Gunnell, D. (2021). Mental health of children and young people during pandemic. *BMJ, 372*, n614. https://doi.org/10.1136/bmj.n614

Franco, L. S., Shanahan, D. F., & Fuller, R. A. (2017). A review of the benefits of nature experiences: More than meets the eye. *International Journal of Environmental Research and Public Health, 14*(8), 864. https://doi.org/10.3390/ijerph14080864

Furuyashiki, A., Tabuchi, K., Norikoshi, K., Kobayashi, T., & Oriyama, S. (2019). A comparative study of the physiological and psychological effects of forest bathing (Shinrin-yoku) on working age people with and without depressive tendencies. *Environmental Health and Preventive Medicine, 24*(1), 46. https://doi.org/10.1186/s12199-019-0800-1

Goldberg, S. B., Tucker, R. P., Greene, P. A., Davidson, R. J., Wampold, B. E., Kearney, D. J., & Simpson, T. L. (2018). Mindfulness-based interventions for psychiatric disorders: A systematic review and meta-analysis. *Clinical Psychology Review, 59*, 52–60. https://doi.org/10.1016/j.cpr.2017.10.011

Gouin, J.-P. (2011). Chronic Stress, Immune Dysregulation, and Health. American Journal of *Lifestyle Medicine, 5*(6), 476–485. https://doi.org/10.1177/1559827610395467

Grosse, L., Hoogenboezem, T., Ambrée, O., Bellingrath, S., Jörgens, S., de Wit, H. J., Wijkhuijs, A. M., Arolt, V., & Drexhage, H. A. (2016). Deficiencies of the T and natural killer cell system in major depressive disorder. *Brain, Behavior, and Immunity, 54*, 38–44. https://doi.org/10.1016/j.bbi.2015.12.003

Guendelman, S., Medeiros, S., & Rampes, H. (2017). Mindfulness and emotion regulation: Insights from neurobiological, psychological, and clinical studies. *Frontiers in Psychology, 8*. https://doi.org/10.3389/fpsyg.2017.00220

Hamilton, J. P., Farmer, M., Fogelman, P., & Gotlib, I. H. (2015). Depressive rumination, the default-mode network, and the dark matter of clinical neuroscience. *Biological Psychiatry, 78*(4), 224–230. https://doi.org/10.1016/j.biopsych.2015.02.020

Han, J.-W., Choi, H., Jeon, Y.-H., Yoon, C.-H., Woo, J.-M., & Kim, W. (2016). The effects of forest therapy on coping with chronic widespread pain: Physiological and psychological differences between participants in a forest therapy program and a control group. *International Journal of Environmental Research and Public Health, 13*(3), 255. https://doi.org/10.3390/ijerph13030255

Hansen, M. M., Jones, R., & Tocchini, K. (2017). Shinrin-Yoku (forest bathing) and nature therapy: A state-of-the-art review. *International Journal of Environmental Research and Public Health, 14*(8), 851. https://doi.org/10.3390/ijerph14080851

Hartmann, R., Schmidt, F. M., Sander, C., & Hegerl, U. (2019). Heart rate variability as indicator of clinical state in depression. *Frontiers in Psychiatry, 9*. https://doi.org/10.3389/fpsyt.2018.00735

Hayes, S. C., Wilson, K. G., Gifford, E. V., Follette, V. M., & Strosahl, K. (1996). Experiential avoidance and behavioral disorders: A functional dimensional approach to diagnosis and treatment. *Journal of Consulting and Clinical Psychology, 64*(6), 1152–1168. https://doi.org/10.1037/0022-006x.64.6.1152

Howren, M. B., Lamkin, D. M., & Suls, J. (2009). Associations of depression with C-reactive protein, IL-1, and IL-6: A meta-analysis. *Psychosomatic Medicine, 71*(2), 171–186. https://doi.org/10.1097/PSY.0b013e3181907c1b

Huynh, T., & Torquati, J. C. (2019). Examining connection to nature and mindfulness at promoting psychological Well-being. *Journal of Environmental Psychology, 66*, 101370.

Jeon, J. Y., Kim, I. O., Yeon, P. S., & Shin, W. S. (2021). The physio-psychological effect of forest therapy programs on juvenile probationers. *International Journal of Environmental Research and Public Health, 18*(10), 5467. https://doi.org/10.3390/ijerph18105467

Jiang, B., Schmillen, R., & Sullivan, W. C. (2018). How to waste a break: Using portable electronic devices substantially counteracts attention enhancement effects of green spaces. *Environment and Behavior, 51*(9–10), 1133–1160. https://doi.org/10.1177/0013916518788603

Kachru, S., & Taylor, Z. (2017). *Nature & well-being: Gratitude*. (n.d.). Mind & Life Institute. https://www.mindandlife.org/insight/nature-well-gratitude/

Kaplan, R., & Kaplan, S. (1989). *The experience of nature: A psychological perspective*. Cambridge University Press.

Kaplan, S., & Talbot, J. F. (1983). Psychological benefits of a wilderness experience. *Human Behavior & Environment: Advances in Theory & Research, 6*, 163–203.

Kemp, A. H., Quintana, D. S., Gray, M. A., Felmingham, K. L., Brown, K., & Gatt, J. M. (2010). Impact of depression and antidepressant treatment on heart rate variability: A review and meta-analysis. *Biological Psychiatry, 67*(11), 1067–1074.

Khoury, B., Sharma, M., Rush, S. E., & Fournier, C. (2015). Mindfulness-based stress reduction for healthy individuals: A meta-analysis. *Journal of Psychosomatic Research, 78*(6), 519–528. https://doi.org/10.1016/j.jpsychores.2015.03.009

Killingsworth, M. A., & Gilbert, D. T. (2010). A wandering mind is an unhappy mind. *Science (New York, N.Y.), 330*(6006), 932. https://doi.org/10.1126/science.1192439

Kim, J. G., Jeon, J., & Shin, W. S. (2021). The influence of forest activities in a university campus forest on student's psychological effects. *International Journal of Environmental Research and Public Health, 18*(5), 2457. https://doi.org/10.3390/ijerph18052457

Kim, T., Song, B., Cho, K. S., & Lee, I.-S. (2020). Therapeutic potential of volatile terpenes and terpenoids from forests for inflammatory diseases. *International Journal of Molecular Sciences, 21*(6), 2187. https://doi.org/10.3390/ijms21062187

Kobayashi, H., Song, C., Ikei, H., Park, B.-J., Lee, J., Kagawa, T., & Miyazaki, Y. (2018). Forest walking affects autonomic nervous activity: A population-based study. *Frontiers in Public Health, 6*. https://doi.org/10.3389/fpubh.2018.00278

Kotera, Y., Richardson, M., & Sheffield, D. (2020). Effects of Shinrin-Yoku (forest bathing) and nature therapy on mental health: A systematic review and meta-analysis. *International Journal of Mental Health and Addiction*. https://doi.org/10.1007/s11469-020-00363-4

Kovess-Masféty, V., Alonso, J., de Graaf, R., & Demyttenaere, K. (2005). A European approach to rural—Urban differences in mental health: The ESEMeD 2000 comparative study. *The Canadian Journal of Psychiatry, 50*(14), 926–936. https://doi.org/10.1177/070674370505001407

Kring, A. M. (2008). Emotion disturbances as transdiagnostic processes in psychopathology. In M. Lewis, J. M. Haviland-Jones, & L. Feldman-Barrett (Eds.), *Handbook of emotions* (3rd ed., pp. 691–705). Guilford Press.

Kushner, R. F., & Mechanick, J. I. (2015). Lifestyle medicine-an emerging new discipline. *US Endocrinology, 11*(1), 36–40.

Langer, A. I., Schmidt, C., & Krogh, C. (2017). Mindfulness meditation and the perception of beauty: Implications for an ecological well-being. In M. P. Levine (Ed.), *Perception of Beauty*. IntechOpen. https://doi.org/10.5772/intechopen.69529

Langer, A. I., Solano, E., Bacigalupe, L., Soto, B. Asenjo, A., Navarrete, I., Cifuentes, A., Vergara, R., & Steinebach, S. (Under preparation). Forest activities and mental health prevention on undergraduates students: A pilot randomized controlled trial.

Lee, I., Choi, H., Bang, K.-S., Kim, S., Song, M., & Lee, B. (2017). Effects of forest therapy on depressive symptoms among adults: A systematic review. *International Journal of Environmental Research and Public Health, 14*(3). https://doi.org/10.3390/ijerph14030321

Lee, I., Kim, S., Bang, K.-S., Choi, H., Ko, C., Kim, J., & Kim, S. (2014). An analysis of health promotion programs utilizing forests based on Korea's regional healthcare program plans. *Perspectives in Nursing Science, 11*(1), 10. https://doi.org/10.16952/pns.2014.11.1.10

Li, Q., Kobayashi, M., Inagaki, H., Hirata, Y., Li, Y. J., Hirata, K., Shimizu, T., Suzuki, H., Katsumata, M., Wakayama, Y., Kawada, T., Ohira, T., Matsui, N., & Kagawa, T. (2010). A day trip to a forest park increases human natural killer activity and the expression of anti-cancer proteins in male subjects. *Journal of Biological Regulators and Homeostatic Agents, 24*(2), 157–165.

Li, Q., Morimoto, K., Nakadai, A., Inagaki, H., Katsumata, M., Shimizu, T., Hirata, Y., Hirata, K., Suzuki, H., Miyazaki, Y., Kagawa, T., Koyama, Y., Ohira, T., Takayama, N., Krensky, A. M., & Kawada, T. (2007). Forest bathing enhances human natural killer activity and expression of anti-cancer proteins. *International Journal of Immunopathology and Pharmacology, 20*(2 Suppl 2), 3–8. https://doi.org/10.1177/03946320070200S202

Lyu, B., Zeng, C., Xie, S., Li, D., Lin, W., Li, N., Jiang, M., Liu, S., & Chen, Q. (2019). Benefits of a three-day bamboo forest therapy session on the psychophysiology and immune system responses of male college students. *International Journal of Environmental Research and Public Health, 16*(24), 4991. https://doi.org/10.3390/ijerph16244991

Maas, J., Verheij, R. A., de Vries, S., Spreeuwenberg, P., Schellevis, F. G., & Groenewegen, P. P. (2009). Morbidity is related to a green living environment. *Journal of Epidemiology and Community Health, 63*(12), 967–973. https://doi.org/10.1136/jech.2008.079038

Macháčková, K., Dudík, R., Zelený, J., Kolářová, D., Vinš, Z., & Riedl, M. (2021). Forest manners exchange: Forest as a place to remedy risky behaviour of adolescents: Mixed methods approach. *International Journal of Environmental Research and Public Health, 18*(11), 5725. https://doi.org/10.3390/ijerph18115725

Mao, G. X., Lan, X. G., Cao, Y. B., Chen, Z. M., He, Z. H., Lv, Y. D., Wang, Y. Z., Hu, X. L., Wang, G. F., & Yan, J. (2012). Effects of short-term forest bathing on human health in a broad-leaved evergreen forest in Zhejiang Province, China. *Biomedical and Environmental Sciences: BES, 25*(3), 317–324. https://doi.org/10.3967/0895-3988.2012.03.010

McCullough, M. E., Emmons, R. A., & Tsang, J.-A. (2002). The grateful disposition: A conceptual and empirical topography. *Journal of Personality and Social Psychology, 82*(1), 112–127. https://doi.org/10.1037//0022-3514.82.1.112

McEwen, B. S. (2008). Central effects of stress hormones in health and disease: Understanding the protective and damaging effects of stress and stress mediators. *European Journal of Pharmacology, 583*(2–3), 174–185. https://doi.org/10.1016/j.ejphar.2007.11.071

McEwen, B. S. (2017). Neurobiological and systemic effects of chronic stress. *Chronic Stress (Thousand Oaks, Calif), 1*, 2470547017692328. https://doi.org/10.1177/2470547017692328

Medeiros, S., Crempien, C., Vásquez-Rosati, A., Duarte, J., Andreu, C., Langer, I., Ibaceta, M., Silva, J. R., & Cosmelli, S. D. (2021). Assessing subjective processes and vulnerability in mindfulness-based interventions: A mixed methods exploratory study. *Constructivist Foundations, 16*(2), 203–220. https://constructivist.info/16/2/203

Medeiros, S., & Guendelman, S. (2019). A socio-cognitive, developmentally informed perspective for contemplative practices in adolescence: Towards resilient communities. In C. Steinebach & A. I. Langer (Eds.), *Enhancing resilience in youth: Mindfulness-based interventions in positive environments* (pp. 175–187). Springer. https://doi.org/10.1007/978-3-030-25513-8_11

Meherali, S., Punjani, N., Louie-Poon, S., Abdul Rahim, K., Das, J. K., Salam, R. A., & Lassi, Z. S. (2021). Mental health of children and adolescents amidst COVID-19 and past pandemics: A rapid systematic review. *International Journal of Environmental Research and Public Health, 18*(7), 3432. https://doi.org/10.3390/ijerph18073432

Mellick, W. H., Mills, J. A., Kroska, E. B., Calarge, C. A., Sharp, C., & Dindo, L. N. (2019). Experiential avoidance predicts persistence of major depressive disorder and generalized anxiety disorder in late adolescence. *The Journal of Clinical Psychiatry, 80*(6), 18m12265. https://doi.org/10.4088/JCP.18m12265

Miller, G. E., & Cole, S. W. (2012). Clustering of depression and inflammation in adolescents previously exposed to childhood adversity. *Biological Psychiatry, 72*(1), 34–40. https://doi.org/10.1016/j.biopsych.2012.02.034

Mind and Life Education Research Network (MLERN). (2012). Contemplative practices and mental training: Prospects for American education. *Child Development Perspectives, 6*(2), 146–153. https://doi.org/10.1111/j.1750-8606.2012.00240.x

Mygind, L., Kjeldsted, E., Hartmeyer, R., Mygind, E., Bølling, M., & Bentsen, P. (2019). Mental, physical and social health benefits of immersive nature-experience for children and adolescents: A systematic review and quality assessment of the evidence. *Health & Place, 58*, 102136. https://doi.org/10.1016/j.healthplace.2019.05.014

Nhất Hạnh. (2013). *Love letter to the earth*. Parallax Press.

Nisbet, E. K., Zelenski, J. M., & Grandpierre, Z. (2019). Mindfulness in nature enhances connectedness and mood. *Ecopsychology, 11*(2), 81–91. https://doi.org/10.1089/eco.2018.0061

Ochiai, H., Ikei, H., Song, C., Kobayashi, M., Takamatsu, A., Miura, T., Kagawa, T., Li, Q., Kumeda, S., Imai, M., & Miyazaki, Y. (2015). Physiological and psychological effects of forest therapy on middle-aged males with high-Normal Blood pressure. *International Journal of Environmental Research and Public Health, 12*(3), 2532–2542. https://doi.org/10.3390/ijerph120302532

Oh, B., Lee, K., Zaslawski, C., Yeung, A., Rosenthal, D., Larkey, L., & Back, M. (2017). Health and Well-being benefits of spending time in forests: Systematic review. *Environmental Health and Preventive Medicine, 22*(1). https://doi.org/10.1186/s12199-017-0677-9

Oliver, A., Pile, V., Elm, D., & Lau, J. Y. F. (2019). The cognitive neuropsychology of depression in adolescents. *Current Behavioral Neuroscience Reports, 6*(4), 227–235. https://doi.org/10.1007/s40473-019-00187-0

Owens, M., & Bunce, H. L. I. (2022). The potential for outdoor nature-based interventions in the treatment and prevention of depression. *Frontiers in Psychology, 13*. https://doi.org/10.3389/fpsyg.2022.740210

Park, B. J., Tsunetsugu, Y., Kasetani, T., Kagawa, T., & Miyazaki, Y. (2009). The physiological effects of Shinrin-yoku (taking in the forest atmosphere or forest bathing): Evidence from field experiments in 24 forests across Japan. *Environmental Health and Preventive Medicine, 15*(1), 18–26. https://doi.org/10.1007/s12199-009-0086-9

Pritchard, A., Richardson, M., Sheffield, D., & McEwan, K. (2020). The relationship between nature connectedness and eudaimonic well-being: A meta-analysis. *Journal of Happiness Studies, 21*(3), 1145–1167. https://doi.org/10.1007/s10902-019-00118-6

Quintana, D. S., Alvares, G. A., & Heathers, J. A. J. (2016). Guidelines for reporting articles on psychiatry and heart rate variability (GRAPH): Recommendations to advance research communication. *Translational Psychiatry, 6*(5), e803. https://doi.org/10.1038/tp.2016.73

Rajoo, K. S., Karam, D. S., & Abdul Aziz, N. A. (2019). Developing an effective forest therapy program to manage academic stress in conservative societies: A multi-disciplinary approach. *Urban Forestry & Urban Greening, 43*, 126353. https://doi.org/10.1016/j.ufug.2019.05.015

Rohleder, N. (2019). Stress and inflammation – The need to address the gap in the transition between acute and chronic stress effects. *Psychoneuroendocrinology, 105*, 164–171. https://doi.org/10.1016/j.psyneuen.2019.02.021

Rosenkranz, M. A., Davidson, R. J., Maccoon, D. G., Sheridan, J. F., Kalin, N. H., & Lutz, A. (2013). A comparison of mindfulness-based stress reduction and an active control in modulation of neurogenic inflammation. *Brain, Behavior, and Immunity, 27*(1), 174–184. https://doi.org/10.1016/j.bbi.2012.10.013

Sadowski, I., Böke, N., Mettler, J., Heath, N., & Khoury, B. (2020). Naturally mindful? The role of mindfulness facets in the relationship between nature relatedness and subjective well-being. *Current Psychology*, 1–16. https://doi.org/10.1007/s12144-020-01056-w

Sansone, R. A., & Sansone, L. A. (2010). Gratitude and well being. *Psychiatry (Edgmont), 7*(11), 18–22.

Sawyer, K. B., Thoroughgood, C. N., Stillwell, E. E., Duffy, M. K., Scott, K. L., & Adair, E. A. (2021). Being present and thankful: A multi-study investigation of mindfulness, gratitude, and employee helping behavior. *Journal of Applied Psychology. Advance Online Publication*. https://doi.org/10.1037/apl0000903

Shaffer, F., McCraty, R., & Zerr, C. (2014). A healthy heart is not a metronome: An integrative review of the heart's anatomy and heart rate variability. *Frontiers in Psychology, 5*. https://doi.org/10.3389/fpsyg.2014.01040

Song, C., Ikei, H., & Miyazaki, Y. (2016). Physiological effects of nature therapy: A review of the research in Japan. *International Journal of Environmental Research and Public Health, 13*(8), 781. https://doi.org/10.3390/ijerph13080781

Stier-Jarmer, M., Throner, V., Kirschneck, M., Immich, G., Frisch, D., & Schuh, A. (2021). The psychological and physical effects of forests on human health: A systematic review of systematic reviews and meta-analyses. *International Journal of Environmental Research and Public Health, 18*(4). https://doi.org/10.3390/ijerph18041770

Sung, J., Woo, J. M., Kim, W., Lim, S. K., & Chung, E. J. (2012). The effect of cognitive behavior therapy-based "forest therapy" program on blood pressure, salivary cortisol level, and quality of life in elderly hypertensive patients. *Clinical and Experimental Hypertension (New York, N.Y.: 1993), 34*(1), 1–7. https://doi.org/10.3109/10641963.2011.618195

Tillmann, S., Tobin, D., Avison, W., & Gilliland, J. (2018). Mental health benefits of interactions with nature in children and teenagers: A systematic review. *Journal of Epidemiology and Community Health, 72*(10), 958–966. https://doi.org/10.1136/jech-2018-210436

Timko Olson, E. R., Hansen, M. M., & Vermeesch, A. (2020). Mindfulness and Shinrin-Yoku: Potential for physiological and psychological interventions during uncertain times. *International Journal of Environmental Research and Public Health, 17*(24), 9340. https://doi.org/10.3390/ijerph17249340

Trivedi, J. K., Sareen, H., & Dhyani, M. (2008). Rapid urbanization – Its impact on mental health: A south Asian perspective. *Indian Journal of Psychiatry, 50*(3), 161–165. https://doi.org/10.4103/0019-5545.43623

Ulrich, R. S. (1983). Aesthetic and affective response to natural environment. In I. Altman & F. Wohlwill (Eds.), *Human behavior and the environment. Behavior and the natural environment* (Vol. 6, pp. 85–125). Plenum.

Ulrich, R. S., Simons, R. F., Losito, B. D., Fiorito, E., Miles, M. A., & Zelson, M. (1991). Stress recovery during exposure to natural and urban environments. *Journal of Environmental Psychology, 11*(3), 201–230. https://doi.org/10.1016/S0272-4944(05)80184-7

United Nations. (2018). *2018 revision of world urbanization prospects | multimedia library – United Nations Department of economic and social affairs*. Un.org. https://www.un.org/development/desa/publications/2018-revision-of-world-urbanization-prospects.html

Vanaken, G. J., & Danckaerts, M. (2018). Impact of green space exposure on children's and adolescents' mental health: A systematic review. *International Journal of Environmental Research and Public Health, 15*(12), 2668. https://doi.org/10.3390/ijerph15122668

Wang, J. L. (2004). Rural-urban differences in the prevalence of major depression and associated impairment. *Social Psychiatry and Psychiatric Epidemiology, 39*(1), 19–25. https://doi.org/10.1007/s00127-004-0698-8

White, M. P., Alcock, I., Grellier, J., Wheeler, B. W., Hartig, T., Warber, S. L., Bone, A., Depledge, M. H., & Fleming, L. E. (2019). Spending at least 120 minutes a week in nature is associated with good health and wellbeing. *Scientific Reports, 9*(1), 7730. https://doi.org/10.1038/s41598-019-44097-3

Wolf, K., Krueger, S., & Rozance, M. (2014). Stress, wellness & physiology – A literature review. *Green Cities: Good Health*. Retrieved from http://www.greenhealth.washington.edu

Wood, A. M., Froh, J. J., & Geraghty, A. W. A. (2010). Gratitude and well-being: A review and theoretical integration. *Clinical Psychology Review, 30*(7), 890–905. https://doi.org/10.1016/j.cpr.2010.03.005

Zhang, S., Chen, J. M., Kuang, L., Cao, J., Zhang, H., Ai, M., Wang, W., Zhang, S. D., Wang, S. Y., Liu, S. J., & Fang, W. D. (2016). Association between abnormal default mode network activity and suicidality in depressed adolescents. *BMC Psychiatry, 16*(1), 337. https://doi.org/10.1186/s12888-016-1047-7

Chapter 6
Internet-Based Interventions for Prevention and Early Treatment of Depression in Higher Education Students

Álvaro Jiménez-Molina, Pamela Franco, Scarlett Mac-Ginty, and Vania Martínez

6.1 Higher Education Students and Mental Health

Over the past two decades, the percentage of people accessing higher education has more than doubled worldwide (World Bank, 2018). Access to higher education institutions brings several changes and significant challenges. Many young people must adapt to the transition from a highly structured school model to a context characterized by greater flexibility, autonomy, new academic demands, and learning

Á. Jiménez-Molina
Facultad de Psicología, Universidad Diego Portales, Santiago, Chile

Millennium Institute for Research in Depression and Personality (MIDAP), Santiago, Chile

Millennium Nucleus to Improve the Mental Health of Adolescents and Youths (Imhay), Santiago, Chile

P. Franco
Millennium Institute for Research in Depression and Personality (MIDAP), Santiago, Chile

Doctoral Program in Psychotherapy, Pontificia Universidad Católica de Chile and Universidad de Chile, Santiago, Chile

S. Mac-Ginty
Millennium Nucleus to Improve the Mental Health of Adolescents and Youths (Imhay), Santiago, Chile

Institute of Psychiatry, Psychology & Neuroscience, King's College London, London, UK

V. Martínez (✉)
Millennium Institute for Research in Depression and Personality (MIDAP), Santiago, Chile

Millennium Nucleus to Improve the Mental Health of Adolescents and Youths (Imhay), Santiago, Chile

CEMERA, Facultad de Medicina, Universidad de Chile, Santiago, Chile
e-mail: vmartinezn@uchile.cl

V. Martínez, C. Miranda-Castillo (eds.), *Prevention and Early Treatment of Depression Through the Life Course*, Depression and Personality,
https://doi.org/10.1007/978-3-031-13029-8_6

methods, among other factors (Coertjens et al., 2017). Likewise, individual and family expectations about this period, accompanied by significant changes in interpersonal support networks and high levels of uncertainty about the future, can be sources of psychosocial tress.

Higher education also coincides with a crucial period in the life course called "emerging adulthood" (Arnett, 2000), which is a critical phase that concurs with the age of the onset of most mental disorders (Kessler et al., 2007; McGorry et al., 2011). In addition, some studies have found that higher education students have an increased risk of mental and substance abuse disorders compared to the general population of the same age range (Conley et al., 2015; Evans et al., 2018). Internationally, it is estimated that approximately one-third of higher education students meet the 12-month prevalence criteria for mental disorders, primarily major depressive episodes (18.5%) or generalized anxiety disorder (16.7%) (Auerbach et al., 2019; Bruffaerts et al., 2019). A meta-analysis showed a 12-month prevalence estimate of suicidal ideation, suicide plans, and suicide attempts in higher education students of 10.6%, 3.0%, and 1.2%, respectively (Mortier et al., 2018).

Mental health problems in higher education students have been associated with negative impacts on young people's development (Alonso et al., 2019; Auerbach et al., 2016), poorer academic performance and higher dropout rates (Reavley & Jorm, 2019), and a negative impact on later functioning in the labor market (Ashwood et al., 2016; Goldman-Mellor et al., 2014; Niederkrotenthaler et al., 2014).

There is an imbalance between the high prevalence of mental health problems among higher education students and their levels of access to treatment (Auerbach et al., 2018; Ebert et al. 2019b). Only 36% of students with a lifetime mental disorder and a similar proportion who had suicidal behaviors received some form of treatment during the last 12 months (Bruffaerts et al., 2019). This treatment gap involves structural (financial cost and availability of services) and cultural (stigma) barriers. Negative attitudes and beliefs regarding mental disorders and their treatment are also important barriers to seeking help (Eisenberg et al., 2012; Vidourek et al., 2014). Higher education students often perceive that institutional health services do not meet their needs (Goodman, 2017), and treatment is often not perceived as necessary, with many students preferring to manage the problem individually or within their closest support network (Ebert et al. 2019b). In addition, many students do not perceive themselves as ill because they have difficulty recognizing symptoms (Ebert et al. 2019b).

In this context, several interventions and strategies have been developed to address student mental health in higher education, including (1) contextual interventions for mental health promotion (e.g., enhancement of the built environment, social marketing strategies, curriculum-based strategies) (Fernandez et al., 2016), (2) universal and indicated prevention programs for subjects with subclinical levels of symptoms or at-risk populations (Conley et al., 2015, 2016), and (3) brief psychosocial interventions focused on treating specific diagnoses such as depression and anxiety disorder (Conley et al., 2015; Cuijpers et al., 2016; Winzer et al., 2018). An umbrella review of meta-analyses of randomized trials examining prevention and treatment interventions for depression, anxiety, and stress in higher education students shows that effective interventions are now available at universal, indicated, and treatment levels (Cuijpers et al., 2021). The most promising results have been found for indicated prevention and treatment interventions compared to universal prevention. Although commonly used in prevention programs in educational settings, psychoeducation strategies alone did not seem to bring any significant improvement (Martineau et al., 2018).

Institutions of higher education are relevant sites for the prevention, early detection, and treatment of mental disorders, but the high prevalence of mental health problems among students reduces the likelihood that educational institutions will have sufficient resources to meet the need for mental health services. Therefore, there is a need to implement better methods to identify students at risk of developing a mental disorder and to improve prevention programs and early intervention strategies for timely management of mental health problems in higher education students (Duffy et al., 2019).

6.2 Internet-Based Interventions and Mental Health

Internet-based interventions for the prevention and early treatment of depression deserve special attention as an area of research and development at the intersection of mental health and education. These interventions are usually based on a web platform or a mobile application (app) and can be unguided/self-administered or guided. Unguided programs are generally automated interventions without any human interaction, although they may include some additional form of assistance (e.g., personal monitoring). Guided programs include human support ranging from low-intensity support (e.g., e-mail feedback and encouragement) to synchronous assessments (e.g., chat) or teletherapy, but with considerably less support than face-to-face therapy. Guidance may be related to the therapeutic content itself (e.g., homework) or focused on encouraging adherence to the program (e.g., reinforcement).

Table 6.1 proposes a theoretical classification of Internet-based interventions in mental health.

Given the rapid technological development and proliferation of Internet-based treatments in recent years, there have been several studies conducted to evaluate the effects of Internet-based approaches to depression. A recent meta-analysis shows that there is evidence for the efficacy of Internet-based interventions for the treatment of depression in a variety of populations and age groups and different settings (Moshe et al., 2021). The authors of that study found a greater effect size for participants with higher pretreatment depression severity (Moshe et al., 2021). They found no influence of participant age on outcomes, suggesting that Internet-based interventions may be equally effective for individuals of all age groups.

Table 6.1 Theoretical classification of Internet-based interventions for mental health

Target population	*Prevention*	
	Universal Selective Indicated	Targeted at the entire population Targeted to at-risk population subgroups Targeted at individuals with subthreshold symptoms
	Early intervention	
	Case identification	Identification of individuals with subthreshold or clinically significant symptoms through screening strategies, self-report questionnaires, or interviews with health or education professionals
	Early treatment	Intervention for individuals presenting subthreshold symptoms or clinical intervention for individuals meeting diagnostic criteria
Intervention specificity	Specific	Interventions targeting specific mental symptoms or disorders
	Transdiagnostic	Interventions targeting a set of hypothetical mechanisms shared by a group of mental disorders or syndromes
Intervention strategy	Psychoeducation	Primarily provides information to participants on topics such as stress, coping, and ways to relax
	Cognitive behavioral	Focused on how cognitions can be monitored and used effectively to change behaviors or emotions
	Meditation	Includes various meditation and relaxation techniques, such as mindfulness and yoga
	Social skills training	Focused on the development of interpersonal skills through assertiveness training, role-playing, or interpersonal skills development exercises
	Interpersonal psychotherapy	Assess how changes in social relationships impact psychological functioning
Supervision (human support)	Guided	The instructor or group leader directly monitors individuals' practice of new skills and provides feedback and helpful suggestions to encourage mastery of the skills
	Unguided	Fully automated interventions, without human intervention
Outcomes	Emotional distress	Measures of depression, anxiety, or stress, as well as measures of general psychological distress or well-being
	Social and emotional skills	Different types of cognitive, affective, and social skills such as coping techniques and mindfulness, among others
	Self-perceptions	Primarily measures of self-esteem and self-efficacy
	Interpersonal relationships	Measures of relationship quality and satisfaction, social support and adjustment, conflict and communication styles
	Health status	Measures of physical health status and symptoms, as well as reports of health-related behaviors (drinking, smoking, drug use, exercising, or nutrition)
Delivery format	Technology-delivered	Uses technology as a vehicle for mental healthcare service delivery
	Blended	Combines face-to-face and internet-based approaches

6.3 Internet-Based Interventions for Higher Education Students

Young adults are among the main users of the Internet and new technologies (Antoun, 2015) and are very active in online searching for health information (Hanauer et al., 2004; Rennis et al., 2015). In fact, "stress," "anxiety," and "depression" are among the most searched health topics by higher education students on the Internet (Montagni et al., 2018). Therefore, higher education students represent an ideal target for mental health interventions based on the Internet and digital technologies.

Internet-based interventions for higher education students may target universal or selective prevention, promotion of help-seeking and increased willingness to accept treatment when offered, indicated prevention for those at risk, early intervention for students with subthreshold symptoms, or clinical intervention for students who meet diagnostic criteria (Cuijpers et al., 2018; Harrer et al., 2019). A body of literature on technology-delivered interventions for higher education students suggests that these interventions may be effective in improving mental well-being outcomes (Davies et al., 2014; Farrer et al., 2013; Harrer et al., 2018). However, a meta-analysis by Harrer et al. (2019) on Internet interventions for mental health in college students found smaller effects on depression ($g = 0.18$, 95% CI (0.08, 0.27)) than those found for such interventions in other target groups (SMD = 0.90, 95% CI (0.73, 1.04); Königbauer et al., 2017). Since "effect size" is a statistical concept, it does not necessarily reflect the clinical relevance of interventions. Furthermore, these effects may be related to higher education settings, the age range of the students, or other characteristics of individuals that need to be studied.

6.3.1 Internet-Based Interventions for Depression in Higher Education Students

We selected a set of 18 Internet-based preventive and early treatment interventions for depression in higher education, whose studies have been published in 19 articles within the last decade (2011–2021) (Bantjes et al., 2021; Cavanagh et al., 2013; Day et al., 2013; Dear et al., 2019; El Morr et al., 2020; Ellis et al., 2011; Farrer et al., 2019; Fitzpatrick et al., 2017; Fulmer et al., 2018; Harrer et al., 2021; Kvillemo et al., 2016; Levin et al., 2017; Lintvedt et al., 2013; Melnyk et al., 2015; Mullin et al., 2015; Musiat et al., 2014; Palacios et al., 2018; Ritvo et al., 2021; Salamanca-Sanabria et al., 2020). Most studies have been conducted in North America ($n = 7$), Europe ($n = 5$), or Australia ($n = 4$), and very little research exists in Africa ($n = 1$) and Latin America ($n = 1$). Therefore, most of the interventions were developed in higher education institutions located in the Global North, reflecting the great variability in the degree of digital health penetration in different regions (Jiménez-Molina et al., 2019).

The interventions varied considerably in terms of duration, intensity, guidance, and rationale. The duration of the interventions ranged from 2 to 8 weeks. The vast majority had a modular structure, and half of the programs (9/18) distribute their components between five and seven modules or sessions. This indicates that they are generally short or ultrashort interventions.

Some studies suggest that the duration of digital technology-based programs has a significant influence on the effects of the interventions (Etzelmueller et al., 2020). For example, Richards & Richardson (2012) found that Internet-based interventions with eight sessions or less were more effective than interventions with more than eight sessions, and a meta-analysis concluded that the optimal effect and maximum acceptability were achieved in interventions with approximately seven modules (Moshe et al., 2021). Given that the risk of program dropout increases significantly for longer program lengths, there is a need to better understand the optimal combination between duration and number of modules for interventions targeting young people in higher education.

Most of the interventions were designed as part of universal prevention strategies. Most (13/18) were designed specifically to address depressive symptoms. However, some programs also included psychological distress, anxiety and stress symptoms, life satisfaction, self-efficacy, and academic performance as secondary outcomes.

Regarding the theoretical framework and techniques underpinning the intervention strategies, most of them (11/18) were based on cognitive behavioral theory. These interventions conceptually understand depression as a psychological disorder associated with cognitive, behavioral, and emotional maintenance processes, so they aim to intervene in these processes using techniques based on digital technologies. Internet-based cognitive behavioral therapy (iCBT) has shown moderate to large effects on depression ($g = 1.18$, 95% CI: 1.06–1.29) in usual adult care (Etzelmueller et al., 2020). However, the potential efficacy of this type of intervention for the prevention and early treatment of depression in higher education settings appears to be lower compared to other contexts (Harrer et al., 2019).

One strategy that has been developed in recent years consists of Internet-based programs supported by meditation techniques (e.g., audio files with instructions for mindfulness meditation exercises) (Cavanagh et al., 2013; El Morr et al., 2020; Kvillemo et al., 2016; Ritvo et al., 2021). Unlike traditional cognitive behavioral therapy (CBT), mindfulness-based interventions do not directly target the reduction of a specific set of symptoms, but rather account for a transdiagnostic understanding of mental health problems and address a general way of relating to experiences through the performance of repeated meditation exercises. Typically, mindfulness-based interventions advocate an open and nonreactive perception of events and train the individual to process experiences without attempting to control, suppress, or avoid sensations and situations. These skills trigger cognitive, emotional, and somatic effects linked to self-regulation strategies (Langer et al., 2020). Internet-based mindfulness interventions are effective in the treatment of depression and anxiety disorders (Boettcher et al., 2014), but more studies with higher education students might be necessary to have a better assessment of their benefits in this population.

We also found interventions that combine different strategies: cognitive behavioral strategies with meditation, psychoeducation, interpersonal therapy, and specific skills training, such as stress management, problem-solving, concrete thinking, and coping skills for some aspects related to the difficulties of college life (e.g., procrastination) (Farrer et al., 2019; Fulmer et al., 2018; Harrer et al., 2021; Lintvedt et al., 2013). These types of interventions demonstrate that digitally supported programs can be flexible enough to incorporate strategies that go beyond specific techniques to address symptoms traditionally associated with mental disorders. Likewise, psychoeducation strategies about the underlying causes and mechanism of depression, as well as the provision of information about ways to cope with some of the difficulties of college life and how and where to access available support services, were a cross-cutting component of most interventions.

Most of the interventions reviewed were web-based resources (14/18), including discussion forums, online courses, wellness center/resource library, or a combination of these strategies. One intervention was an online workshop and e-book (Bantjes et al., 2021), two were mobile app-based (Fitzpatrick et al., 2017; Fulmer et al., 2018), and one intervention combined a web platform and a mobile app (Harrer et al., 2021).

Some interventions included a form of guidance, which could be through weekly contact or support with a trained therapist or assistant, either by phone or messaging system or through an online discussion group moderator or well-being coaches. However, more than half of the interventions were unguided or self-administered (13/18). These interventions included some form of automated reminders (e.g., prompts) or automated personalized feedback (e.g., based on questionnaire results). Interestingly, some forms of unguided interventions used chatbots, a system that can interact with human users (Fitzpatrick et al., 2017; Fulmer et al., 2018). For example, the *Woebot* program was associated with a high level of engagement by most individuals who used the bot almost every day, with some users describing the bot as a "fun" and "empathetic" system (Fitzpatrick et al., 2017). In this sense, the developers of this bot suggest that people are willing to disclose personal information to an artificial intelligence (AI) program (Fitzpatrick et al., 2017).

6.3.2 Main Findings of the Interventions

The studies reviewed showed mixed results. On the one hand, a significant number of interventions were effective in reducing depressive symptoms and increasing depression literacy (Bantjes et al., 2021; Cavanagh et al., 2013; Day et al., 2013; Dear et al., 2019; El Morr et al., 2020; Fitzpatrick et al., 2017; Fulmer et al., 2018; Harrer et al., 2021; Levin et al., 2017; Lintvedt et al., 2013; Musiat et al., 2014; Palacios et al., 2018; Ritvo et al., 2021; Salamanca-Sanabria et al., 2020). There was also a significant effect on the reduction of anxiety symptoms and perceived stress in favor of intervention groups compared to control conditions (Bantjes et al., 2021; Ellis et al., 2011; Musiat et al., 2014; Palacios et al., 2018) and improvements related to other secondary outcomes (e.g., behavioral activation) after treatment (Harrer et al., 2021; Levin et al., 2017). Not only were significant improvements in depressive symptoms found from pre- to post-intervention, but some studies showed that these improvements were maintained at 3–6 months of follow-up (Day et al., 2013; Harrer et al., 2021; Salamanca-Sanabria et al., 2020). In some studies, more pronounced reductions in depressive symptoms were found among participants with clinically significant symptoms at baseline (Musiat et al., 2014).

On the other hand, some studies showed no significant effects on depressive symptom reduction in the post-intervention phase or compared to control conditions (Farrer et al., 2019; Kvillemo et al., 2016; Melnyk et al., 2015; Mullin et al., 2015). In this regard, some students may be more likely than others to respond to Internet-based interventions linked to several predictors of intervention response that have yet to be determined. For example, Harrer et al. (2019) show that the effects of Internet-based interventions in university students were greatest when participants were preselected across symptom cutoff points or risk factors. It seems that the effects of Internet-based interventions on depression in higher education students depend on the severity of symptoms at baseline. In this sense, interventions tailored to individuals based on their presenting symptoms may have better outcomes.

6.3.3 Program Adherence and Usability

Adherence to Internet-based programs might be a critical factor in determining their outcomes. As previously suggested, one of the main problems with Internet-based interventions for depression in young people is high levels of nonadherence (Martínez et al., 2021). A recent meta-analysis shows that the mean percentage of the intervention group that completed all modules in Internet-based interventions for depression was 55.3% (Moshe et al., 2021). A study by Karyotaki et al. (2018) suggests that younger adults have a higher risk of dropping out of Internet-based interventions than older adults, while Moshe et al. (2021) found that there was no significant influence of age, gender, or guidance on adherence.

One of the most striking results of the studies reviewed is related to the serious problems of adherence and usability of the interventions that translate into high levels of research attrition and high intervention dropout rates. Some studies operationalized adherence as the proportion of participants who completed all or a certain percentage of the intervention, while others defined it as the mean number of modules completed. Beyond these differences, there is a gap between intervention acceptability and participant satisfaction with program usability and adherence levels. Although some studies report that a large proportion of participants rated the interventions as "very useful" or "useful" and show high levels of participant satisfaction and acceptability, and even report that they would recommend the program to others (Dear et al., 2019; Ellis et al., 2011; Farrer et al., 2019; Mullin et al., 2015;

Musiat et al., 2014; Palacios et al., 2018), in several studies, less than 60% of participants completed all program modules (Cavanagh et al., 2013; Farrer et al., 2019; Kvillemo et al., 2016; Lintvedt et al., 2013; Mullin et al., 2015; Musiat et al., 2014; Palacios et al., 2018). For example, in the study by Kvillemo et al. (2016), less than two-fifths of participants completed the entire program. The authors suggest that program retention and compliance may have been affected because participants were not required to have a certain level of psychological symptoms to be included in the intervention (Kvillemo et al., 2016).

Some studies indicate that many of the potential participants who were approached to join the programs did not initiate the intervention (e.g., in the study by Melnyk et al., 2015, only 17% of the students invited to participate in the study initiated the intervention). In other cases, recruitment was based on offering additional credits to students, making it difficult to determine whether higher education students would be willing to participate in a program purely for mental health reasons, without additional incentives (Levin et al., 2017).

Given the important role that adherence plays in mediating outcomes, there would be benefit from further research on the design factors that influence adherence in higher education students, especially in unguided interventions, where adherence is often lower.

One way to address the problem of low adherence to programs is to improve their attractiveness and allow participants to customize some of their elements. For example, MoodGYM program participants complained about the monotony and redundancy of the resources and the length of the program itself (Ellis et al., 2011). Only one-third of the participants indicated that they enjoyed using the program. In the study by Farrer et al. (2019), some participants noted that the program was "too complex," contained "too much information," or was difficult to navigate. This underscores the need to focus more on providing programs that are relevant and meet the needs of higher education students.

Concerning improving the attractiveness of programs, the use of apps to support the prevention and early treatment of depression may be a particularly useful strategy for young people in higher education. However, several shortcomings of mental health apps have been repeatedly described, such as poor handling of users' personal information, poor adherence to evidence-based techniques, low app credibility, and lack of content personalization (Martinengo et al., 2021). Therefore, future studies with higher education students should examine how different platforms of interventions (web-based, app-based, or a combination of both) are associated with their acceptability, adherence, and effectiveness.

Other strategies to increase adherence, such as the inclusion of user-centered designs, should also be evaluated. Having a participatory design approach (i.e., including end users and other key stakeholders in all stages of the development process) when developing or adapting an Internet-based intervention for depression could help ensure that interventions meet the needs of higher education students and are better tailored to the actual user experience (Schilling et al., 2021). In addition, it is highly recommended to include features of persuasive systems, whereby technology is designed to reinforce, change, and shape attitudes and behaviors (Parada et al., 2020).

6.3.4 Human Support or Guidance

Perhaps one of the most critical issues in the development of Internet-based interventions for mental health is the role of human support or guidance. Previous research suggests that guided Internet-based interventions for university students have higher effect sizes than unguided interventions (Conley et al., 2016; Cuijpers et al., 2018). However, the meta-analysis conducted by Harrer et al. (2019) did not find that the availability of guidance significantly moderated intervention efficacy. A recent meta-analysis of patient data network suggests that baseline depressive symptoms may be an important factor explaining differences in the effectiveness of guided versus unguided interventions (Karyotaki et al., 2021). This study shows that individuals with mild and subthreshold depression were associated with little or no benefit from therapeutic guidance, while guided interventions were associated with more effectiveness in individuals with moderate to severe depression (Karyotaki et al., 2021).

Several studies have also shown that guided interventions result in a higher number of completed modules and lower attrition compared to unguided interventions (Baumeister et al., 2014; Richards & Richardson, 2012). Some studies included in this review suggest that more frequent contact with study coordinators and more reminders as ways to help participants complete daily exercises could increase the likelihood of program success (Kvillemo et al., 2016; Salamanca-Sanabria et al., 2020).

Future studies should explore in detail the importance of human support in Internet-based interventions for depression in higher education students to increase engagement and adherence, as well as to improve outcomes. The most cost-effective options for providing guided interventions are not yet sufficiently understood, and there are many options for innovation in this regard. Given the resources of higher education institutions, there is a need to explore "blended approaches," i.e., combining the strengths of Internet-based and face-to-face interventions (Wentzel et al., 2016). Although interventions adopting this approach in higher education still appear to be scarce, this format represents a good alternative to address the growing need for access to psychological support and treatment of mental disorders in higher education students, without disproportionately increasing the costs of health and care services in these institutions. One way to organize the delivery of these interventions is through "stepped care" models, implementing higher-intensity interventions or face-to-face assistance depending on the severity of depressive symptoms. This is certainly an aspect that future Internet-based programs should address, in particular, the selection of the type of intervention according to the severity of symptoms.

6.3.5 *Studies Design and Quality*

There is a growing number of studies testing the feasibility and acceptability of Internet-based interventions for the prevention and early intervention of depression in higher education students. However, very few studies tested the effectiveness of these interventions through randomized controlled trial (RCT) designs. There is a need for methodological advances in large-scale effectiveness studies, as well as cost-effectiveness and implementation studies.

For the reviewed efficacy studies, a common weakness is that most of them used wait-list control groups as a comparison, which often leads to an overestimation of intervention effects. Also, in most of the studies, the outcomes were generally evaluated in the short term (less than 6-month follow-up), which does not allow for assessing whether the positive effects of the intervention were sustained over time.

Another problem identified is that several studies had relatively small numbers of participants and showed a significant gender imbalance of participants, including mainly women, who in some cases accounted for more than 75% of the sample (Cavanagh et al., 2013; Day et al., 2013; El Morr et al., 2020; Ellis et al., 2011; Farrer et al., 2019; Harrer et al., 2021; Kvillemo et al., 2016; Lintvedt et al., 2013; Melnyk et al., 2015; Ritvo et al., 2021).

Future studies should place more emphasis on comparing online interventions with traditional face-to-face interventions, either alone or in combination. This information is crucial for justifying the scalability of interventions.

Given that previous research has documented the enormous potential of Internet-based interventions for other target groups and application domains (Moshe et al., 2021), more research is needed on how Internet-based interventions should be designed and delivered to maximize these capabilities in higher education settings. For example, much remains to be done in implementing digitally supported programs to promote help-seeking in higher education students and to optimize referral systems for community health services (Ebert et al., 2019a). Specifically, more research is needed to determine which types of interventions are best suited to which students, and in what context, to optimize their effects to fully realize the potential of Internet-based interventions to improve the mental health of higher education students.

6.4 Description of Specific Internet-Based Programs

In this section, we will describe in detail some specific programs for the prevention and early treatment of depression that have been implemented in the context of higher education. This description is mainly intended to outline some trends in the development of interventions and their potential benefits for students. Specifically, we have chosen three programs to highlight interventions that have adopted a transdiagnostic approach, that have developed a process of cultural adaptation of interventions, and that may be particularly useful in distance education contexts. The rationale for this selection is based on three main reasons.

First, different prevalence studies show that there is high comorbidity among mental disorders, especially with regard to depression (Plana-Ripoll et al., 2019). Probably, these high comorbidity rates are not a simple co-occurrence of disorders, but the result of an underlying common basis (Dalgleish et al., 2020; Marshall, 2020). In response to this issue, a transdiagnostic approach to understanding and intervening in mental disorders has grown rapidly (Newby et al., 2015), which targets a set of hypothesized mechanisms shared by a group of mental disorders (Schaeuffele et al., 2021). Recently, these interventions are being adapted to Internet-based strategies for the higher education population.

Second, while enrollment growth in higher education over the past two decades has been greatest in low- and middle-income countries (UNESCO IEPP, 2017), most Internet-based interventions for depression have been developed in high-income Western countries. Given that the inclusion of diverse populations is often underrepresented in the evaluation of these interventions (Cuijpers et al., 2018) and that there are cultural differences in the expression and understanding of depression across cultures (Haroz et al., 2017), greater attention to their cultural sensitivity and ecological validity is needed to maximize their efficacy and contribute to their dissemination across countries. In this context, cultural adaptation of interventions developed in high-income countries that have proven to be effective is key to contributing to the reduction of global inequalities in mental health (Salamanca-Sanabria et al., 2019; Spanhel et al., 2021).

Third, the lockdown and physical distancing measures implemented in the context of the COVID-19 pandemic forced many higher education institutions to implement distance learning modalities. Evidence suggests that distance education students face a high level of stress compared to face-to-face students, most likely due to the need to cope with the demands of multiple social roles, the lower likelihood of social support from peers, and the lack of access to campus mental health services (Apolinário-Hagen et al., 2018). Changes in the higher education system in the context of the COVID-19 pandemic represent an opportunity to advance the implementation of interventions supported by digital technologies (Mac-Ginty et al., 2021). Depression prevention, screening, and early intervention could be enhanced by using the technological infrastructure that institutions have acquired to provide continuity of academic activities in the context of the pandemic. It is also possible that the intensive use of the Internet and digital technology in the context of the pandemic has increased the willingness of students and health professionals to use Internet-based programs.

6.4.1 Transdiagnostic Internet-Based Interventions

Most Internet-based interventions in mental health have been developed and evaluated on specific symptoms and disorders. However, we found five interventions that used a transdiagnostic approach to address depressive symptoms in higher education students (Dear et al., 2019; Farrer et al., 2019; Levin et al., 2017; Mullin et al., 2015; Musiat et al., 2014). The development of this type of interventions seems to be still scarce, but growing in recent years.

Transdiagnostic approaches assume that individuals suffering from mental disorders share specific behavioral and cognitive processes (e.g., selective attention, interpretive bias, recurrent negative thinking, avoidance behaviors, etc.) that contribute to the development and maintenance of these disorders (Newby et al., 2015). This approach could provide very useful tools for higher education students who must deal with a range of problems simultaneously.

A good example of Internet-based transdiagnostic interventions is "PLUS" (Personality and Living of University Students), which focused on the prevention of common mental disorders in university students (Musiat et al., 2014). "PLUS" consists of five cognitive behavioral modules, which can be completed in any order. Each module focuses on the potentially negative impact of personality traits on certain aspects of life and how users can overcome them. The objective of the modules is to help users recognize and reduce unhelpful behaviors and thoughts resulting from certain personality-related factors. As an unguided intervention, it has the potential to be widely applied without the need for additional infrastructure.

The introductory module of "PLUS" presents the principles of the cognitive behavioral model and reports on the impact of personality on behavior. Then, the module "Perfectionism" addresses the positive and negative aspects of perfectionism and provides tools to identify and challenge perfectionist thoughts and behaviors. The module "Self-esteem" addresses strategies for overcoming low self-esteem, while the module "anxiety and worry" focuses on developing strategies to identify and reduce the impact of anxiety and worry. The fifth module, "Dealing with difficult emotions," addresses the consequences of emotional instability (neuroticism) and some strategies for emotional regulation.

In a first evaluation of the program, high attrition was observed (half of the participants dropped out after a 6-week follow-up) (Musiat et al., 2014). For analyses of the impact of the intervention, students were grouped into high and low risk of developing mental health problems according to their personality characteristics (and not their symptoms). The intervention was effective in increasing self-esteem and reducing depressive and anxious symptoms in the high-risk group compared to the control condition (three online modules addressing relevant student life issues). An RCT to evaluate the efficacy and cost-effectiveness of PLUS is currently underway in four countries (the United Kingdom, Republic of Ireland, Austria, and Germany), representing one of the largest trials of an Internet-based mental health intervention in higher education (Musiat et al., 2019).

Overall, the PLUS program supports the idea of preventing mental disorders by acting on underlying vulnerability factors in high-risk students. However, the current evidence from transdiagnostic programs is still too preliminary to indicate whether this approach is useful for the range of problems for which students in higher education generally seek treatment and whether it is more effective than disorder-specific approaches.

6.4.2 Cultural Adaptation of Internet-Based Interventions

Given that low- and middle-income countries have poor access to mental health services, Internet-based interventions could help close the treatment gap in these countries (Jiménez-Molina et al., 2019). Considering the paucity of studies in these countries, cultural adaptation of Internet-based interventions that have proven effective in other contexts can be very useful to accelerate the adoption process of these strategies. Cultural adaptation includes methodologies to achieve functional, conceptual, and linguistic equivalence of interventions in different cultural and socioeconomic communities (Spanhel et al., 2021). This method facilitated the adaptation of programs while maintaining the original treatment components (fidelity) and supports the inclusion of community members in the adaptation process as an essential component to increase its validity (Helms, 2015).

A study by Salamanca-Sanabria et al. (2019) attempted to integrate a cultural sensitivity and ecological validity framework to adapt "Space from Depression," a seven-module iCBT program for the treatment of depression (Richards et al., 2015), to the specific needs of Colombian college students. This program includes self-monitoring, behavioral activation, cognitive restructuring, and questioning core beliefs. All modules consist of questionnaires, videos, educational content, and activities with homework suggestions. In addition, users are provided with an assistant, who gives feedback and monitors the users' evolution every week (Richards et al., 2015). The original program has been evaluated by users as acceptable and was effective compared to a control group (waiting list) in an Irish community sample (Richards et al., 2015, 2016).

The culturally adapted version of the "Space from Depression" program ("*Yo Puedo Sentirme Bien*," Spanish version) contains an initial module that introduces the basic premises of CBT for depression and encourages users to identify their current difficulties. The second module aims to track mood and invites users to explore different aspects of emotions, physical reactions, action, and inaction. The third module motivates users to track their thoughts and explore the connection between their cognitions and mood. The fourth module promotes behavior change to improve mood, including behavioral activation ideas. Users can plan activities and plot their relationship to their mood. The fifth module is intended for the user to learn how to challenge distorted negative thought patterns. The sixth module describes the role that deeply held core beliefs may play in mood and depression. This module also contains a series of interactive activities to identify and challenge unhelpful core beliefs. In the last module, users are encouraged to bring together all the skills and ideas acquired through the program, note their personal warning signs, and develop a plan to maintain a state of well-being.

"*Yo Puedo Sentirme Bien*" was evaluated in an RCT to examine its efficacy and feasibility in Colombian university students with depressive symptoms (Salamanca-Sanabria et al., 2020). Although research attrition and treatment dropouts were high, the results showed significant effects on the reduction of depressive symptoms for the treatment group, and these effects were maintained at a 3-month follow-up (Salamanca-Sanabria et al., 2020).

6.4.3 Internet-Based Stress Intervention for Distance Learning Students

The "StudiCare Fernstudierende" (Harrer et al., 2021) is an Internet- and app-based intervention to prevent depression in university students that adjusted the "StudiCare Stress" program (Harrer et al., 2018) to the needs of university distance learners. Specifically, it is a two-part intervention consisting of seven modules plus a booster module in which cognitive behavioral coping methods are used to manage personal difficulties and minimize stress factors. The first part of the intervention focuses on problem-oriented coping, while the second part focuses on emotion-oriented coping using emotion regulation strategies. Completing a module requires between 30 and 90 minutes, and participants are encouraged to work on no more than two modules per week. Therefore, the intervention is expected to last between 5 and 7 weeks.

The introductory module includes psychoeducational material and information on stress, as well as a description of the progress plan for the following sessions. The next two modules are devoted to stress management and systematic problem-solving strategies, and to providing information on the basic principles of muscle and breathing relaxation, including audio exercises for daily use. The fourth module is dedicated to self-criticism management and contains mindfulness exercises. The next two modules incorporate exercises on acceptance and tolerance of unpleasant emotions and strategies aimed at self-compassion and self-support, as well as strategies for overcoming dysfunctional perfectionistic thought-action patterns. Another module is devoted to recognizing physiological warning signs and creating a master plan for the future. The booster module allows repeating some previous exercises and includes information on self-help and psychotherapy, as well as a recapitulation of all the modules. Also, optional mini-modules are offered to participants, which address specific topics such as social support, rumination and worry, time management, concentration and procrastination, sleep, motivation, nutrition and exercise, and coping with writer's block (Harrer et al., 2019).

Evaluation of "StudiCare Fernstudierende" has shown substantial effects on reducing the severity of depressive symptoms, as well as positive effects on behavioral activation, perceived stress, anxiety, and other post-intervention outcomes. Compared to the active control group (psychoeducation), the intervention was found to be more helpful for depressive symptoms. These effects were maintained at a 3-month follow-up (Harrer et al., 2021). In addition, significant effects of the intervention on participants' academic outcomes were found.

Overall, this program shows that Internet-based interventions aimed at stress reduction can not only be effective in reducing perceived stress but can also provide significant effects on depressive symptoms. In addition, this program demonstrates that higher education students in distance learning modalities can benefit significantly from digitally supported interventions that allow for flexible use of available resources without time and location restrictions.

6.5 Conclusion

Internet-based interventions for the prevention and early treatment of depression in higher education students are growing rapidly, especially in high-income countries. Accumulating evidence shows promising results, but with important challenges. A wide range of factors could be influencing the effectiveness of these interventions, such as participant characteristics, intervention design, intervention duration or number of modules, the intensity of support or human guidance, and program adherence. To address some of these challenges, the development of interventions should be informed by the youth themselves.

Despite the limitations and challenges identified, we conclude that Internet-based interventions for the prevention and early treatment of depression in higher education students can have a beneficial impact on student functioning. Furthermore, integrating these programs into higher education settings offers several advantages. First, students would be able to access these programs at any time and from anywhere with an Internet connection, which helps to significantly reduce barriers to accessing mental health services. Second, Internet-based programs allow for a rapid scale-up effect of prevention and treatment interventions, in contrast to face-to-face care. Third, the relative anonymity and privacy of Internet-based interventions reduce the stigma of receiving professional treatment for depression. Thus, these interventions may help overcome cultural and attitudinal barriers to seeking treatment, such as fear of social judgment.

Overall, these advantages make these programs a highly scalable and potentially more cost-effective form of preventive and early intervention for depression than other forms of mental health treatment (Moshe et al., 2021). Internet-based interventions may be especially beneficial in overcoming logistical and financial barriers that burden both health services and users, holding promise for low-cost interventions with positive outcomes (Paganini et al., 2018). Indeed, students' concern about the high cost of health services strongly influences their decision to seek health information online (Rennis et al., 2015).

Given the rapid technological development and proliferation of Internet-based treatments in recent years, a more comprehensive understanding of the effects of Internet-based approaches to address depression in higher education students is needed.

Conflict of Interest The authors declare that they have no conflict of interest.

Acknowledgments This manuscript was supported by ANID – Millennium Science Initiative Program–ICS13_005 and NCS2021_081, and by ANID–FONDECYT N°1221230. Á.J.-M. received funding from ANID/FONDECYT POSTDOCTORADO/2020-3200944. PF received funding from ANID/PFCHA/BECA DOCTORADO NACIONAL/2019-21190745. SM-G received funding from ANID/PFCHA/BECA DOCTORADO EN EL EXTRANJERO BECAS CHILE/2019-72200092.

References

Alonso, J., Vilagut, G., Mortier, P., Auerbach, R. P., Bruffaerts, R., Cuijpers, P., Demyttenaere, K., Ebert, D. D., Ennis, E., Gutiérrez-García, R. A., Green, J. G., Hasking, P., Lee, S., Bantjes, J., Nock, M. K., Pinder-Amaker, S., Sampson, N. A., Zaslavsky, A. M., Kessler, R. C., & Collaborators, W. H. O. W. M. H.-I. C. S. (2019). The role impairment associated with mental disorder risk profiles in the WHO world mental health international college student initiative. *International Journal of Methods in Psychiatric Research, 28*(2), e1750. https://doi.org/10.1002/mpr.1750

Antoun, C. (2015). Who are the internet users, mobile internet users, and mobile-mostly internet users? Demographic differences across internet-use subgroups in the U.S. In D. Toninelli, R. Pinter, & P. de Pedraza (Eds.), *Mobile research methods: Opportunities and challenges of mobile research methodologies* (pp. 99–117). Ubiquity Press.

Apolinário-Hagen, J., Groenewold, S. D., Fritsche, L., Kemper, J., Krings, L., & Salewski, C. (2018). Die Gesundheit Fernstudierender stärken. *Prävention und Gesundheitsförderung, 13*(2), 151–158. https://doi.org/10.1007/s11553-017-0620-3

Arnett, J. J. (2000). Emerging adulthood. A theory of development from the late teens through the twenties. *The American Psychologist, 55*(5), 469–480. https://doi.org/10.1037/0003-066X.55.5.469

Ashwood, J. S., Stein, B. D., Briscombe, B., Sontag-Padilla, L., Woodbridge, M. W., May, E., Seelam, R., & Burnam, M. A. (2016). Payoffs for California college students and taxpayers from investing in student mental health. *RAND Health Quarterly, 5*(4), 11.

Auerbach, R. P., Alonso, J., Axinn, W. G., Cuijpers, P., Ebert, D. D., Green, J. G., Hwang, I., Kessler, R. C., Liu, H., Mortier, P., Nock, M. K., Pinder-Amaker, S., Sampson, N. A., Aguilar-Gaxiola, S., Al-Hamzawi, A., Andrade, L. H., Benjet, C., Caldas-de-Almeida, J. M., Demyttenaere, K., Florescu, S., et al. (2016). Mental disorders among college students in the World Health Organization world mental health surveys. *Psychological Medicine, 46*(14), 2955–2970. https://doi.org/10.1017/S0033291716001665

Auerbach, R. P., Mortier, P., Bruffaerts, R., Alonso, J., Benjet, C., Cuijpers, P., Demyttenaere, K., Ebert, D. D., Green, J. G., Hasking, P., Lee, S., Lochner, C., McLafferty, M., Nock, M. K., Petukhova, M. V., Pinder-Amaker, S., Rosellini, A. J., Sampson, N. A., Vilagut, G., Zaslavsky, A. M., et al. (2019). Mental disorder comorbidity and suicidal thoughts and behaviors in the World Health Organization world mental health surveys international college student initiative. *International Journal of Methods in Psychiatric Research, 28*(2), e1752. https://doi.org/10.1002/mpr.1752

Auerbach, R. P., Mortier, P., Bruffaerts, R., Alonso, J., Benjet, C., Cuijpers, P., Demyttenaere, K., Ebert, D. D., Green, J. G., Hasking, P., Murray, E., Nock, M. K., Pinder-Amaker, S., Sampson, N. A., Stein, D. J., Vilagut, G., Zaslavsky, A. M., Kessler, R. C., & WHO WMH-ICS Collaborators. (2018). WHO world mental health surveys international college student project: Prevalence and distribution of mental disorders. *Journal of Abnormal Psychology, 127*(7), 623–638. https://doi.org/10.1037/abn0000362

Bantjes, J., Kazdin, A. E., Cuijpers, P., Breet, E., Dunn-Coetzee, M., Davids, C., Stein, D. J., & Kessler, R. C. (2021). A web-based group cognitive behavioral therapy intervention for symptoms of anxiety and depression among university students: Open-label, pragmatic trial. *JMIR Mental Health, 8*(5), e27400. https://doi.org/10.2196/27400

Baumeister, H., Reichler, L., Munzinger, M., & Lin, J. (2014). The impact of guidance on internet-based mental health interventions—A systematic review. *Internet Interventions, 1*(4), 205–215. https://doi.org/10.1016/j.invent.2014.08.003

Boettcher, J., Aström, V., Påhlsson, D., Schenström, O., Andersson, G., & Carlbring, P. (2014). Internet-based mindfulness treatment for anxiety disorders: A randomized controlled trial. *Behavior Therapy, 45*(2), 241–253. https://doi.org/10.1016/j.beth.2013.11.003

Bruffaerts, R., Mortier, P., Auerbach, R. P., Alonso, J., Hermosillo De la Torre, A. E., Cuijpers, P., Demyttenaere, K., Ebert, D. D., Green, J. G., Hasking, P., Stein, D. J., Ennis, E., Nock, M. K., Pinder-Amaker, S., Sampson, N. A., Vilagut, G., Zaslavsky, A. M., Kessler, R. C., & WHO WMH-ICS Collaborators. (2019). Lifetime and 12-month treatment for mental disorders and suicidal thoughts and behaviors among first year college students. *International Journal of Methods in Psychiatric Research, 28*(2), e1764. https://doi.org/10.1002/mpr.1764

Cavanagh, K., Strauss, C., Cicconi, F., Griffiths, N., Wyper, A., & Jones, F. (2013). A randomised controlled trial of a brief online mindfulness-based intervention. *Behaviour Research and Therapy, 51*(9), 573–578. https://doi.org/10.1016/j.brat.2013.06.003

Coertjens, L., Brahm, T., Trautwein, C., & Lindblom-Ylänne, S. (2017). Students' transition into higher education from an international perspective. *Higher Education, 73*(3), 357–369. https://doi.org/10.1007/s10734-016-0092-y

Conley, C. S., Durlak, J. A., & Kirsch, A. C. (2015). A meta-analysis of universal mental health prevention programs for higher education students. *Prevention Science: The Official Journal of the Society for Prevention Research, 16*(4), 487–507. https://doi.org/10.1007/s11121-015-0543-1

Conley, C. S., Durlak, J. A., Shapiro, J. B., Kirsch, A. C., & Zahniser, E. (2016). A meta-analysis of the impact of universal and indicated preventive technology-delivered interventions for higher education students. *Prevention Science: The Official Journal of the Society for Prevention Research, 17*(6), 659–678. https://doi.org/10.1007/s11121-016-0662-3

Cuijpers, P., Cristea, I. A., Ebert, D. D., Koot, H. M., Auerbach, R. P., Bruffaerts, R., & Kessler, R. C. (2016). Psychological treatment of depression in college students: A Metaanalysis. *Depression and Anxiety, 33*(5), 400–414. https://doi.org/10.1002/da.22461

Cuijpers, P., Karyotaki, E., Reijnders, M., Purgato, M., & Barbui, C. (2018). Psychotherapies for depression in low- and middle-income countries: A meta-analysis. *World Psychiatry: Official Journal of the World Psychiatric Association (WPA), 17*(1), 90–101. https://doi.org/10.1002/wps.20493

Cuijpers, P., Miguel, C., Ciharova, M., Aalten, P., Batelaan, N., Salemink, E., Spinhoven, P., Struijs, S., de Wit, L., Gentili, C., Ebert, D., Harrer, M., Bruffaerts, R., Kessler, R. C., & Karyotaki, E. (2021). Prevention and treatment of mental health and psychosocial problems in college students: An umbrella review of meta-analyses. *Clinical Psychology: Science and Practice, 28*(3), 229–244. https://doi.org/10.1037/cps0000030

Dalgleish, T., Black, M., Johnston, D., & Bevan, A. (2020). Transdiagnostic approaches to mental health problems: Current status and future directions. *Journal of Consulting and Clinical Psychology, 88*(3), 179–195. https://doi.org/10.1037/ccp0000482

Davies, E. B., Morriss, R., & Glazebrook, C. (2014). Computer-delivered and web-based interventions to improve depression, anxiety, and psychological well-being of university students: A systematic review and meta-analysis. *Journal of Medical Internet Research, 16*(5), e130. https://doi.org/10.2196/jmir.3142

Day, V., McGrath, P. J., & Wojtowicz, M. (2013). Internet-based guided self-help for university students with anxiety, depression and stress: A randomized controlled clinical trial. *Behaviour Research and Therapy, 51*(7), 344–351. https://doi.org/10.1016/j.brat.2013.03.003

Dear, B. F., Johnson, B., Singh, A., Wilkes, B., Brkic, T., Gupta, R., Jones, M. P., Bailey, S., Dudeney, J., Gandy, M., Fogliati, R., & Titov, N. (2019). Examining an internet-delivered intervention for anxiety and depression when delivered as a part of routine care for university students: A phase IV trial. *Journal of Affective Disorders, 256*, 567–577. https://doi.org/10.1016/j.jad.2019.06.044

Duffy, A., Saunders, K., Malhi, G. S., Patten, S., Cipriani, A., McNevin, S. H., MacDonald, E., & Geddes, J. (2019). Mental health care for university students: A way forward? *The Lancet. Psychiatry, 6*(11), 885–887. https://doi.org/10.1016/S2215-0366(19)30275-5

Ebert, D. D., Franke, M., Kählke, F., Küchler, A. M., Bruffaerts, R., Mortier, P., Karyotaki, E., Alonso, J., Cuijpers, P., Berking, M., Auerbach, R. P., Kessler, R. C., Baumeister, H., & WHO World Mental Health – International College Student Collaborators. (2019a). Increasing intentions to use mental health services among university students. Results of a pilot randomized controlled trial within the World Health Organization's World Mental Health International College Student Initiative. *International Journal of Methods in Psychiatric Research, 28*(2), e1754. https://doi.org/10.1002/mpr.1754

Ebert, D. D., Mortier, P., Kaehlke, F., Bruffaerts, R., Baumeister, H., Auerbach, R. P., Alonso, J., Vilagut, G., Martínez, K. I., Lochner, C., Cuijpers, P., Kuechler, A. M., Green, J., Hasking, P., Lapsley, C., Sampson, N. A., Kessler, R. C., & WHO World Mental Health – International College Student Initiative Collaborators. (2019b). Barriers of mental health treatment utilization among first-year college students: First cross-national results from the WHO World Mental Health International College Student Initiative. *International Journal of Methods in Psychiatric Research, 28*(2), e1782. https://doi.org/10.1002/mpr.1782

Eisenberg, D., Hunt, J., & Speer, N. (2012). Help seeking for mental health on college campuses: Review of evidence and next steps for research and practice. *Harvard Review of Psychiatry, 20*(4), 222–232. https://doi.org/10.3109/10673229.2012.712839

El Morr, C., Ritvo, P., Ahmad, F., Moineddin, R., & Team, M. V. C. (2020). Effectiveness of an 8-week web-based mindfulness virtual community intervention for university students on symptoms of stress, anxiety, and depression: Randomized controlled trial. *JMIR Mental Health, 7*(7), e18595. https://doi.org/10.2196/18595

Ellis, L. A., Campbell, A. J., Sethi, S., & ODea, B. M. (2011). Comparative randomized trial of an online cognitive-behavioral therapy program and an online support group for depression and anxiety. *Journal of Cybertherapy and Rehabilitation, 4*(4), 461–467. https://link.gale.com/apps/doc/A321336263/AONE?u=anon~f4604693&sid=googleScholar&xid=2d31718f

Etzelmueller, A., Vis, C., Karyotaki, E., Baumeister, H., Titov, N., Berking, M., Cuijpers, P., Riper, H., & Ebert, D. D. (2020). Effects of internet-based cognitive behavioral therapy in routine care for adults in treatment for depression and anxiety: Systematic review and meta-analysis. *Journal of Medical Internet Research, 22*(8), e18100. https://doi.org/10.2196/18100

Evans, T. M., Bira, L., Gastelum, J. B., Weiss, L. T., & Vanderford, N. L. (2018). Evidence for a mental health crisis in graduate education. *Nature Biotechnology, 36*(3), 282–284. https://doi.org/10.1038/nbt.4089

Farrer, L., Gulliver, A., Chan, J. K., Batterham, P. J., Reynolds, J., Calear, A., Tait, R., Bennett, K., & Griffiths, K. M. (2013). Technology-based interventions for mental health in tertiary students: Systematic review. *Journal of Medical Internet Research, 15*(5), e101. https://doi.org/10.2196/jmir.2639

Farrer, L. M., Gulliver, A., Katruss, N., Fassnacht, D. B., Kyrios, M., & Batterham, P. J. (2019). A novel multi-component online intervention to improve the mental health of university students: Randomised controlled trial of the Uni virtual clinic. *Internet Interventions, 18*, 100276. https://doi.org/10.1016/j.invent.2019.100276

Fernandez, A., Howse, E., Rubio-Valera, M., Thorncraft, K., Noone, J., Luu, X., Veness, B., Leech, M., Llewellyn, G., & Salvador-Carulla, L. (2016). Setting-based interventions to promote mental health at the university: A systematic review. *International Journal of Public Health, 61*(7), 797–807. https://doi.org/10.1007/s00038-016-0846-4

Fitzpatrick, K. K., Darcy, A., & Vierhile, M. (2017). Delivering cognitive behavior therapy to young adults with symptoms of depression and anxiety using a fully automated conversational agent (Woebot): A randomized controlled trial. *JMIR Mental Health, 4*(2), e19. https://doi.org/10.2196/mental.7785

Fulmer, R., Joerin, A., Gentile, B., Lakerink, L., & Rauws, M. (2018). Using psychological artificial intelligence (Tess) to relieve symptoms of depression and anxiety: Randomized controlled trial. *JMIR Mental Health, 5*(4), e64. https://doi.org/10.2196/mental.9782

Goldman-Mellor, S. J., Caspi, A., Harrington, H., Hogan, S., Nada-Raja, S., Poulton, R., & Moffitt, T. E. (2014). Suicide attempt in young people: A signal for long-term health care and social needs. *JAMA Psychiatry, 71*(2), 119–127. https://doi.org/10.1001/jamapsychiatry.2013.2803

Goodman, L. (2017). Mental health on university campus and the needs of students they seek to serve. *Building Healthy Academic Communities Journal, 1*(2), 31–44. https://doi.org/10.18061/bhac.v1i2.6056

Hanauer, D., Dibble, E., Fortin, J., & Col, N. F. (2004). Internet use among community college students: Implications in designing healthcare interventions. *Journal of American College Health, 52*(5), 197–202. https://doi.org/10.3200/JACH.52.5.197-202

Haroz, E. E., Ritchey, M., Bass, J. K., Kohrt, B. A., Augustinavicius, J., Michalopoulos, L., Burkey, M. D., & Bolton, P. (2017). How is depression experienced around the world? A systematic review of qualitative literature. *Social Science & Medicine (1982), 183*, 151–162. https://doi.org/10.1016/j.socscimed.2016.12.030

Harrer, M., Adam, S. H., Baumeister, H., Cuijpers, P., Karyotaki, E., Auerbach, R. P., Kessler, R. C., Bruffaerts, R., Berking, M., & Ebert, D. D. (2019). Internet interventions for mental health in university students: A systematic review and meta-analysis. *International Journal of Methods in Psychiatric Research, 28*(2), e1759. https://doi.org/10.1002/mpr.1759

Harrer, M., Adam, S. H., Fleischmann, R. J., Baumeister, H., Auerbach, R., Bruffaerts, R., Cuijpers, P., Kessler, R. C., Berking, M., Lehr, D., & Ebert, D. D. (2018). Effectiveness of an internet- and app-based intervention for college students with elevated stress: Randomized controlled trial. *Journal of Medical Internet Research, 20*(4), e136. https://doi.org/10.2196/jmir.9293

Harrer, M., Apolinário-Hagen, J., Fritsche, L., Salewski, C., Zarski, A. C., Lehr, D., Baumeister, H., Cuijpers, P., & Ebert, D. D. (2021). Effect of an internet- and app-based stress intervention compared to online psychoeducation in university students with depressive symptoms: Results of a randomized controlled trial. *Internet Interventions, 24*, 100374. https://doi.org/10.1016/j.invent.2021.100374

Helms, J. E. (2015). An examination of the evidence in culturally adapted evidence-based or empirically supported interventions. *Transcultural Psychiatry, 52*(2), 174–197. https://doi.org/10.1177/1363461514563642

Jiménez-Molina, Á., Franco, P., Martínez, V., Martínez, P., Rojas, G., & Araya, R. (2019). Internet-based interventions for the prevention and treatment of mental disorders in Latin America: A scoping review. *Frontiers in Psychiatry, 10*, 664. https://doi.org/10.3389/fpsyt.2019.00664

Karyotaki, E., Ebert, D. D., Donkin, L., Riper, H., Twisk, J., Burger, S., Rozental, A., Lange, A., Williams, A. D., Zarski, A. C., Geraedts, A., van Straten, A., Kleiboer, A., Meyer, B., Ünlü Ince, B. B., Buntrock, C., Lehr, D., Snoek, F. J., Andrews, G., Andersson, G., et al. (2018). Do guided internet-based interventions result in clinically relevant changes for patients with depression? An individual participant data meta-analysis. *Clinical Psychology Review, 63*, 80–92. https://doi.org/10.1016/j.cpr.2018.06.007

Karyotaki, E., Efthimiou, O., Miguel, C., Bermpohl, F., Furukawa, T. A., Cuijpers, P., & Individual Patient Data Meta-Analyses for Depression (IPDMA-DE) Collaboration, Riper, H., Patel, V., Mira, A., Gemmil, A. W., Yeung, A. S., Lange, A., Williams, A. D., Mackinnon, A., Geraedts, A., van Straten, A., Meyer, B., Björkelund, C., Knaevelsrud, C., … Forsell, Y. (2021). Internet-based cognitive behavioral therapy for depression: A systematic review and individual patient data network meta-analysis. *JAMA Psychiatry, 78*(4), 361–371. https://doi.org/10.1001/jamapsychiatry.2020.4364

Kessler, R. C., Angermeyer, M., Anthony, J. C., De Graaf, R., Demyttenaere, K., Gasquet, I., De Girolamo, G., Gluzman, S., Gureje, O., Haro, J. M., Kawakami, N., Karam, A., Levinson, D., Medina Mora, M. E., Oakley Browne, M. A., Posada-Villa, J., Stein, D. J., Adley Tsang, C. H., Aguilar-Gaxiola, S., Alonso, J., et al. (2007). Lifetime prevalence and age-of-onset distributions of mental disorders in the World Health Organization's World Mental Health Survey Initiative. *World Psychiatry: Official Journal of the World Psychiatric Association (WPA), 6*(3), 168–176.

Königbauer, J., Letsch, J., Doebler, P., Ebert, D., & Baumeister, H. (2017). Internet- and mobile-based depression interventions for people with diagnosed depression: A systematic review and meta-analysis. *Journal of Affective Disorders, 223*, 28–40. https://doi.org/10.1016/j.jad.2017.07.021

Kvillemo, P., Brandberg, Y., & Bränström, R. (2016). Feasibility and outcomes of an internet-based mindfulness training program: A pilot randomized controlled trial. *JMIR Mental Health, 3*(3), e33. https://doi.org/10.2196/mental.5457

Langer, Á. I., Medeiros, S., Valdés-Sánchez, N., Brito, R., Steinebach, C., Cid-Parra, C., Magni, A., & Krause, M. (2020). A qualitative study of a mindfulness-based intervention in educational contexts in Chile: An approach based on Adolescents' voices. *International Journal of Environmental Research and Public Health, 17*(18), 6927. https://doi.org/10.3390/ijerph17186927

Levin, M. E., Haeger, J. A., Pierce, B. G., & Twohig, M. P. (2017). Web-based acceptance and commitment therapy for mental health problems in college students: A randomized controlled trial. *Behavior Modification, 41*(1), 141–162. https://doi.org/10.1177/0145445516659645

Lintvedt, O. K., Griffiths, K. M., Sørensen, K., Østvik, A. R., Wang, C. E., Eisemann, M., & Waterloo, K. (2013). Evaluating the effectiveness and efficacy of unguided internet-based self-help intervention for the prevention of depression: A randomized controlled trial. *Clinical Psychology & Psychotherapy, 20*(1), 10–27. https://doi.org/10.1002/cpp.770

Mac-Ginty, S., Jiménez-Molina, A., & Martínez, V. (2021). Impacto de la pandemia por COVID-19 en la salud mental de estudiantes universitarios en Chile. *Revista Chilena de Psiquiatría y Neurología de la Infancia y la Adolescencia, 32*(1), 23–37.

Marshall, M. (2020). The hidden links between mental disorders. *Nature, 581*(7806), 19–21. https://doi.org/10.1038/d41586-020-00922-8

Martineau, M., Beauchamp, G., & Marcotte, D. (2018). Efficacité des interventions en prévention et en promotion de la santé mentale dans les établissements d'enseignement postsecondaire. *Santé Mentale au Québec, 42*(1), 165–182. https://doi.org/10.7202/1040249ar

Martinengo, L., Stona, A. C., Griva, K., Dazzan, P., Pariante, C. M., von Wangenheim, F., & Car, J. (2021). Self-guided cognitive behavioral therapy apps for depression: Systematic assessment of features, functionality, and congruence with evidence. *Journal of Medical Internet Research, 23*(7), e27619. https://doi.org/10.2196/27619

Martínez, V., Espinosa-Duque, D., Jiménez-Molina, Á., Rojas, G., Vöhringer, P. A., Fernández-Arcila, M., Luttges, C., Irarrázaval, M., Bauer, S., & Moessner, M. (2021). Feasibility and acceptability of "Cuida tu Ánimo" (take care of your mood): An internet-based program for prevention and early intervention of adolescent depression in Chile and Colombia. *International Journal of Environmental Research and Public Health, 18*(18), 9628. https://doi.org/10.3390/ijerph18189628

McGorry, P. D., Purcell, R., Goldstone, S., & Amminger, G. P. (2011). Age of onset and timing of treatment for mental and substance use disorders: Implications for preventive intervention strategies and models of care. *Current Opinion in Psychiatry, 24*(4), 301–306. https://doi.org/10.1097/YCO.0b013e3283477a09

Melnyk, B. M., Amaya, M., Szalacha, L. A., Hoying, J., Taylor, T., & Bowersox, K. (2015). Feasibility, acceptability, and preliminary effects of the COPE online cognitive-behavioral skill-building program on mental health outcomes and academic performance in Freshmen college students: A randomized controlled pilot study. *Journal of Child and Adolescent Psychiatric Nursing: Official Publication of the Association of Child and Adolescent Psychiatric Nurses, Inc, 28*(3), 147–154. https://doi.org/10.1111/jcap.12119

Montagni, I., Cariou, T., Feuillet, T., Langlois, E., & Tzourio, C. (2018). Exploring digital health use and opinions of university students: Field survey study. *JMIR mHealth and uHealth, 6*(3), e65. https://doi.org/10.2196/mhealth.9131

Mortier, P., Cuijpers, P., Kiekens, G., Auerbach, R. P., Demyttenaere, K., Green, J. G., Kessler, R. C., Nock, M. K., & Bruffaerts, R. (2018). The prevalence of suicidal thoughts and behaviours among college students: A meta-analysis. *Psychological Medicine, 48*(4), 554–565. https://doi.org/10.1017/S0033291717002215

Moshe, I., Terhorst, Y., Philippi, P., Domhardt, M., Cuijpers, P., Cristea, I., Pulkki-Råback, L., Baumeister, H., & Sander, L. B. (2021). Digital interventions for the treatment of depression: A meta-analytic review. *Psychological Bulletin, 147*(8), 749–786. https://doi.org/10.1037/bul0000334

Mullin, A., Dear, B. F., Karin, E., Wootton, B. M., Staples, L. G., Johnston, L., Gandy, M., Fogliati, V., & Titov, N. (2015). The UniWellbeing course: A randomised controlled trial of a transdiagnostic internet-delivered cognitive behavioural therapy (CBT) programme for university students with symptoms of anxiety and depression. *Internet Interventions, 2*(2), 128–136. https://doi.org/10.1016/j.invent.2015.02.002

Musiat, P., Conrod, P., Treasure, J., Tylee, A., Williams, C., & Schmidt, U. (2014). Targeted prevention of common mental health disorders in university students: Randomised controlled trial of a transdiagnostic trait-focused web-based intervention. *PLoS One, 9*(4), e93621. https://doi.org/10.1371/journal.pone.0093621

Musiat, P., Potterton, R., Gordon, G., Spencer, L., Zeiler, M., Waldherr, K., Kuso, S., Nitsch, M., Adamcik, T., Wagner, G., Karwautz, A., Ebert, D. D., Dodd, A., Dooley, B., Harrison, A., Whitt, E., Haselgrove, M., Sharpe, H., Smith, J., Tressler, R., et al. (2019). Web-based indicated prevention of common mental disorders in university students in four European countries – Study protocol for a randomised controlled trial. *Internet Interventions, 16*, 35–42. https://doi.org/10.1016/j.invent.2018.02.004

Newby, J. M., McKinnon, A., Kuyken, W., Gilbody, S., & Dalgleish, T. (2015). Systematic review and meta-analysis of transdiagnostic psychological treatments for anxiety and depressive disorders in adulthood. *Clinical Psychology Review, 40*, 91–110. https://doi.org/10.1016/j.cpr.2015.06.002

Niederkrotenthaler, T., Tinghög, P., Alexanderson, K., Dahlin, M., Wang, M., Beckman, K., Gould, M., & Mittendorfer-Rutz, E. (2014). Future risk of labour market marginalization in young suicide attempters – A population-based prospective cohort study. *International Journal of Epidemiology, 43*(5), 1520–1530. https://doi.org/10.1093/ije/dyu155

Paganini, S., Teigelkötter, W., Buntrock, C., & Baumeister, H. (2018). Economic evaluations of internet- and mobile-based interventions for the treatment and prevention of depression: A systematic review. *Journal of Affective Disorders, 225*, 733–755. https://doi.org/10.1016/j.jad.2017.07.018

Palacios, J. E., Richards, D., Palmer, R., Coudray, C., Hofmann, S. G., Palmieri, P. A., & Frazier, P. (2018). Supported internet-delivered cognitive behavioral therapy programs for depression, anxiety, and stress in university students: Open, non-randomised trial of acceptability, effectiveness, and satisfaction. *JMIR Mental Health, 5*(4), e11467. https://doi.org/10.2196/11467

Parada, F., Martínez, V., Espinosa, H. D., Bauer, S., & Moessner, M. (2020). Using persuasive systems design model to evaluate "Cuida tu Ánimo": An internet-based pilot program for prevention and early intervention of adolescent depression. *Telemedicine Journal and e-Health: The Official Journal of the American Telemedicine Association, 26*(2), 251–254. https://doi.org/10.1089/tmj.2018.0272

Plana-Ripoll, O., Pedersen, C. B., Holtz, Y., Benros, M. E., Dalsgaard, S., de Jonge, P., Fan, C. C., Degenhardt, L., Ganna, A., Greve, A. N., Gunn, J., Iburg, K. M., Kessing, L. V., Lee, B. K., Lim, C., Mors, O., Nordentoft, M., Prior, A., Roest, A. M., Saha, S., et al. (2019). Exploring comorbidity within mental disorders among a Danish National Population. *JAMA Psychiatry, 76*(3), 259–270. https://doi.org/10.1001/jamapsychiatry.2018.3658

Reavley, N., & Jorm, A. F. (2019). Prevention and early intervention to improve mental health in higher education students: A review. *Early Intervention in Psychiatry, 4*(2), 132–142. https://doi.org/10.1111/j.1751-7893.2010.00167.x

Rennis, L., McNamara, G., Seidel, E., & Shneyderman, Y. (2015). Google it!: Urban community college students' use of the internet to obtain self-care and personal health information. *College Student Journal, 49*(3), 414–426.

Richards, D., Murphy, T., Viganó, N., Timulak, L., Doherty, G., Sharry, J., & Hayes, C. (2016). Acceptability, satisfaction and perceived efficacy of "*space from depression*" an internet-delivered treatment for depression. *Internet Interventions, 5*, 12–22. https://doi.org/10.1016/j.invent.2016.06.007

Richards, D., & Richardson, T. (2012). Computer-based psychological treatments for depression: A systematic review and meta-analysis. *Clinical Psychology Review, 32*(4), 329–342. https://doi.org/10.1016/j.cpr.2012.02.004

Richards, D., Timulak, L., O'Brien, E., Hayes, C., Vigano, N., Sharry, J., & Doherty, G. (2015). A randomized controlled trial of an internet-delivered treatment: Its potential as a low-intensity community intervention for adults with symptoms of depression. *Behaviour Research and Therapy, 75*, 20–31. https://doi.org/10.1016/j.brat.2015.10.005

Ritvo, P., Ahmad, F., El Morr, C., Pirbaglou, M., Moineddin, R., & Team, M. V. C. (2021). A mindfulness-based intervention for student depression, anxiety, and stress: Randomized controlled trial. *JMIR Mental Health, 8*(1), e23491. https://doi.org/10.2196/23491

Salamanca-Sanabria, A., Richards, D., & Timulak, L. (2019). Adapting an internet-delivered intervention for depression for a Colombian college student population: An illustration of an integrative empirical approach. *Internet Interventions, 15*, 76–86. https://doi.org/10.1016/j.invent.2018.11.005

Salamanca-Sanabria, A., Richards, D., Timulak, L., Connell, S., Mojica Perilla, M., Parra-Villa, Y., & Castro-Camacho, L. (2020). A culturally adapted cognitive behavioral internet-delivered intervention for depressive symptoms: Randomized controlled trial. *JMIR Mental Health, 7*(1), e13392. https://doi.org/10.2196/13392

Schaeuffele, C., Schulz, A., Knaevelsrud, C., Renneberg, B., & Boettcher, J. (2021). CBT at the crossroads: The rise of transdiagnostic treatments. *International Journal of Cognitive Therapy, 14*(1), 86–113. https://doi.org/10.1007/s41811-020-00095-2

Schilling, S. H., Carreño, A., Tapia, E., Mascayano, F., Pitronello, R., Santander, F., Jorquera, M. J., Burrone, M. S., & Alvarado, R. V. (2021). Experts by experience: Qualitative evaluation of adolescent participation in the development of a technological intervention to prevent youth suicide in Chile. *Frontiers in Psychiatry, 11*, 522057. https://doi.org/10.3389/fpsyt.2020.522057

Spanhel, K., Balci, S., Feldhahn, F., Bengel, J., Baumeister, H., & Sander, L. B. (2021). Cultural adaptation of internet- and mobile-based interventions for mental disorders: A systematic review. *NPJ Digital Medicine, 4*(1), 128. https://doi.org/10.1038/s41746-021-00498-1

UNESCO IEPP. (2017). Six ways to ensure higher education leaves no one behind. *Policy Paper*, 1–10. https://unesdoc.unesco.org/ark:/48223/pf0000247862

Vidourek, R. A., King, K. A., Nabors, L. A., & Merianos, A. L. (2014). Students' benefits and barriers to mental health help-seeking. *Health Psychology and Behavioral Medicine, 2*(1), 1009–1022. https://doi.org/10.1080/21642850.2014.963586

Wentzel, J., van der Vaart, R., Bohlmeijer, E. T., & van Gemert-Pijnen, J. E. (2016). Mixing online and face-to-face therapy: How to benefit from blended Care in Mental Health Care. *JMIR Mental Health, 3*(1), e9. https://doi.org/10.2196/mental.4534

Winzer, R., Lindberg, L., Guldbrandsson, K., & Sidorchuk, A. (2018). Effects of mental health interventions for students in higher education are sustainable over time: A systematic review and meta-analysis of randomized controlled trials. *PeerJ, 6*, e4598. https://doi.org/10.7717/peerj.4598

World Bank. (2018). *World development indicators. School enrollment, tertiary (% gross)* [Data file]. https://data.worldbank.org/indicator/SE.TER.ENRR

Part II
Adults and Older Adults

Chapter 7
Interventions for Adult Depression in Primary Health-Care Clinics

Pablo Martínez and Graciela Rojas

7.1 The Global Burden of Adult Depression

Depression has been one of the most relevant public health problems in recent decades. According to the Global Burden of Disease (GBD) Study 2019, led by the Institute for Health Metrics and Evaluation (IHME), 279 million people worldwide suffer from depressive disorders – equivalent to 3.8% of the world's population (GBD 2019 Mental Disorders Collaborators, 2022). A closer inspection of the data provided by the IHME notes that the prevalence of depression increases during adulthood, reaching a peak of 6.0% immediately before older adulthood (Global Burden of Disease Collaborative Network, 2020). Depression mainly affects people during the most productive years of their lives, producing more significant declines in health than chronic physical illnesses such as arthritis or diabetes (Moussavi et al., 2007). Importantly, the health loss attributed to depression occurs earlier than those ascribed to these chronic physical diseases (Global Burden of Disease

P. Martínez
Faculté de Médecine et des Sciences de la Santé, Université de Sherbrooke, Longueuil, QC, Canada

Centre de Recherche Charles-Le Moyne (CRCLM), Longueuil, QC, Canada

Millennium Institute for Depression and Personality Research (MIDAP), Santiago, Chile

Millennium Nucleus to Improve the Mental Health of Adolescents and Youths (Imhay), Santiago, Chile

G. Rojas (✉)
Millennium Institute for Depression and Personality Research (MIDAP), Santiago, Chile

Millennium Nucleus to Improve the Mental Health of Adolescents and Youths (Imhay), Santiago, Chile

Hospital Clínico Universidad de Chile, Santiago, Chile

V. Martínez, C. Miranda-Castillo (eds.), *Prevention and Early Treatment of Depression Through the Life Course*, Depression and Personality,
https://doi.org/10.1007/978-3-031-13029-8_7

Collaborative Network, 2020). The patterning of the decrements in health produced by depression makes it one of the leading causes of years lived with disability, particularly in the 20–59 age group (GBD 2019 Mental Disorders Collaborators, 2022).

Depression is also associated with one of the most significant causes of death globally – suicide. The World Health Organization's (WHO) Global Health Estimates (2017) report that more than 800,000 people die by suicide worldwide every year. Notably, depression is responsible for nearly half (46.1%) of the suicide burden attributed to mental and substance use disorders (Ferrari et al., 2014). Moreover, according to a recent systematic review and meta-regression, people with major depression are nearly eight times more likely than those not having this disorder to die by suicide (Moitra et al., 2021). Complementarily, there is very suggestive evidence of a possible association between depression and excess mortality in cancer, heart failure, and acute myocardial infarction, which would be mediated by pathological and physiological mechanisms and alterations in the behavior of the disease (Machado et al., 2018).

Depression does not affect the adult population equally. The IHME data suggests that, as older adulthood approaches, the prevalence of depression is twice as high in adults living in low-income vs. high-income countries (Global Burden of Disease Collaborative Network, 2020). The same source of information shows that for every depressed man, there are 1.5 depressed women in adulthood, regardless of the income level of the nation (Global Burden of Disease Collaborative Network, 2020). Furthermore, the GBD Study 2019 and WHO estimates found higher health losses attributable to depression in countries with increased rates of childhood sexual abuse, intimate partner violence, and conflict and war (Charlson et al., 2019; GBD 2019 Risk Factors Collaborators, 2020), highlighting population-level vulnerabilities to depression and its health consequences due to differential exposure to psychosocial risk factors. Notably, a recent systematic analysis of the prevalence of major depressive disorders during the ongoing COVID-19 pandemic noticed that the locations hardest hit by the pandemic had the most significant increases in the burden of depressive disorders (Santomauro et al., 2021).

7.2 Adult Depression in Primary Health Care

In the 1990s, the WHO led a relevant international study on psychological problems in general health care (Üstün & Sartorius, 1995). Primary health-care facilities in 14 culturally and economically diverse countries participated in the study. The diagnostic criteria of the International Classification of Diseases, Tenth Edition (ICD-10), were used to determine diagnoses for depression, anxiety disorders, and alcoholism, among others (Üstün & Sartorius, 1995). The WHO primary health-care study established that depression was the most prevalent mental disorder among the consulting population (10.4%), being more frequent in women (female/male ratio of 1.9) and patients with lesser education (Üstün & Sartorius, 1995). In four primary health-care centers (Santiago de Chile, Rio de Janeiro, Paris, and Bangalore), the female rate of depression was significantly higher than the male rate (Üstün & Sartorius, 1995). In addition, the WHO primary health-care study showed that psychiatric comorbidity of depression was consistently associated with severe limitations in daily activities and poorer health perception (Üstün & Sartorius, 1995).

More recently, a meta-analysis of 41 studies totaling 50,371 patients in mainly urban primary health-care clinics from more than ten countries explored the accuracy of unassisted diagnoses of depression by general practitioners (Mitchell et al., 2009). The studies included in Mitchell et al.'s meta-analysis identified cases of depression through psychiatric expert diagnosis or validated structured or semi-structured interviews. When studies recruiting adult patients aged 18–65 years were considered, the prevalence of depression in primary health care was 18.4% (Mitchell et al., 2009). Mitchell et al. (2009) estimated a depression prevalence of 17.2% for ICD-based studies, differing from the WHO primary health-care study, which reported a depression prevalence of 10.4% through the same method (Üstün & Sartorius, 1995). Such discrepancies might be driven by variations in sampling procedures or differences across primary health-care centers – e.g., the meta-analysis by Mitchell et al. (2009) relied mainly on primary health-care clinics from Western developed countries.

Large primary health-care cohorts in Australia ($n = 7620$ patients) (Gunn et al., 2012), England ($n = 403{,}985$) (Cassell et al., 2018), and Scotland ($n = 1{,}751{,}841$) (Smith et al., 2014) have established that comorbid depression and chronic physical conditions are the rules and not the exception. Depressed individuals in primary health care were more likely than nondepressed individuals to have physical comorbidities (Smith et al., 2014). Moreover, nearly half of depressed patients suffer multimorbidity, which is the presence of multiple diseases or conditions (Gunn et al., 2012; Smith et al., 2014). The most typical comorbidities found in depressed patients were painful conditions, stroke, and irritable bowel syndrome (Cassell et al., 2018; Gunn et al., 2012; Smith et al., 2014). Notably, one of the studies reported a dose-response relationship between the number of chronic physical diseases and the severity of depressive symptoms (Gunn et al., 2012). Multimorbidity in depressed patients was associated with socioeconomic deprivation (Cassell et al., 2018; Smith et al., 2014), considerable health losses (Gunn et al., 2012; Smith et al., 2014), and health services utilization (Cassell et al., 2018).

Well-designed prospective cohort studies have identified the main risk factors for depression in primary health-care adult patients. The WHO primary health-care study found that psychological problems (e.g., recurrent suicidal thoughts and previous depressive episodes), as well as poor health status, predicted new depressive episodes at 12-month follow-up (Barkow et al., 2002). The same study noticed that sociodemographic factors (i.e., low formal education and unemployment) appeared to be more salient for sustained non-remission of a depressive episode (Barkow et al., 2003). The PredictD international study developed a predictive algorithm for depression in primary health care based on data from 10,045 attendees in Europe and Chile. Psychosocial and clinical variables (e.g., difficulties in paid and unpaid work, lifetime depression, family history of psychological problems, poor physical and mental health status) were consistently selected in the PredictD algorithm (King et al., 2008).

Thus, depression appears to be particularly frequent in Western urban primary health-care facilities, and it is commonly associated with both physical and psychiatric comorbidities, generating significant degrees of disability. As in the general non-consultant population, depression mainly affects women, with psychosocial, psychological, and clinical variables leading to an increased propensity to depression in primary health-care attendees. Interestingly, secondary analyses of the PredictD data expand our understanding of the interplay between sex and risk factors for the onset of depression in primary health-care attendees (Stegenga et al., 2012). According to this study, women were not only more exposed than men to known risk factors, but they also faced enhanced susceptibility to depression resulting from exposure to these risk factors (Stegenga et al., 2012). Women were particularly affected by poor neighborhood conditions, whereas men were significantly impacted by living alone (Stegenga et al., 2012).

7.3 Integrating Mental Health into Primary Health Care

The WHO primary health-care study revealed that general practitioners acted as first contact care and gatekeepers for more than 75% of patients with mental health problems (Üstün & Sartorius, 1995). Complementarily, analyses of the WHO World Mental Health Surveys 2000–2005 described the use of mental health services for anxiety, mood, and substance disorders (Wang et al., 2007). The study found that among 84,850 participants in 17 low-, middle-, and high-income countries, the general practitioners were the largest source of mental health services (Wang et al., 2007). These findings confirm that primary health care plays a relevant role in the management of mental disorders, especially depression. Thus, it is necessary for general practitioners and allied health professionals in primary health care to timely and adequately detect, diagnose, and manage depression.

International organizations such as the WHO and its Regional Office for the Americas (PAHO), with support from the United Nations Children's Fund (UNICEF), have been instrumental in advancing the political and technical case for mental health integration into primary health care, with a particular emphasis on the Region of the Americas. As a point of reference, the Third Special Meeting of the Americas' Ministers of Health, held in Chile in 1972, summarized the health sector's challenges and achievements (Organización Panamericana de la Salud, 1972). Regarding mental health care, the 1972 meeting recognized the critical state of mental health services in the Region, with virtually no coverage for a then vast rural population and the severe insufficiency to meet the needs of a comprehensive mental health program (Organización Panamericana de la Salud, 1972). The 1972 meeting envisioned the necessary changes to address the mental health services crisis, such as integrating psychiatric care into primary health care and primary mental health promotion and prevention activities into general health care (Organización Panamericana de la Salud, 1972).

The highly influential International Conference on Primary Health Care in Alma-Ata took place just 6 years after the 1972 meeting. The International Conference on Primary Health Care was jointly sponsored by the WHO and UNICEF, in which 134 countries and 67 international organizations participated (World Health Organization, 1978). The Conference recognized the urgent need to act on the grave inequalities in the global state of health and exhorted promotion and protection actions to realize the right to health (World Health Organization, 1978). According to the Conference, a primary health-care approach was deeply needed to achieve equity in health for all the people of the world (World Health Organization, 1978). Primary health care was considered essential health care that is universally accessible, acceptable, and affordable, "bringing health care close to where people live and work" (World Health Organization, 1978). The Conference emphasized that primary health care was the cornerstone of the health-care system and one of the foundations for social and economic development (World Health Organization, 1978).

The International Conference on Primary Health Care broadly recommended a set of priority contents for primary health care, such as the promotion of food supply and proper nutrition, the provision of maternal and child health care, and immunization against major infectious diseases (World Health Organization, 1978). The inclusion of mental health promotion was stressed among these subjects, an initial expression of the willingness and relevance of integrating mental health into primary health care (World Health Organization, 1978). This seminal disposition would find the definitive political and technical impetus with the Conference for the Restructuring of Psychiatric Care in Latin America, held in Caracas in 1990 (Levav et al., 1994). Although mainly regional in scope, with the participation of 11 Latin American countries (Levav et al., 1994), the Caracas Declaration has been recognized as a very influential milestone in global mental health (Patel et al., 2018).

The Caracas Declaration became a reference for mental health services reform processes, enshrining the commitment of Latin American governments to the development of community-based alternatives to psychiatric hospitals while respecting human rights (Levav et al., 1994). The Caracas Declaration explicitly states that restructuring psychiatric care should be based on primary health care, emphasizing decentralization, social participation and inclusion, and a preventive approach (Levav et al., 1994). Subsequent PAHO/WHO Executive Committee Resolutions have urged Latin American and Caribbean member states to adopt and deepen the principles set by the Caracas Declaration. Specifically, the Strategy and Plan of Action on Mental Health, among its recommendations, stresses the need to "review the organization of mental health services and carry out needed changes, emphasizing decentralization and strengthening the mental health component of primary health care" (Pan American Health Organization, 2009). This document also recognizes depression as a priority condition for which essential interventions should be available in primary health care (Pan American Health Organization, 2009).

Gathering much of the experience accumulated in Latin America, the WHO and the World Organization of Family Doctors (WONCA) provide a series of arguments for integrating mental health into primary health care (World Health Organization & World Organization of Family Doctors, 2008). Most reasons for primary mental health care are directly linked to the principles highlighted by the International Conference on Primary Health Care: an accessible, acceptable, affordable, and holistic approach to mental health care, taking advantage of the embeddedness of primary health care in local communities (World Health Organization & World Organization of Family Doctors, 2008). Furthermore, the WHO and WONCA recognized that primary mental health care minimizes stigma and discrimination and prevents human rights violations as they typically occur in psychiatric hospitals (World Health Organization & World Organization of Family Doctors, 2008).

The WHO/WONCA document also states that the integration of mental health into primary health care should be made explicit in all the areas of action of mental health policies and plans, safeguarding continued financial and human resources (World Health Organization & World Organization of Family Doctors, 2008). As for human resources, the WHO/WONCA document underlines that primary health-care workers need undergraduate and in-service training and supervision to perform specific and well-defined mental health tasks adequately (World Health Organization & World Organization of Family Doctors, 2008). Essential psychotropic medications should be directly available to patients in primary health-care facilities, and specialized mental health resources should be available to primary health-care patients and workers. Advocacy is required to sensitize political leaders, health authorities, and primary health-care workers on the relevance of primary mental health care. Thus, to ensure clear and continued commitments and investments to the integration processes from government health and non-health and nongovernment sectors. Finally, health and intersectoral coordination are fundamental in helping primary health-care patients integrate fully into their communities (World Health Organization & World Organization of Family Doctors, 2008).

The following paragraphs are dedicated to detailing a successful example for developing and integrating a mental health component into primary health care, which particularly applies to the case of adult depression. The Chilean case aligns very well with the principles stated in the WHO/WONCA framework. Following the restoration of democracy in Chile, psychiatric reform found the political will to expand community mental health care (Minoletti et al., 2012). In 1993, the first national mental health plan was published, emphasizing the importance of developing a mental health component in primary health care as one of its priority areas. This plan was accompanied by attempts to provide ongoing mental health training to human resources and integrate psychosocial practitioners (e.g., psychologists) into traditionally biomedical health teams. The deinstitutionalization process was complemented and significantly aided by establishing community mental health facilities and day hospitals (Minoletti et al., 2012).

The National Mental Health and Psychiatry Plan was created in 2000 in response to the limitations identified following the first national mental health plan's experiences and to lessen the prevalence of impairment linked with mental diseases (Gobierno de Chile, 2020). This new mental health strategy established a model for mental health services networks and specified the roles of health teams. It also incorporated sectoral and intersectoral efforts in mental health (e.g., in education, housing, and justice) and identified seven programmatic priorities: depression, alcohol and drug misuse and dependency, attention deficit hyperactivity disorder, victims of violence, schizophrenia, and dementia are among the topics covered in this section (Ministerio de Salud de Chile, 2000). The National Depression Program exemplifies how a mental health component can be integrated into primary health care among the programmatic aims.

Araya et al. (2003) conducted one of the first randomized clinical trials in a middle-income country in the early 2000s. In Chile, the authors evaluated the effectiveness of a stepwise improvement program for treating depression in primary health-care attendees. Given the substantial proportion of women affected by depression in primary health care, this study enrolled 240 adult women diagnosed with major depression using the Diagnostic and Statistical Manual of Mental Disorders, Fourth Edition (DSM-IV) criteria. Women were randomly assigned to receive usual care for depression or a stepped-care program, a highly structured, multicomponent intervention consisting of the following components: (1) a manualized, group-based psychoeducational intervention, (2) systematic monitoring of clinical evolution, and (3) a pre-established relapse prevention strategy (Araya et al., 2003).

The results of this clinical trial were highly positive: at 3 and 6 months, 49% and 70% of women who received the stepped-care program experienced recovery from depression, as measured by a Hamilton Depression Scale score of less than 8, respectively, compared to 15% and 32% of women who received usual treatment (Araya et al., 2003). This clinical trial was notable for the reorganization of primary health-care resources, with most actions carried out by nonmedical health professionals, and for the increased adherence of users in their treatment, which had a significant impact on the structure of the National Depression Program (Araya et al., 2003).

The National Depression Program began with a pilot phase in 2001, following the second National Mental Health and Psychiatry Plan adoption, and by 2003 had expanded to virtually every Chilean territory. The National Depression Program includes the following components (Alvarado et al., 2012):

1. On-site diagnostic evaluation of patients with a suspected depressive episode by a general practitioner or psychologist, based on the diagnostic criteria for depression in the ICD.
2. Indication of stepped-care treatment, according to severity level, incorporating (1) comprehensive evaluation by the primary health-care team, (2) treatment with antidepressant drugs, (3) individual psychotherapy and psychoeducational group intervention, and (4) visits to monitor the patient's clinical progress.
3. Patients with mild to moderate depression are managed in primary health-care clinics. The more severe cases are referred to specialized and outpatient mental health facilities for evaluation by a psychiatrist. If the clinical response to initial treatment is not favorable, the patient is reassessed by a psychiatrist at the primary health-care facility and, if necessary, referred to specialty care.

In September 2004, the Regime of Explicit Health Guarantees became law, mandating public and private health-care providers to guarantee access, quality, timeliness, and financial coverage for health care for prioritized health conditions (Araya et al., 2009). At the end of 2005, the second Regime of Explicit Health Guarantees came into force, which incorporated depression among the prioritized health conditions, and established that (1) all beneficiaries aged 15 years and over, with diagnostic confirmation, will have access to treatment; (2) for beneficiaries with mild or moderate depressions, treatment must be promptly initiated from the diagnostic confirmation, and, in more severe cases, consultation with a specialist must be made within 30 days from referral; (3) financial protection corresponds to a maximum co-payment of 20%; and (4) quality is defined by the provision of specific benefits for depression by an accredited or certified provider (Ministerio de Salud de Chile, 2006).

The Clinical Guidelines for Depression in People Aged 15 Years and Over currently direct the National Depression Program (Ministerio de Salud de Chile, 2013). The Clinical Guidelines stated objectives are to facilitate the active detection of depressive disorders, the reduction of their complications through comprehensive and continuous management, and to promote the rational use of available resources. Its successive editions and other regulatory documents, such as the Guidelines for Network Planning and Programming 2019 (Ministerio de Salud de Chile, 2019), have emphasized the management of major depression in primary health care, assisted referral to specialized mental health care in those cases with high suicidal risk, bipolar disorder, or treatment resistance (Ministerio de Salud de Chile, 2013), and the administration of individual psychotherapy in specialized mental health facilities (Ministerio de Salud de Chile, 2019).

7.4 Barriers to the Treatment of Depression in Primary Health Care

The Lancet Commission on Global Mental Health and Sustainable Development stresses that mental health is a public good necessary for sustainable development (Patel et al., 2018). However, the low priority given to mental health is one of the main macrostructural barriers that threaten access to this public good and sustainable development (Patel et al., 2018). An influential review on resources for mental health care found that scarcity, inequity, and inefficiency of such resources are the main obstacles to better mental health (Saxena et al., 2007). These severe limitations mean that the populations most vulnerable and in greatest need of mental health care have the least access to these services (Saxena et al., 2007). While mental health policies, plans, and laws exist in many countries, they are often outdated and poorly aligned with human rights standards to protect people with mental disorders (Saxena et al., 2007). As referred below, these structural barriers affect the quality of mental health services in primary health care.

The WHO Mental Health Atlas 2020 reported that the median global public expenditure on mental health was a meager 2.1% of total government health expenditure (World Health Organization, 2021). Moreover, most countries (81%) allocated less than a fifth of this expenditure to primary health care (World Health Organization, 2021). The WHO Mental Health Atlas 2020 assessed the functional integration of mental health into primary health care, considering the adoption of guidelines, the availability of pharmacological and psychosocial interventions, and training and supervision of primary health-care professionals (World Health Organization, 2021). Only 15% of countries met all criteria for functional integration of mental health into primary health care, whereas 31% met most criteria (World Health Organization, 2021). Notably, a low proportion of countries informed the provision of pharmacological (39%) and psychosocial (21%) interventions in primary health-care centers (World Health Organization, 2021).

Although 80% of countries noted that training was available for primary health-care professionals, the WHO Mental Health Atlas does not report details such as type, duration, or coverage (World Health Organization, 2021). An assessment of the mental health systems of 42 low- and middle-income countries made by the WHO offers a complementary view (World Health Organization, 2009). The evaluation showed that the proportion of total undergraduate training hours devoted to mental health is negligible for primary health-care professionals; the same occurs with refresher courses and in-service training (World Health Organization, 2009). In general, the higher the income level, the greater the training opportunities reported for primary health-care professionals (World Health Organization, 2009). The scarce training opportunities may affect primary health-care professionals' ability to manage depression. For instance, despite Chile's successful integration of mental health into primary health care, a recent study found that nurses, midwives, and general practitioners had difficulties in depression screening and diagnosis (Martínez et al., 2019).

International studies led by the WHO have shown that general practitioners in primary health care are the first and foremost source of mental health care (Üstün & Sartorius, 1995; Wang et al., 2007). However, the WHO primary health-care study and Mitchell et al.'s meta-analysis observed that nearly half of depressed patients (47.3–54.2%) were correctly recognized by general practitioners, signaling the need for improved diagnosis (Mitchell et al., 2009; Üstün & Sartorius, 1995). The detection of depression by primary health-care clinicians in low- and middle-income countries is considerably lower, with rates typically in the ranges of 0–12% (Fekadu et al., 2020). Low detection rates might be influenced by illness behavior, as patients usually present somatic symptoms instead of psychological complaints (Üstün & Sartorius, 1995). Organizational factors might also shape detection accuracies, such as increased performance monitoring, periodic review of clinical outcomes, presence of an appointment system, and general practitioners assuming responsibility for coordination of patient care (Mitchell et al., 2011; Üstün & Sartorius, 1995).

A return on investment analysis for depression and anxiety disorders in 36 countries estimated that between 80% and 95% of depressed people do not receive basic psychosocial treatments or antidepressants, the usual primary health-care treatments for depression, when available (Chisholm et al., 2016). Complementarily, Pence et al. conducted a literature review to study the depression treatment continuum in primary health care (Pence et al., 2012). The authors determined that of all primary health-care patients with a major depressive episode, 24% received any treatment, 9% were adequately treated, and 6% achieved remission (Pence et al., 2012). They also projected that improving the adequacy of treatment would have the largest single impact on remission rates. It is relevant to address the barriers to managing depression in primary health care because early detection and treatment of depressive disorders facilitates the treatment response and remission of mood symptoms and reduces the risk of a chronic course of illness (Ghio et al., 2014).

Several syntheses of qualitative and quantitative studies have explored the barriers to managing depression in primary health care (Barley et al., 2011; Carlsen et al., 2007; Holm & Severinsson, 2012; McPherson & Armstrong, 2012; Schumann et al., 2012). These syntheses underscore that one of the main issues primary health-care clinicians face is understanding depression either as social distress or as a chemical imbalance (Barley et al., 2011; McPherson & Armstrong, 2012; Schumann et al., 2012). Acknowledging the social origins of depression leads primary health-care clinicians to confront the limits of their capabilities, feeling powerless in managing the disease (e.g., should social problems be medicalized?), whereas a “true” depression conforms to a biomedical disease model (Barley et al., 2011; McPherson & Armstrong, 2012; Schumann et al., 2012). Another primary concern is detecting and diagnosing depression. General practitioners refer to depression as puzzling, usually masked in physical symptoms (Barley et al., 2011; McPherson & Armstrong, 2012; Schumann et al., 2012). Making the diagnosis of depression requires a personalized assessment of patients, demanding time (a rare commodity), watchful waiting, and active listening (Barley et al., 2011; McPherson & Armstrong, 2012; Schumann et al., 2012). Addressing patients’ stigma and fears toward mental illness and having a good doctor-patient relationship are essential to overcoming the difficulties found in these processes (Barley et al., 2011; McPherson & Armstrong, 2012; Schumann et al., 2012).

Regarding therapeutic options available, general practitioners admit that active listening, emotional support, and empathy are their best assets when treating depression (Barley et al., 2011; McPherson & Armstrong, 2012; Schumann et al., 2012). These resources also help them negotiate antidepressant use with patients (Barley et al., 2011). However, the management of depression in primary health care is further complicated by organizational factors. For instance, primary health-care clinicians complain about the lack of clear role definitions, difficulties in the coordination of teamwork, and the poor availability of specialized mental health care, perceived as burdened with patients having severe mental disorders (Barley et al., 2011; Carlsen et al., 2007; Holm & Severinsson, 2012; McPherson & Armstrong, 2012). These barriers are complemented by the perception of clinical guidelines for depression as not readily applicable to real clinical contexts and as a threat to the judicialization of the doctor-patient relationship (Carlsen et al., 2007; Holm & Severinsson, 2012). Finally, even when clinicians recognize the need for training in depression management, negative experiences with previous depression training programs and prioritization of training in addressing physical health problems are limitations to furthering their skills (Barley et al., 2011; McPherson & Armstrong, 2012).

7.5 Evidence-Based Interventions for Adult Depression in Primary Health Care

In this section, the main findings of recent systematic reviews and meta-analyses on the effectiveness of psychological and pharmacological interventions that have been tested in primary health care are reviewed. Furthermore, acknowledging the relevance of combined psychological and pharmacological interventions, wc introduce the principles of the collaborative care model. The collaborative care model is a complex, highly effective, and influential approach to treating depression in primary health care. We finalize with a brief mention of the integration of information technologies into the primary health-care treatment of depression.

Antidepressants are acceptable and more effective than placebo in adults with major depression (Cipriani et al., 2018). However, most of the evidence cannot be directly applied to primary health care: studies have been conducted in different settings and recruited individuals with moderate to severe depressive symptoms (Cipriani et al., 2018). Few clinical trials have evaluated the efficacy of antidepressants in primary health care, despite the availability of psychotropics being a principle in primary mental health care (World Health Organization & World Organization of Family Doctors, 2008). Arroll et al.'s (2016) meta-analysis found 17 studies comparing antidepressants to placebo in primary health care. In general, these studies enrolled patients with mild to moderate depressive symptoms and explored short-term outcomes. The authors concluded that tricyclic antidepressants (e.g., amitriptyline) and selective serotonin reuptake inhibitors (e.g., sertraline and escitalopram) provided significant benefits in terms of response (i.e., >50% reduction in depressive symptoms from baseline) (Arroll et al., 2016). However, they caution that their data does not shed light as to when, who, and for how long antidepressants should be used in primary health-care attendees (Arroll et al., 2016).

Cognitive behavioral therapy and problem-solving therapy are the most studied psychological treatments for adult depression in primary health care (Cuijpers et al., 2019; Zhang et al., 2019). While cognitive behavioral therapy aims to change dysfunctional thoughts and cognitive distortions (Hofmann et al., 2013), problem-solving therapy trains patients in adaptive problem-solving attitudes and skills (Bell & D'Zurilla, 2009). Cuijpers et al. (2019) found that psychotherapies for depression in primary health care are effective and that face-to-face comparisons revealed no significant differences between them. Moreover, the same evidence synthesis showed that psychotherapies for depression could be delivered by general practitioners and allied health-care workers (Cuijpers et al., 2019). The authors argue that such finding is relevant to scale-up primary health-care depression treatment in low- and middle-income countries (Cuijpers et al., 2019). Interestingly, research has shown that psychotherapies' effectiveness for depression in primary health care is moderated by treatment modality: individual interventions and outside primary health-care facilities (i.e., closer to patients' homes) are more effective (Zhang et al., 2019).

More recently, a network meta-analysis by Cuijpers et al. (2021) provided the first comparison between pharmacological, psychological, and combined interventions for depression in primary health care. Cuijpers et al.'s network meta-analysis (2021) included 58 studies, totaling 9301 mostly adult primary health-care attendees. The authors found that the three types of treatments explored were more effective than treatment as usual and waitlist controls (Cuijpers et al., 2021). However, a clear preference for combined pharmacological and psychological interventions was evidenced, achieving better response, remission, and improvement in depressive symptoms (Cuijpers et al., 2021). Notably, the network meta-analysis found no significant differences in the acceptability of these interventions, underlining the relevance of adapting treatment offer to patients' preferences (Cuijpers et al., 2021).

The collaborative care model might be thought of as a model for the integration of combined interventions for managing depression in primary health care. A group of researchers in the United States, led by Wayne Katon et al. (1995, 1996, 1997, 1999), developed the collaborative care model based on chronic and recurrent illness care. This model provided a multicomponent intervention, with increased patient engagement and education, more regular treatment in the acute phase of the illness, and more intensive treatment for more severe patients (i.e., stepped treatment). This was complemented by strict monitoring of treatment adherence, training for primary care physicians in the management of depression, and closer collaboration between treating physicians and psychiatrists (i.e., mental health consultancies). Collaborative care proved feasible to implement in primary health care, acceptable to patients and general practitioners, effective in reducing depressive symptoms, and cost-effective (Katon et al., 1995, 1996, 1997, 1999).

Currently, the collaborative care model has robust evidence for its benefits: decreased depressive symptoms, increased adherence and response to treatment, improvements in quality of life and satisfaction with care, and economic efficiency, in a wide range of depressed patients (Miller et al., 2013; Vanderlip et al., 2016). According to Vanderlip et al. (2016), the collaborative care model involves:

(i) A general practitioner who leads a multidisciplinary health-care team in coordination with a case manager (e.g., a nurse). The primary health-care team receives consultation from a mental health specialist.
(ii) Improving the quality of care and health outcomes of a population, through a systematic review of cases periodically to redirect health resources, and analysis of aggregated patient data to identify and act on gaps in care in the population.
(iii) Health care is based on timely measurements for assessing progress in patients' health status through reliable, change-sensitive, and simple-to-apply instruments (e.g., the Patient Health Questionnaire-9, PHQ-9, in the case of depression).

(iv) The provision of evidence-based interventions, structured in a stepped manner (e.g., greater intensity of interventions as the case's complexity increases), and with instruments to support clinical decision making (e.g., mental health consultancies, clinical guidelines with standardized management algorithms, among others).

A panel of experts studied the effectiveness of the collaborative care model in clinical trials published between 2004 and 2009, reporting the finding of robust evidence for significant improvements in depressive symptoms, adherence, and response to treatment, quality of life, and satisfaction with care in a wide range of depressed patients (Thota et al., 2012). Complementarily, a systematic review of the economic efficiency of the collaborative care model (Jacob et al., 2012), conducted by the same expert panel, found positive economic benefits, lower programmatic costs, willingness-to-pay exceeding expenses, and greater cost-effectiveness in sites receiving the intervention.

Finally, scientific innovations in the management of depression in primary health care from developed countries have been presented, raising questions about the feasibility of implementing such models in under-resourced settings in developing countries. In this regard, Patel et al. (2009) reviewed the evidence on the efficacy of treatments and the provision of interventions for the management of depression in low- and middle-income countries. They proposed a "package" of care for depression in these settings (Patel et al., 2009). The authors concluded that a basic package for depression management should include routine use of culturally adapted instruments to improve depression screening; patient education about their health problem and treatment alternatives; context-specific antidepressant treatments and psychotherapy, such as generic antidepressants and problem-solving therapy; and that task shifting to nonspecialist health workers, who provide first-line care and are supervised by specialists, is essential to integrate this package into routine care in community services (Patel et al., 2009).

7.6 Conclusion

Depression is a very important public health problem worldwide. It is frequent in people who attend primary care clinics, and it is frequently associated with chronic diseases and psychiatric comorbidities.

The primary care team can play a crucial role in depression management. Therefore, it is necessary for the development of a mental health component in primary care based on the principles of the collaborative care model that has demonstrated a highly effective and influential approach to treating depression in primary health care.

Acknowledgments This work was supported by ANID – Millennium Science Initiative Program – ICS13_005, ANID – FONDECYT – 1180224, and U Redes Consolidación (Grant URC 007/18).

References

Alvarado, R., Rojas, G., Minoletti, A., Alvarado, F., & Domínguez, C. (2012). Depression program in primary health care. *International Journal of Mental Health, 41*(1), 38–47. https://doi.org/10.2753/IMH0020-7411410103

Araya, R., Alvarado, R., & Minoletti, A. (2009). Chile: An ongoing mental health revolution. *Lancet (London, England), 374*(9690), 597–598. https://doi.org/10.1016/S0140-6736(09)61490-2

Araya, R., Rojas, G., Fritsch, R., Gaete, J., Rojas, M., Simon, G., & Peters, T. J. (2003). Treating depression in primary care in low-income women in Santiago, Chile: A randomised controlled trial. *Lancet (London, England), 361*(9362), 995–1000. https://doi.org/10.1016/S0140-6736(03)12825-5

Arroll, B., Chin, W.-Y., Martis, W., Goodyear-Smith, F., Mount, V., Kingsford, D., Humm, S., Blashki, G., & MacGillivray, S. (2016). Antidepressants for treatment of depression in primary care: A systematic review and meta-analysis. *Journal of Primary Health Care, 8*(4), 325–334. https://doi.org/10.1071/HC16008

Barkow, K., Maier, W., Ustün, T. B., Gänsicke, M., Wittchen, H. U., & Heun, R. (2002). Risk factors for new depressive episodes in primary health care: An international prospective 12-month follow-up study. *Psychological Medicine, 32*(4), 595–607. https://doi.org/10.1017/s0033291702005263

Barkow, K., Maier, W., Ustün, T. B., Gänsicke, M., Wittchen, H.-U., & Heun, R. (2003). Risk factors for depression at 12-month follow-up in adult primary health care patients with major depression: An international prospective study. *Journal of Affective Disorders, 76*(1–3), 157–169. https://doi.org/10.1016/s0165-0327(02)00081-2

Barley, E. A., Murray, J., Walters, P., & Tylee, A. (2011). Managing depression in primary care: A meta-synthesis of qualitative and quantitative research from the UK to identify barriers and facilitators. *BMC Family Practice, 12*, 47. https://doi.org/10.1186/1471-2296-12-47

Bell, A. C., & D'Zurilla, T. J. (2009). Problem-solving therapy for depression: A meta-analysis. *Clinical Psychology Review, 29*(4), 348–353. https://doi.org/10.1016/j.cpr.2009.02.003

Carlsen, B., Glenton, C., & Pope, C. (2007). Thou shalt versus thou shalt not: A meta-synthesis of GPs' attitudes to clinical practice guidelines. *The British Journal of General Practice, 57*(545), 971–978.

Cassell, A., Edwards, D., Harshfield, A., Rhodes, K., Brimicombe, J., Payne, R., & Griffin, S. (2018). The epidemiology of multimorbidity in primary care: A retrospective cohort study. *British Journal of General Practice, 68*(669), e245–e251. https://doi.org/10.3399/bjgp18X695465

Charlson, F., van Ommeren, M., Flaxman, A., Cornett, J., Whiteford, H., & Saxena, S. (2019). New WHO prevalence estimates of mental disorders in conflict settings: A systematic review and meta-analysis. *Lancet (London, England), 394*(10194), 240–248. https://doi.org/10.1016/S0140-6736(19)30934-1

Chisholm, D., Sweeny, K., Sheehan, P., Rasmussen, B., Smit, F., Cuijpers, P., & Saxena, S. (2016). Scaling-up treatment of depression and anxiety: A global return on investment analysis. *The Lancet Psychiatry, 3*(5), 415–424. https://doi.org/10.1016/S2215-0366(16)30024-4

Cipriani, A., Furukawa, T. A., Salanti, G., Chaimani, A., Atkinson, L. Z., Ogawa, Y., Leucht, S., Ruhe, H. G., Turner, E. H., Higgins, J. P. T., Egger, M., Takeshima, N., Hayasaka, Y., Imai, H., Shinohara, K., Tajika, A., Ioannidis, J. P. A., & Geddes, J. R. (2018). Comparative efficacy and acceptability of 21 antidepressant drugs for the acute treatment of adults with major depressive disorder: A systematic review and network meta-analysis. *Lancet (London, England), 391*(10128), 1357–1366. https://doi.org/10.1016/S0140-6736(17)32802-7

Cuijpers, P., Oud, M., Karyotaki, E., Noma, H., Quero, S., Cipriani, A., Arroll, B., & Furukawa, T. A. (2021). Psychologic treatment of depression compared with pharmacotherapy and combined treatment in primary care: A network meta-analysis. *The Annals of Family Medicine, 19*(3), 262–270. https://doi.org/10.1370/afm.2676

Cuijpers, P., Quero, S., Dowrick, C., & Arroll, B. (2019). Psychological treatment of depression in primary care: Recent developments. *Current Psychiatry Reports, 21*(12), 129. https://doi.org/10.1007/s11920-019-1117-x

Fekadu, A., Demissie, M., Berhane, R., Medhin, G., Bitew, T., Hailemariam, M., Minaye, A., Habtamu, K., Milkias, B., Petersen, I., Patel, V., Cleare, A. J., Mayston, R., Thornicroft, G., Alem, A., Hanlon, C., & Prince, M. (2020). *Under detection of depression in primary care settings in low and middle-income countries: A systematic review and meta-analysis* (p. 2020.03.20.20039628). https://doi.org/10.1101/2020.03.20.20039628

Ferrari, A. J., Norman, R. E., Freedman, G., Baxter, A. J., Pirkis, J. E., Harris, M. G., Page, A., Carnahan, E., Degenhardt, L., Vos, T., & Whiteford, H. A. (2014). The burden attributable to mental and substance use disorders as risk factors for suicide: Findings from the global burden of disease study 2010. *PLoS One, 9*(4), e91936. https://doi.org/10.1371/journal.pone.0091936

GBD 2019 Mental Disorders Collaborators. (2022). Global, regional, and national burden of 12 mental disorders in 204 countries and territories, 1990–2019: A systematic analysis for the Global Burden of Disease Study 2019. *The Lancet Psychiatry, 9*(2), 137–150. https://doi.org/10.1016/S2215-0366(21)00395-3

GBD 2019 Risk Factors Collaborators. (2020). Global burden of 87 risk factors in 204 countries and territories, 1990-2019: A systematic analysis for the Global Burden of Disease Study 2019. *Lancet (London, England), 396*(10258), 1223–1249. https://doi.org/10.1016/S0140-6736(20)30752-2

Ghio, L., Gotelli, S., Marcenaro, M., Amore, M., & Natta, W. (2014). Duration of untreated illness and outcomes in unipolar depression: A systematic review and meta-analysis. *Journal of Affective Disorders, 152–154*, 45–51. https://doi.org/10.1016/j.jad.2013.10.002

Global Burden of Disease Collaborative Network. (2020). *Global Burden of Disease Study 2019 (GBD 2019) results*. Institute for Health Metrics and Evaluation (IHME). http://ghdx.healthdata.org/gbd-results-tool/result

Gobierno de Chile. (2020). *Política Nacional para la Reducción del Riesgo de Desastres: Plan Estratégico Nacional 2020-2030* (p. 176). ONEMI – Ministerio del Interior y Seguridad Pública.

Gunn, J. M., Ayton, D. R., Densley, K., Pallant, J. F., Chondros, P., Herrman, H. E., & Dowrick, C. F. (2012). The association between chronic illness, multimorbidity and depressive symptoms in an Australian primary care cohort. *Social Psychiatry and Psychiatric Epidemiology, 47*(2), 175–184. https://doi.org/10.1007/s00127-010-0330-z

Hofmann, S. G., Asmundson, G. J. G., & Beck, A. T. (2013). The science of cognitive therapy. *Behavior Therapy, 44*(2), 199–212. https://doi.org/10.1016/j.beth.2009.01.007

Holm, A. L., & Severinsson, E. (2012). Chronic care model for the management of depression: Synthesis of barriers to, and facilitators of, success. *International Journal of Mental Health Nursing, 21*(6), 513–523. https://doi.org/10.1111/j.1447-0349.2012.00827.x

Jacob, V., Chattopadhyay, S. K., Sipe, T. A., Thota, A. B., Byard, G. J., Chapman, D. P., & Community Preventive Services Task Force. (2012). Economics of collaborative care for management of depressive disorders: A community guide systematic review. *American Journal of Preventive Medicine, 42*(5), 539–549. https://doi.org/10.1016/j.amepre.2012.01.011

Katon, W., Robinson, P., Von Korff, M., Lin, E., Bush, T., Ludman, E., Simon, G., & Walker, E. (1996). A multifaceted intervention to improve treatment of depression in primary care. *Archives of General Psychiatry, 53*(10), 924–932. https://doi.org/10.1001/archpsyc.1996.01830100072009

Katon, W., Von Korff, M., Lin, E., Simon, G., Walker, E., Bush, T., & Ludman, E. (1997). Collaborative management to achieve depression treatment guidelines. *The Journal of Clinical Psychiatry, 58*(Suppl 1), 20–23.

Katon, W., Von Korff, M., Lin, E., Simon, G., Walker, E., Unützer, J., Bush, T., Russo, J., & Ludman, E. (1999). Stepped collaborative care for primary care patients with persistent symptoms of depression: A randomized trial. *Archives of General Psychiatry, 56*(12), 1109–1115. https://doi.org/10.1001/archpsyc.56.12.1109

Katon, W., Von Korff, M., Lin, E., Walker, E., Simon, G. E., Bush, T., Robinson, P., & Russo, J. (1995). Collaborative management to achieve treatment guidelines. Impact on depression in primary care. *JAMA, 273*(13), 1026–1031.

King, M., Walker, C., Levy, G., Bottomley, C., Royston, P., Weich, S., Bellón-Saameño, J. A., Moreno, B., Svab, I., Rotar, D., Rifel, J., Maaroos, H.-I., Aluoja, A., Kalda, R., Neeleman, J., Geerlings, M. I., Xavier, M., Carraça, I., Gonçalves-Pereira, M., et al. (2008). Development and validation of an international risk prediction algorithm for episodes of major depression in general practice attendees: The PredictD study. *Archives of General Psychiatry, 65*(12), 1368–1376. https://doi.org/10.1001/archpsyc.65.12.1368

Levav, I., Restrepo, H., & de Macedo, C. G. (1994). The restructuring of psychiatric care in Latin America: A new policy for mental health services. *Journal of Public Health Policy, 15*(1), 71–85. https://doi.org/10.2307/3342608

Machado, M. O., Veronese, N., Sanches, M., Stubbs, B., Koyanagi, A., Thompson, T., Tzoulaki, I., Solmi, M., Vancampfort, D., Schuch, F. B., Maes, M., Fava, G. A., Ioannidis, J. P. A., & Carvalho, A. F. (2018). The association of depression and all-cause and cause-specific mortality: An umbrella review of systematic reviews and meta-analyses. *BMC Medicine, 16*(1), 112. https://doi.org/10.1186/s12916-018-1101-z

Martínez, P., Rojas, G., Martínez, V., Marín, R., Cornejo, J. P., & Gómez, V. (2019). Measuring primary health care clinicians' skills for depression management. *Frontiers in Psychiatry, 10*, 570. https://doi.org/10.3389/fpsyt.2019.00570

McPherson, S., & Armstrong, D. (2012). General practitioner management of depression: A systematic review. *Qualitative Health Research, 22*(8), 1150–1159. https://doi.org/10.1177/1049732312448540

Miller, C. J., Grogan-Kaylor, A., Perron, B. E., Kilbourne, A. M., Woltmann, E., & Bauer, M. S. (2013). Collaborative chronic care models for mental health conditions: Cumulative meta-analysis and metaregression to guide future research and implementation. *Medical Care, 51*(10), 922–930. https://doi.org/10.1097/MLR.0b013e3182a3e4c4

Ministerio de Salud de Chile. (2000). *Plan Nacional de Salud Mental y Psiquiatría*. Gobierno de Chile.

Ministerio de Salud de Chile. (2006). *Segundo Régimen de Garantías Explícitas en Salud*. Gobierno de Chile.

Ministerio de Salud de Chile. (2013). *Guía Clínica Depresión en personas de 15 años y más*. Gobierno de Chile.

Ministerio de Salud de Chile. (2019). *Orientaciones para la planificación y programación en red*. Gobierno de Chile.

Minoletti, A., Rojas, G., & Horvitz-Lennon, M. (2012). Mental health in primary care in Chile: Lessons for Latin America. *Cadernos Saúde Coletiva, 20*, 440–447.

Mitchell, A. J., Rao, S., & Vaze, A. (2011). International comparison of clinicians' ability to identify depression in primary care: Meta-analysis and meta-regression of predictors. *British Journal of General Practice, 61*(583), e72–e80. https://doi.org/10.3399/bjgp11X556227

Mitchell, A. J., Vaze, A., & Rao, S. (2009). Clinical diagnosis of depression in primary care: A meta-analysis. *Lancet (London, England), 374*(9690), 609–619. https://doi.org/10.1016/S0140-6736(09)60879-5

Moitra, M., Santomauro, D., Degenhardt, L., Collins, P. Y., Whiteford, H., Vos, T., & Ferrari, A. (2021). Estimating the risk of suicide associated with mental disorders: A systematic review and meta-regression analysis. *Journal of Psychiatric Research, 137*, 242–249. https://doi.org/10.1016/j.jpsychires.2021.02.053

Moussavi, S., Chatterji, S., Verdes, E., Tandon, A., Patel, V., & Ustun, B. (2007). Depression, chronic diseases, and decrements in health: Results from the World Health Surveys. *Lancet (London, England), 370*(9590), 851–858. https://doi.org/10.1016/S0140-6736(07)61415-9

Organización Panamericana de la Salud. (1972). *Informe sobre la III reunión especial de Ministros de Salud y medidas necesarias para dar cumplimiento a las decisiones adoptadas.* Organización Panamericana de la Salud – Organización Mundial de la Salud. https://iris.paho.org/handle/10665.2/5926

Pan American Health Organization. (2009). *Strategy and plan of action on mental health.* PAHO/WHO. https://iris.paho.org/handle/10665.2/33930

Patel, V., Saxena, S., Lund, C., Thornicroft, G., Baingana, F., Bolton, P., Chisholm, D., Collins, P. Y., Cooper, J. L., Eaton, J., Herrman, H., Herzallah, M. M., Huang, Y., Jordans, M. J. D., Kleinman, A., Medina-Mora, M. E., Morgan, E., Niaz, U., Omigbodun, O., et al. (2018). The Lancet Commission on global mental health and sustainable development. *Lancet (London, England), 392*(10157), 1553–1598. https://doi.org/10.1016/S0140-6736(18)31612-X

Patel, V., Simon, G., Chowdhary, N., Kaaya, S., & Araya, R. (2009). Packages of care for depression in low- and middle-income countries. *PLoS Medicine, 6*(10), e1000159. https://doi.org/10.1371/journal.pmed.1000159

Pence, B. W., O'Donnell, J. K., & Gaynes, B. N. (2012). The depression treatment cascade in primary care: A public health perspective. *Current Psychiatry Reports, 14*(4), 328–335. https://doi.org/10.1007/s11920-012-0274-y

Santomauro, D. F., Herrera, A. M. M., Shadid, J., Zheng, P., Ashbaugh, C., Pigott, D. M., Abbafati, C., Adolph, C., Amlag, J. O., Aravkin, A. Y., Bang-Jensen, B. L., Bertolacci, G. J., Bloom, S. S., Castellano, R., Castro, E., Chakrabarti, S., Chattopadhyay, J., Cogen, R. M., Collins, J. K., et al. (2021). Global prevalence and burden of depressive and anxiety disorders in 204 countries and territories in 2020 due to the COVID-19 pandemic. *The Lancet, 398*(10312), 1700–1712. https://doi.org/10.1016/S0140-6736(21)02143-7

Saxena, S., Thornicroft, G., Knapp, M., & Whiteford, H. (2007). Resources for mental health: Scarcity, inequity, and inefficiency. *Lancet (London, England), 370*(9590), 878–889. https://doi.org/10.1016/S0140-6736(07)61239-2

Schumann, I., Schneider, A., Kantert, C., Löwe, B., & Linde, K. (2012). Physicians' attitudes, diagnostic process and barriers regarding depression diagnosis in primary care: A systematic review of qualitative studies. *Family Practice, 29*(3), 255–263. https://doi.org/10.1093/fampra/cmr092

Smith, D. J., Court, H., McLean, G., Martin, D., Martin, J. L., Guthrie, B., Gunn, J., & Mercer, S. W. (2014). Depression and multimorbidity: A cross-sectional study of 1,751,841 patients in primary care. *The Journal of Clinical Psychiatry, 75*(11), 4205. https://doi.org/10.4088/JCP.14m09147

Stegenga, B. T., King, M., Grobbee, D. E., Torres-González, F., Švab, I., Maaroos, H.-I., Xavier, M., Saldivia, S., Bottomley, C., Nazareth, I., & Geerlings, M. I. (2012). Differential impact of risk factors for women and men on the risk of major depressive disorder. *Annals of Epidemiology, 22*(6), 388–396. https://doi.org/10.1016/j.annepidem.2012.04.011

Thota, A. B., Sipe, T. A., Byard, G. J., Zometa, C. S., Hahn, R. A., McKnight-Eily, L. R., Chapman, D. P., Abraido-Lanza, A. F., Pearson, J. L., Anderson, C. W., Gelenberg, A. J., Hennessy, K. D., Duffy, F. F., Vernon-Smiley, M. E., Nease, D. E., Williams, S. P., & Community Preventive Services Task Force. (2012). Collaborative care to improve the management of depressive disorders: A community guide systematic review and meta-analysis. *American Journal of Preventive Medicine, 42*(5), 525–538. https://doi.org/10.1016/j.amepre.2012.01.019

Üstün, T. B., & Sartorius, N. (1995). *Mental illness in general health care: An international study.* John Wiley & Sons.

Vanderlip, E. R., Rundell, J., Avery, M., Alter, C., Engel, C., Fortney, J., & Williams, M. (2016). *Dissemination of integrated care within adult primary care settings: The collaborative care model*. American Psychiatric Association and Academy of Psychosomatic Medicine.

Wang, P. S., Aguilar-Gaxiola, S., Alonso, J., Angermeyer, M. C., Borges, G., Bromet, E. J., Bruffaerts, R., de Girolamo, G., de Graaf, R., Gureje, O., Haro, J. M., Karam, E. G., Kessler, R. C., Kovess, V., Lane, M. C., Lee, S., Levinson, D., Ono, Y., Petukhova, M., et al. (2007). Use of mental health services for anxiety, mood, and substance disorders in 17 countries in the WHO world mental health surveys. *Lancet (London, England), 370*(9590), 841–850. https://doi.org/10.1016/S0140-6736(07)61414-7

World Health Organization. (1978). *Primary health care: Report of the international conference on Primary Health Care, Alma-Ata, USSR, 6–12 September 1978: Jointly sponsored by the World Health Organization and the United Nations Children's Fund*. WHO.

World Health Organization. (2009). *Mental health systems in selected low- and middle-income countries: A WHO-AIMS cross-national analysis* (p. 103). World Health Organization. https://apps.who.int/iris/handle/10665/44151

World Health Organization. (2017). *Depression and other common mental disorders: Global health estimates*. World Health Organization.

World Health Organization. (2021). *Mental health atlas 2020*. World Health Organization. https://apps.who.int/iris/handle/10665/345946

World Health Organization, & World Organization of Family Doctors. (2008). *Integrating mental health into primary care: A global perspective*. WHO/WONCA.

Zhang, A., Franklin, C., Jing, S., Bornheimer, L. A., Hai, A. H., Himle, J. A., Kong, D., & Ji, Q. (2019). The effectiveness of four empirically supported psychotherapies for primary care depression and anxiety: A systematic review and meta-analysis. *Journal of Affective Disorders, 245*, 1168–1186. https://doi.org/10.1016/j.jad.2018.12.008

Chapter 8
The Potential of Internet-Based Psychological Interventions for Perinatal Depression Prevention and Treatment

Pamela Franco, Marcia Olhaberry, Antonia Muzard, María Asunción Lara, and Pim Cuijpers

8.1 Perinatal Depression Prevalence, Etiology, and Infant Consequences

According to the Diagnostic and Statistical Manual of Mental Disorders (DSM), PND shares the characteristics of depression in other stages of the life cycle, with the peculiarity that its onset occurs during pregnancy or during the 4 weeks following delivery (American Psychiatric Association, 2013; Ferrari et al., 2013). However, in clinical practice and research, PND is defined as depression occurring during pregnancy (antenatal depression) and up to 1 year (O'Hara & McCabe, 2013) or 2 years after giving birth (postpartum depression) (Cuijpers et al., 2021). Studies show an overall PND prevalence of 11.9%, with a higher prevalence in low- and middle-income countries (Woody et al., 2017) or countries with high wealth disparities (Hahn-Holbrook et al., 2018). Between 6% and 38% of women develop

P. Franco (✉) · A. Muzard
Doctoral Program in Psychotherapy, Pontificia Universidad Católica de Chile and Universidad de Chile, Santiago, Chile

Millennium Institute for Research in Depression and Personality (MIDAP), Santiago, Chile
e-mail: pvfranco@uc.cl

M. Olhaberry
Millennium Institute for Research in Depression and Personality (MIDAP), Santiago, Chile

School of Psychology, Pontificia Universidad Católica de Chile, Santiago, Chile

M. A. Lara
Ramón de la Fuente Muñiz National Institute of Psychiatry, Mexico City, Mexico

P. Cuijpers
Department of Clinical, Neuro and Developmental Psychology, Amsterdam Public Health Research Institute, Vrije Universiteit Amsterdam, Amsterdam, the Netherlands

V. Martínez, C. Miranda-Castillo (eds.), *Prevention and Early Treatment of Depression Through the Life Course*, Depression and Personality,
https://doi.org/10.1007/978-3-031-13029-8_8

antenatal depression (Field, 2011), and between 3% and 38% develop postpartum depression (Fisher et al., 2012; Hahn-Holbrook et al., 2018). Approximately half of PND episodes spring during pregnancy (American Psychiatric Association, 2013; Raskin et al., 2016; Wisner et al., 2013), and evidence shows that depression at this stage is linked to a greater probability of developing postpartum depression (Figueiredo & Conde, 2011; Koutra et al., 2014; Toohey, 2012). Suicidal thoughts may affect approximately 20% of women with PND, and some of them also report thinking of harming their children (Wisner et al., 2013). Indeed, in some countries, suicide is a leading cause of maternal death (Knight et al., 2019; PMMRC, 2016).

Studies have shown that PND has a multicausal etiology. Risk factors include unplanned or unwanted pregnancies, ambivalence concerning motherhood (Bowen & Muhajarine, 2006), low income, absence of a support network, extreme ages (teenagers or >40 years), lack of a partner, insecure attachment pattern, a history of depression (Faisal-Cury & Rossi Menezes, 2007; Field, 2017a, b; Olhaberry et al., 2014), and adverse or traumatic experiences during childhood (Buist & Janson, 2001; Nelson et al., 2002). Stress, drug use, conflicts with a partner, domestic violence, and a low educational level have also been associated with PND (Field, 2017a, b).

One of PND's most relevant and worrying characteristics is its negative impact on both the mother and the baby (Clatworthy, 2012; Field, 2011; Slomian et al., 2019). When comparing non-depressed pregnant women with antenatal depression, evidence shows more frequent preterm deliveries and newborns with increased cardiac activity, smaller stature, or lower weight (Diego et al., 2009; Emory & Dieter, 2006; Fekadu Dadi et al., 2020; Hompoth et al., 2020). Negative consequences on children of mothers with PND have also been reported regarding their affective, cognitive, and behavioral development (Grace et al., 2003; Milgrom et al., 2008; Pearson et al., 2012), along with the greater risk of suffering from depression throughout life (Fox & Borelli, 2015; Pawlby et al., 2009; Slomian et al., 2019). Some of these negative consequences for children of depressed mothers can be explained by symptoms during pregnancy, regardless of the presence or absence of postpartum depression (Deave et al., 2008; Stein et al., 2014).

Evidence shows a larger presence of insecure and disorganized attachments in children of depressed mothers (Hayes et al., 2013; Martins & Gaffan, 2000), especially when mothers present severe and chronic depression (McMahon et al., 2006). Postpartum depression has also been linked to maternal anxiety symptoms and stress, which heightens PND influence on mother-baby dyadic adjustment (Rollè et al., 2017; Vismara et al., 2016), intensifying negative affect and reducing the maternal sensitive response to the baby's needs (Behrendt et al., 2019; Lefkovics et al., 2018). Given all this, postpartum depression is considered one of the most relevant risk factors for the quality of mother-baby interactions and infant development (Campbell et al., 2004; Stein et al., 2014; Slomian et al., 2019). Moreover, a negative impact on the quality of mother-baby interactions has been reported even when depressive symptomatology is subclinical (Tronick & Reck, 2009). The latter highlights the need to intervene early.

8.2 Perinatal Depression Prevention and Treatment

The United States Preventive Services Task Force recommends routine depression screening for all perinatal women (American College of Obstetricians and Gynecologists, 2014). Other countries around the world have also implemented routine perinatal depression screening (beyondblue, 2011; MINSAL, 2014). However, specific issues have been reported regarding PND detection and diagnosis since symptoms such as irritability, low mood, emotional lability, anxiety, and sleep disorders are commonly experienced during the perinatal period (Halbreich & Karkun, 2006). In contrast, depressive symptoms are normalized by perinatal women, their families, and caregivers, who attribute them to being part of the psychological adjustment to pregnancy and having a new baby (Sword et al., 2008). Additionally, being outspoken about depression is embarrassing for many women because of the cultural belief that defines the perinatal time as "a period of happiness" (Dennis & Chung-Lee, 2006). All of these facts hinder early screening and timely treatment.

Interventions to prevent or treat PND can include one or a combination of the following strategies: pharmacological treatments such as antidepressant medication; psychoeducation; psychological treatments such as cognitive behavioral or interpersonal therapy, individually or group-administered; maternal-child interaction guidance for bond promotion such as video-feedback; psychosocial interventions such as nondirective counseling; peer support such as periodic group reunions with other mothers; and other non-pharmacological/non-psychological treatments such as bright light therapy, acupuncture, exercise, and massage (Field, 2017a, b; Fitelson et al., 2010; Ladyman et al., 2020; Letourneau et al., 2017; Lucena et al., 2020; Olhaberry, Escobar, et al., 2015, Olhaberry, León, et al. 2015; Werner et al., 2015). Interventions for PND prevention are conducted during pregnancy or the postpartum period. They may target either all women (i.e., universal) or those with specific characteristics (e.g., at risk for depression) (Sockol et al., 2013).

Psychotherapy is recommended as the first-line approach for PND and may be combined with pharmacotherapy, depending on depression severity, available options, women's acceptance, and perinatal period (pregnancy or postpartum) (Molenaar et al., 2018). Among the theoretical models supporting psychological interventions, cognitive behavioral models are the most frequently applied (Cuijpers et al., 2021). Interventions may include psychoeducation on PND, identification of support networks, promotion of positive thoughts and pleasant activities, and the provision of written material (Huynh-Nhu et al., 2013; Kozinsky et al., 2012; Lara et al., 2010; Milgrom et al., 2011; O'Connor et al., 2016). Although the literature links PND with bonding difficulties between the mother and her baby (Martins & Gaffan, 2000), most psychological interventions on PND seek to reduce its symptoms and do not necessarily aim to improve the quality of the bond (Olhaberry et al., 2013). Interventions that simultaneously address PND symptomatology and the mother-baby bond use varied strategies, from psychodynamic approaches that seek to relate the mother's attachment patterns with the type of relationship she has with her baby, to the promotion of strategies for increasing maternal sensitivity and mentalization (Santelices et al., 2010; Svanberg et al., 2010).

Pregnancy and postnatal periods provide PND screening, prevention, and intervention opportunities because of the increased assistance to health-care services for routine checkups (Sockol et al., 2013). However, PND is globally both underrecognized and undertreated (Pearlstein et al., 2009). Even when detected, women frequently do not receive assistance or do not adhere to treatments (Dennis & Chung-Lee, 2006; Rojas et al., 2015, 2018). Barriers to addressing perinatal depression have been identified at different levels (Byatt et al., 2012, 2013; Dennis & Chung-Lee, 2006; Goodman, 2009; Rojas et al., 2015). At the patient level, negative beliefs about PND and psychological treatments, stigma, fear of being judged as an unfit parent, lack of time or energy, childcare issues, lack of confidence in health-care professionals, and economic barriers have been identified. At the perinatal health-care professionals' level, lack of time, training, and knowledge on mental health have been identified. There is limited access to mental health care at the health-care system level, a long wait for appointments, and a lack of communication and continuity between perinatal and mental health providers. Therefore, there is an urgent need for friendly, easily accessible, low-cost, evidence-based interventions to reduce the burden of PND (Lee et al., 2016). To effectively address PND, the design of intervention modalities should consider treatment access barriers, mothers' preferences, available evidence, and the mother-child relationship.

8.3 Perinatal Women's Use of Internet Resources for Health Information and Advice

Worldwide, women are increasingly using the Internet as a source of health information during pregnancy and postpartum, regardless of their socioeconomic status (Guerra-Reyes et al., 2016; Osma et al., 2016; Slomian et al., 2017). Some key factors influencing information-seeking reported by perinatal women are dissatisfaction with the information provided by health professionals, lack of time to ask health professionals questions (Lagan et al., 2010), and the desire to find information "on their own" (Slomian et al., 2017). Nevertheless, studies have shown that many women perceive that the information they find on websites is not always reliable (Goetz et al., 2017). Some mothers have turned to social media, such as Facebook, to find social support (Morris, 2014) and share supposedly evidence-based information. In such cases, there is still the risk of accessing poor quality or inaccurate information (which can also quickly go viral) that may be evaluated mistakenly by women as evidence-based information and used to make health-care decisions (Dekker et al., 2016).

Studies have shown that most perinatal women, whether sampled from general populations or populations with PND symptomatology, have searched online for information on mental health (mostly on PND) and self-help strategies at least once

(Fonseca et al., 2016; Maloni et al., 2013). In the case of women with PND, peer-to-peer online forums have been found to provide social support and improve women's disclosure to health-care providers by enabling the expression of their self-stigmatization (Moore et al., 2017). Websites can also provide education about PND and its treatment, which is a significant help-seeking facilitator (Dennis & Chung-Lee, 2006). Nonetheless, studies in which experts have evaluated the content of websites that provide information on PND show a fair share of sites containing incomplete, not helpful, and even incorrect information (Moore & Ayers, 2011; Summers & Logsdon, 2005). On the other hand, the preference for websites or peer-to-peer forums has been related to women's education level. College graduates tend to gravitate toward specific websites linked to professional or academic organizations, while mothers with lower education levels tend to gravitate toward peer-to-peer forum sites (Guerra-Reyes et al., 2016). This preference might be related to women's levels of health literacy (Shieh et al., 2009).

The globally widespread presence of mobile phones has also prompted attention to smartphone apps' potential to provide information and interventions (Lal, 2019). Some advantages of these apps include the convenience of completing app assignments or other activities in people's day-to-day lives (Webb et al., 2017). An online survey conducted in Australia with women who were pregnant or had given birth to at least one child in the previous 3 years showed that almost 75% of respondents had used at least one pregnancy app, with 50% reporting using at least one parenting app (Lupton & Pedersen, 2016). In the wake of this trend, the market for health-related apps has proliferated. In China, an app store inspection allowed the detection of 6153 apps developed for maternal and child health care (Zhang et al., 2018). In Canada, a similar study found 1054 depression-related apps (Shen et al., 2015). However, available apps claiming to provide psychological psychoeducation or intervention have not usually been tested for efficacy (Schueller, 2018). The lack of evidence becomes evident when systematic reviews of studies that assess the effectiveness of apps for perinatal care or depression management identify only a small number of studies.

Thus, the Internet and digital technologies have the potential to reach an enormous number of women who are already seeking information online. Furthermore, the increasing use of Internet resources for health information is aligned with a trend today: patients are more invested in their health care, and this growing importance of "participatory health" requires innovative support (van Gemert-Pijnen et al., 2018).

8.4 Internet-Based Interventions for Mental Health Care

In response to the need to support and improve mental health conditions and mental health care and take advantage of the spread of technology, clinicians and researchers have taken advantage of the benefits of information and communication technologies. In particular, the many technologies related to the Internet are referred to as "e-mental health" (Riper et al., 2010). E-mental health involves the use of digital technologies and new media for screening, health promotion, prevention, early intervention, treatment, and relapse prevention, as well as for improving health-care provision (e.g., electronic patient files), professional education (e-learning), and online research in the field of mental health (Riper et al., 2010). Technologies that have been leveraged for e-mental health services and interventions include, among others, websites, social media, videoconferencing solutions, virtual reality, chatbots, smartphone apps (i.e., software applications developed for mobile devices), and wearable devices with sensors (Lal, 2019).

This chapter will focus on psychological interventions delivered through the Internet (i.e., Internet-based interventions (IBIs)) for e-mental health prevention and treatment. During an IBI, patients typically log into a website or smartphone app to read, watch, hear, and download materials arranged into a series of modules (Andersson, 2018; Ebert et al., 2018). They often include homework assignments and the completion of self-administered questionnaires relevant to the presenting problems, allowing to monitor their progress and outcomes (Andersson et al., 2019). IBIs can be automated (i.e., unguided) or may include some form of human support from a clinician (i.e., guided). When interventions are guided, support is usually provided through a messaging system, email, or chat.

IBIs have the potential to overcome logistical and financial barriers for the benefit of both health-care providers and patients, allowing for cost-effective interventions (Krausz et al., 2019; Paganini et al., 2018). IBIs enable patients to access at any time and from anywhere with an Internet connection; may provide a high level of anonymity and privacy (helpful in particular for people who feel stigmatized); can improve continuity of care and patient empowerment; offer flexibility in terms of standardization and personalization; and provide opportunities for easy translatability and cultural adaptability (Lal & Adair, 2014; Schröder et al., 2016). Over the past decade, this field has grown in high-income countries (Lal, 2019) and has slowly but progressively increased its presence in low- and middle-income countries (Jiménez-Molina et al., 2019; Martínez et al., 2018).

8.5 Internet-Based Interventions for Perinatal Depression Care

Over the last few years, there has been a growing effort to develop and test IBIs for PND prevention and treatment with positive outcomes. Preliminary findings from meta-analyses suggest that IBIs may effectively reduce depressive symptomatology in perinatal women. Mu et al.'s (2021) meta-analysis, which is the most recently published meta-analysis, showed that IBIs can decrease the prevalence of PND and alleviate depressive symptoms in perinatal women (overall effect size of $d = 0.64$). Their meta-analysis included seven studies, six using treatment-as-usual controls and one using a waitlist. Only one intervention was unguided, and it was the only intervention that failed to reduce depressive symptomatology. Previous meta-analyses have shown similar effect sizes, with values of 0.60 (Loughnan, Joubert, et al., 2019) and 0.59 (Lau et al., 2017). These effect sizes are similar to those reported in meta-analyses on face-to-face intervention for reducing PND symptoms (Cuijpers et al., 2007, 2021; Sockol et al., 2011). However, the number of studies identified in the meta-analyses on perinatal depression IBIs is small, and the methodological quality of those studies is mixed (Mu et al., 2021). Therefore, more studies are needed to draw more robust conclusions about their efficacy.

Women are reported as willing to participate in perinatal IBIs, independent of their age, race, income level, or having a child at home (Peragallo Urrutia et al., 2015). The same has been found when surveying women with PND (Maloni et al., 2013). Moreover, women who have participated in IBIs designed to prevent or treat PND usually find interventions helpful and positively evaluate their flexibility, accessibility, and convenience (O'Mahen et al., 2015; Pugh et al., 2016; Sawyer et al., 2019). When interventions are guided, women value therapists' assistance and are even able to perceive a strong therapeutic relationship (Pugh et al., 2016).

Nearly all efficacy studies on PND IBIs to date have been conducted in high-income countries. Most of those PND IBIs have a cognitive behavioral approach (Barrera et al., 2015; Fonseca et al., 2020; Forsell et al., 2017; Jannati et al., 2020; Loughnan, Butler, et al., 2019; Loughnan, Sie, et al., 2019; Milgrom et al., 2016; Pugh et al., 2016). Other therapeutic approaches include behavioral activation (O'Mahen, Richards, et al., 2013; O'Mahen, Woodford, et al., 2013), mindfulness (Yang et al., 2019; Sun et al., 2021), problem-solving therapy (Heller et al., 2020), or a combination of different therapeutic approaches (Haga et al., 2018; Sawyer et al., 2019). Some interventions have been adapted from existing IBIs for depression that was not perinatal specific (Heller et al., 2020; Loughnan, Butler, et al., 2019; Loughnan, Sie, et al., 2019; Pugh et al., 2016). Approximately half of the interventions are unguided (Barrera et al., 2015; Haga et al., 2018; Loughnan, Butler, et al., 2019, Loughnan, Sie, et al., 2019; Fonseca et al., 2020; Jannati et al., 2020; Sun et al., 2021). When guided, support is usually provided by a clinical psychologist. Interventions are typically divided into sequential modules (to be completed weekly) with multimedia-presented therapeutic content, accompanied by homework assignments for rehearsing the learned skills. Case examples are commonly included to illustrate therapeutic concepts. Recruitment for trials is usually carried out by advertisements on parenting websites and social media. Most interventions show promising results for reducing depressive symptoms with good levels of participant satisfaction (O'Mahen, Woodford, et al., 2013; Milgrom et al., 2016; Pugh et al., 2016; Forsell et al., 2017; Haga et al., 2018; Loughnan, Butler, et al., 2019; Loughnan, Sie, et al., 2019; Yang et al., 2019; Fonseca et al., 2020; Jannati et al., 2020; Sun et al., 2021). However, many studies showed high intervention attrition (O'Mahen, Richards, et al., 2013; Barrera et al., 2015; Forsell et al., 2017; Haga et al., 2018; Fonseca et al., 2020; Heller et al., 2020; Sun et al., 2021).

8.6 Recommendations for Researchers, Clinicians, and Policymakers

8.6.1 Internet-Based Interventions' Development Process

Although IBIs for PND have proven to be effective, attrition rates are often high and problematic even when the intervention is guided (Forsell et al., 2017; Lau et al., 2017; Lee et al., 2016; O'Mahen, Richards, et al., 2013; O'Mahen, Woodford, et al., 2013). IBIs' attrition is a common problem. A recent meta-analysis of IBIs for depression found that, on average, only 55.3% of participants completed the full intervention (Moshe et al., 2021). One issue identified to work on is how to appropriately tailor the IBI design to ensure usability, acceptability, and engagement among target users while retaining clinical effectiveness (Nicholas et al., 2017). Development methods that are only theory or expert driven have been indicated as possible causes for attrition and adoption problems (van Gemert-Pijnen et al., 2011). These methods do not include the potential end user in the development process of the IBI.

Recent research on intervention development suggests integrating theory- and expert-based approaches with other methods that promote the involvement of the user (and other possible key stakeholders) from an early stage of intervention development and throughout the different stages of the process (van Gemert-Pijnen et al., 2011). The same has been suggested by studies that have assessed mothers' use and preferences for eHealth (Guerra-Reyes et al., 2016; Ramphos et al., 2019; Walker et al., 2017). An intervention development process that creates a good fit between technological, human, and contextual factors may increase the chances of reaching its goals (van Gemert-Pijnen et al., 2011). For example, some PND IBIs were included in their development process interviews, focus groups, and usability tests with postpartum women (Danaher et al., 2012; O'Mahen et al., 2012). Likewise, future studies need to clearly describe the developmental process of the IBIs that are tested for efficacy (Lee et al., 2016). Disclosing the developmental process enhances the intervention's reproducibility, increases the validity of the study findings, and serves as a guide to other researchers who plan to develop similar interventions (Hoddinott, 2015).

The need to involve the potential end user (and other possible key stakeholders) from an early stage of intervention development not only applies to interventions delivered from scratch. It is also very important when adapting an existing evidence-based face-to-face intervention for PND to an IBI. For example, the "Mothers and Babies Course" has been evaluated in several randomized controlled trials, with evidence suggesting that it is a successful evidence-based intervention for PND prevention (Muñoz, Pineda et al., 2021). However, the IBI version of the intervention study showed high attrition and failed to demonstrate a significant reduction in PND. A subsample of participants from the clinical trial was then invited to provide feedback on the IBI to improve it (Ramphos et al., 2019). The authors of the qualitative study conclude that users have valuable input. Nevertheless, for the benefit of time and economic resources, the sooner the involvement of key stakeholders, the better. Later, the intervention can still be updated or adapted (which is a strength of IBIs), but significant changes may imply high costs.

On the other hand, designing IBIs with a persuasive systems approach is highly recommended (for a meta-analysis of the relationship between persuasive technology principles, adherence, and the effect of IBIs on mental health, see Wildeboer et al., 2016). In the persuasive systems approach, the technology is designed to reinforce, change, and shape attitudes, behaviors, or both without coercion or deception (Oinas-Kukkonen & Harjumaa, 2009). Some examples of persuasive features are the reduction and tunneling of therapeutic content (reducing online content into simple tasks, leading users), self-monitoring, and the possibility to tailor the content.

Thus, how can formative work be best guided when designing a hopefully successful intervention? The choice of methods depends on the research questions and goals of each individual project. To aid eHealth intervention developers, van Gemert-Pijnen et al. (2018) developed "the CeHRes Roadmap," a guide that offers practical and valuable suggestions derived from evidence-based strategies (including designing from user-based and persuasive approaches). The roadmap is not a prescriptive theory or approach but provides a multidisciplinary framework in which different methods and approaches can be used.

8.6.2 Cultural Adaptation of Internet-Based Interventions

Newly developing interventions for each population require significant effort. A more resource-saving possibility could be using an evidence-based existing intervention and culturally adapting it for the new target group. In such cases, evidence on traditional treatments shows that culturally adapted interventions are more effective than non-adapted versions of the intervention (Hall et al., 2016). Likewise, a greater extent of cultural adaptation seems to lead to higher effectiveness (Soto et al., 2018). IBIs have been mostly developed and evaluated in high-income countries, so for them to be implemented in low- and middle-income countries (or any culturally differing target group), they should go through a structured process of cultural adaptation. One of the benefits of IBIs is their easy cultural adaptability (Schröder et al., 2016). However, research on the cultural adaptation of IBIs for mental disorders is in its early stages, and there is a lack of studies on a direct comparison of a culturally adapted IBI with a non-adapted IBI (Spanhel et al., 2021). Nevertheless, Spanhel et al. (2021) reviewed the literature on cultural adaptations of IBIs for mental disorders and extracted 17 content, methodological, and procedural components that may provide a valuable base for future researchers to adapt IBIs systematically.

Including the end user in PND IBI development, cultural adaptation, or perinatal content adaptation (when using an existing IBI for depression that is not specific to perinatal women) is particularly relevant when addressing this target group. When addressing perinatal women at risk or with PNDs, we face not only the specific group's beliefs surrounding depression (and its treatment) but also their beliefs and expected behaviors related to motherhood and parenting. Cultural variations in motherhood and parenting beliefs and behaviors can be striking, whether observed among different groups in one society or across societies (Bornstein, 2012).

8.6.3 *The Role of Guidance in Internet-Based Interventions*

Perhaps the most significant and consistent finding regarding the impact of IBIs for depression on effectiveness is the role of guidance (Moshe et al., 2020). Karyotaki et al.'s (2021) recent "individual participant data" network meta-analysis that included 39 randomized controlled trials on IBIs for depression (including PND) demonstrated that both guided and unguided IBIs are associated with a greater reduction in depressive symptoms than treatment-as-usual and waitlist at posttreatment. Differences were maintained at 6 months and 12 months following randomization (Karyotaki et al., 2021). However, guided interventions lead to larger effect sizes than unguided interventions (Karyotaki et al., 2021). Several randomized controlled trials and meta-analyses support this finding (Baumeister et al., 2014; Moshe et al., 2021; Richards & Richardson, 2012). Indeed, guided interventions' effectiveness has been shown to be comparable to face-to-face, group, or telephone interventions, but this comparability has not been found for unguided interventions (Cuijpers et al., 2019).

One explanation for why guided interventions lead to greater therapeutic outcomes than unguided interventions is the higher level of adherence found in the first ones. Studies have found that guided interventions result in a higher number of completed modules and lower attrition than unguided interventions (Baumeister et al., 2014). Likewise, adherence has a significant influence on effect size (Moshe et al., 2021). On the other hand, for guidance to be beneficial, it seems that it is not necessary for the supporter to spend much time with each participant (contact can be minimal), to communicate synchronously, or to have much expertise (Baumeister et al., 2014; Shim et al., 2017). However, as technology further develops, improvements in automated support strategies may help to increase the adherence and effectiveness of unguided interventions (van Gemert-Pijnen et al., 2018). For example, the use of chatbots (a system that can converse and interact with human users) for mental health is an emerging promising research field (see Abd-Alrazaq et al., 2019, for a scoping review on chatbots for mental health).

Nevertheless, baseline depression is an important modifier of the relative association for the efficacy of guided vs. unguided IBIs. Karyotaki et al.'s (2021) meta-analysis found that differences between unguided and guided IBIs in people with baseline symptoms of subthreshold depression (PHQ-9 scores 5–9) were small, while guided IBIs were associated with overall better outcomes in patients with baseline moderate and severe symptoms (PHQ-9 greater than 9). These findings open new avenues for treatment decision-making. Given that individuals with mild depressive symptoms may benefit comparably from guided and unguided IBIs, the latter could be disseminated to a large number of people experiencing mild depressive symptoms at a favorable cost, with therapeutic guidance being prioritized for patients with moderate and severe symptoms (Karyotaki et al., 2021).

Moreover, unguided interventions have the potential to benefit the global community (Muñoz, Le, et al., 2021; Paganini et al., 2018). Providing face-to-face or guided IBIs for prevention or treatment all over a nation or the world to every woman at risk or presenting PND is not feasible (Muñoz, 2019). Consumable interventions are costly (Muñoz, Pineda, et al., 2021). However, unguided IBIs can be used repeatedly by an unlimited number of people anytime, anywhere, without losing their therapeutic or preventive power (Muñoz, Le, et al., 2021). Unguided IBIs could be provided at no charge to every expectant or new mother in the world as "massive open online interventions" (MOOIs), following the example of massive open online courses (MOOCs) (Muñoz et al., 2016). MOOCs are online courses available to anyone in the world, usually for free. In communities where few people have access to the Internet, health clinics could provide resource rooms where people could access MOOIs, and in remote locations where there are no clinics, local providers could use tablets, laptops, or mobile phones to share MOOIs with the people they assist (Muñoz, 2019).

8.6.4 Internet-Based Interventions' Characteristics

Therapeutic Approach IBIs for depression show no significant differences in effect sizes between different therapeutic approaches (Moshe et al., 2021). A recent meta-analysis on face-to-face, group, and guided self-help (including Internet-based) psychological interventions for PND showed the same result (Cuijpers et al., 2021). Most likely, the personalization of the components and content of the intervention is more likely to make a difference. In cognitive behavioral-based IBIs for depression, some components are more helpful than others. For example, evidence suggests that behavioral activation may be beneficial and that relaxation might be harmful (for more information about optimizing and personalizing cognitive behavioral-based IBIs for depression, see Furukawa et al., 2021). Personalization of the intervention according to the user's characteristics and specific needs can also be carried out in other ways, for example, by designing a particular group (e.g., an IBI for first-time mothers and college students), by tailoring the messages users receive, or by designing the intervention in such a way that it can be changed or set up to match user preferences (Ludden et al., 2015).

The Mother-Baby Relationship Research on face-to-face psychological interventions shows that a reduction or remission of depressive symptoms does not necessarily improve the mother-baby relationship (Murray et al., 2003, 2014; Olhaberry et al., 2013) or child development (Tsivos et al., 2015). However, when interventions for PND are aimed at improving the quality of the mother-baby interaction, significant improvements in maternal sensitivity and baby attachment may be observed (Kersten-Alvarez et al., 2011; Olhaberry, León, et al., 2015). Nevertheless, the literature shows that interventions for the prevention or treatment of PND tend to focus on depressive symptomatology reduction without including the baby or mother-baby relationship or by including them in a very minimal way (Olhaberry et al., 2013). The same has been observed with most IBIs for the prevention or treatment of PND. Considering the severe consequences of PND on the baby's affective, cognitive, and behavioral development, there is the need to stress the importance of intervening, including a mother-baby dyad approach. Moreover, this approach should be included in pregnancy, as the presence of antenatal depressive symptoms has been shown to influence the subsequent mother-infant interaction style (Binda et al., 2020). If future research concludes that IBIs for PND effectively improve the mother-baby relationship and were massively implemented, improvements in public health outcomes would be significant.

Peer-Based Support Peer support interventions have shown promising results for reducing PND symptoms and incidence of the disorder (Huang et al., 2020), even when support is provided through technology-based channels such as email or WhatsApp (Shorey et al., 2019). Transitioning to motherhood itself can cause significant disruption to social life (Lee et al., 2016), and a weak support system and social isolation are identified as predisposing factors for developing and maintaining PND (Hawes, 2020). A couple of PND IBIs have integrated peer-based support into the intervention, giving the possibility to interact with other mothers through chat or forums (Milgrom et al., 2016; O'Mahen, Woodford, et al., 2013). However, more research is needed to determine if the inclusion of this kind of support adds to the clinical efficacy of IBIs, which channels are best for interaction, and if moderation by a clinician is needed.

Intervention Length The number of intervention modules on IBIs for depression has a significant influence on effect size and adherence. A recent meta-analysis concluded that an optimal effect and maximum acceptability were achieved in interventions with approximately seven modules (Moshe et al., 2021). Longer interventions risk having higher dropout rates, and therefore, the desired outcome may be compromised. On the other hand, because a high proportion of users do not invest as much effort in IBIs as intended by their developers, some researchers have started to study shorter and more focused interventions. These kinds of interventions are called "microinterventions" (for a conceptualization of "microinterventions," see Baumel et al., 2020), and they are usually single-session interventions. They provide new ways of delivering mental health interventions to perinatal women who have difficulties engaging in longer interventions or when a highly focused objective is intended to be achieved (e.g., how to respond to a crying baby). Microinterventions could also be delivered through tablets (or other devices) in maternity hospital waiting rooms or during hospitalization after childbirth.

8.6.5 Design and Quality of Clinical Trials for Evaluating Internet-Based Interventions

More high-quality randomized controlled trials with larger samples and an examination of long-term effects are required to further assess the effectiveness of IBIs for PND (Loughnan, Joubert, et al., 2019; Zhou et al., 2020). Moshe et al. (2021) reviewed the last three decades of the Internet- and computer-based interventions for the treatment of depression (including PND) and found that nearly half of the studies were underpowered because of small sample sizes and suggested the need for 106 participants (53 in each condition) to detect a statistically significant difference with a power of 80% (t-test, alpha 5%, 1:1 allocation ratio assumed).

Additionally, the results of Moshe et al.'s (2021) meta-analysis highlight the need to use treatment-as-usual as a control (instead of the waiting list), to conduct more effective trials, to use current standards for missing data handling (e.g., using multiple imputations, mixed-effects models, or full information maximum likelihood) to lower the risk of bias, and to conduct further research into processes mediating adherence. Regarding the latter, future studies on mediators and moderators are needed to inform who benefits most from PND IBIs and who is most likely to drop out.

8.6.6 Integration of Internet-Based Interventions in Routine Care Settings

A challenge with IBIs is knowing how to integrate them into the existing pathways of care. One possibility is integrating them into a stepped-care approach (Mental Health Commission of Canada, 2014). Within stepped-care approaches, the degree of support patients receive depends on their actual individual needs. Universal screening for PND should be provided to all pregnant and postpartum women. Based on PND risk or severity and the presence of comorbidities, a decision tree can be developed with different approaches to care. IBIs could be included in the base of the chain for women at risk of developing PND and at the early stages of the disorder. Additionally, an IBI can be offered as preparation for face-to-face treatment (e.g., providing PND psychoeducation or key information about the treatment), as an adjunct to face-to-face treatment (i.e., "blended treatment"), or for relapse prevention when the treatment is completed (Newby et al., 2021). In blended treatments, patients can access the IBI between sessions, combining the strengths of both approaches (Erbe et al., 2017). Blended treatment for PND is a new field (Branquinho et al., 2020), so more research is needed to determine its benefits and for whom and in what scenarios it is suitable.

When offering an IBI, women should be provided with information that may improve the acceptance of such tools (Fonseca et al., 2016). Dissemination actions directed toward potential users include information about the benefits, costs, and efficacy results of IBIs but may also include providing the opportunity to experiment with the technology and clarify doubts about their use (Fonseca et al., 2016).

Future studies should seek to understand how IBIs can complement existing screening, diagnosis, and treatment resources for PND in health-care services, how to best implement them in such contexts, and what type of changes would be needed, for example, training for therapists (Arnberg et al., 2014; Fonseca et al., 2016).

8.7 Conclusion

Access to the Internet is growing worldwide. However, as mentioned in the previous sections, most evidence on IBIs for PND is based on high-income countries. This fact is not specific to PND, as insights from a few high-income countries account for the majority of scientific literature on e-mental health (Zale et al., 2021). Variances in economic resources, digital inequities, science investment, and cultural affinity for technology are possible explanations for the geographical distribution of the studies (Zale et al., 2021). However, in low- and middle-income countries, PND is highly prevalent and has the most significant treatment gap (Gelaye et al., 2016). Efforts are needed so that these countries can also take advantage of IBIs' benefits. One possible way to address this problem is with international collaborative research (Zale et al., 2021). More broadly, increased demand and interest due to the COVID-19 pandemic may accelerate the growth of e-mental health worldwide, resulting in a paradigm shift in the field of psychology, moving from mostly face-to-face treatments to a majority of interventions assisted by or conducted exclusively through digital means (Zale et al., 2021).

Finally, it is essential to emphasize the importance of universal screening, prevention, and early intervention strategies. Screening should focus not only on depressive symptoms but also on risk factors for identifying women who do not have detectable symptoms but are at higher risk than average. Suppose that IBIs for PND prevention and early intervention were massively implemented and that this implementation was cost-effective. In that case, the overall impact in absolute terms could be substantial, resulting in dramatic improvements in public health outcomes such as mental health, quality of life, disease burden, and cost (Rigabert et al., 2020). Tackling mental disorders before they arise in pregnant women and new mothers would aid the overall health of populations, contributing to the healthy development of their children and, conversely, the healthy development of the generations that follow (Muñoz, 2019).

Acknowledgments This work was supported by ANID – Millennium Science Initiative Program – ICS13_005. PF received funding from the Chilean National Agency for Research and Development (ANID)/Scholarship Program/DOCTORADO NACIONAL/2019–21190745. AM received funding from the Chilean National Agency for Research and Development (ANID)/Scholarship Program/DOCTORADO NACIONAL/2020–21200074.

References

Abd-Alrazaq, A. A., Alajlani, M., Alalwan, A. A., Bewick, B. M., Gardner, P., & Househ, M. (2019). An overview of the features of chatbots in mental health: A scoping review. *International Journal of Medical Informatics, 132*, 103978. https://doi.org/10.1016/j.ijmedinf.2019.103978

American College of Obstetricians and Gynecologists. (2014). *Screening for depression during and after pregnancy*. ACOG website: http://www.acog.org/

American Psychiatric Association. (2013). *Diagnostic and statistical manual of mental disorders, 5th ed.: DSM-V*. American Psychiatric Publishing.

Andersson, G. (2018). Internet interventions: Past, present and future. *Internet Interventions, 12*, 181–188. https://doi.org/10.1016/j.invent.2018.03.008

Andersson, G., Titov, N., Dear, B. F., Rozental, A., & Carlbring, P. (2019). Internet-delivered psychological treatments: From innovation to implementation. *World Psychiatry, 18*(1), 20–28. https://doi.org/10.1002/wps.20610

Arnberg, F. K., Linton, S. J., Hultcrantz, M., Heintz, E., & Jonsson, U. (2014). Internet-delivered psychological treatments for mood and anxiety disorders: A systematic review of their efficacy, safety, and cost-effectiveness. *PLoS One, 9*(5), e98118. https://doi.org/10.1371/journal.pone.0098118

Barrera, A. Z., Wickham, R. E., & Muñoz, R. F. (2015). Online prevention of postpartum depression for Spanish- and English-speaking pregnant women: A pilot randomized controlled trial. *Internet Interventions, 2*, 257–265. https://doi.org/10.1016/j.invent.2015.06.002

Baumeister, H., Reichler, L., Munzinger, M., & Lin, J. (2014). The impact of guidance on Internet-based mental health interventions – A systematic review. *Internet Interventions, 1*(4), 205–215. https://doi.org/10.1016/j.invent.2014.08.003

Baumel, A., Fleming, T., & Schueller, S. M. (2020). Digital micro interventions for behavioral and mental health gains: Core components and conceptualization of digital micro intervention care. *Journal of Medical Internet Research, 22*(10), e20631. https://doi.org/10.2196/20631

Behrendt, H. F., Scharke, W., Herpertz-Dahlmann, B., Konrad, K., & Firk, C. (2019). Like mother, like child? Maternal determinants of children's early social-emotional development. *Infant Mental Health Journal, 40*(2), 234–247. https://doi.org/10.1002/imhj.21765

beyondblue. (2011). Clinical practice guidelines for depression and related disorders – Anxiety, bipolar disorder and puerperal psychosis – in the perinatal period. In *A guideline for primary care health professionals*. beyondblue: The National Depression Initiative.

Binda, V., Figueroa, F., & Olhaberry, M. (2020). Antenatal and postnatal depressive symptoms: Association with quality of mother–infant interaction. *Infant Behavior and Development, 57*, 1–12. https://doi.org/10.1016/j.infbeh.2019.101386

Bornstein, M. H. (2012). Cultural approaches to parenting. *Parenting, 12*(2–3), 212–221. https://doi.org/10.1080/15295192.2012.683359

Bowen, A., & Muhajarine, N. (2006). Prevalence of antenatal depression in women enrolled in an outreach program in Canada. *Journal of Obstetric, Gynecologic, and Neonatal Nursing, 35*(4), 491–498. https://doi.org/10.1111/j.1552-6909.2006.00064.x

Branquinho, M., Canavarro, M. C., & Fonseca, A. (2020). A blended cognitive-behavioral intervention for the treatment of postpartum depression: Study protocol for a randomized controlled trial. *International Journal of Environmental Research and Public Health, 17*(22), 8631. https://doi.org/10.3390/ijerph17228631

Buist, A., & Janson, H. (2001). Child sexual abuse, parenting and postpartum depression – A-3-year follow up study. *Child Abuse and Neglect, 25*(7), 909–921. https://doi.org/10.1016/S0145-2134(01)00246-0

Byatt, N., Biebel, K., Friedman, L., Debordes-Jackson, G., Ziedonis, D., & Pbert, L. (2013). Patient's views on depression care in obstetric settings: How do they compare to the views of perinatal health care professionals? *General Hospital Psychiatry, 35*(6), 598–604. https://doi.org/10.1016/j.genhosppsych.2013.07.011

Byatt, N., Biebel, K., Lundquist, R. S., Moore Simas, T. A., Debordes-Jackson, G., Allison, J., & Ziedonis, D. (2012). Patient, provider, and system-level barriers and facilitators to addressing perinatal depression. *Journal of Reproductive and Infant Psychology, 30*(5), 436–449. https://doi.org/10.1080/02646838.2012.743000

Campbell, S. B., Brownell, C. A., Hungerford, A., Spieker, S. I., Mohan, R., & Blessing, J. S. (2004). The course of maternal sensitivity as predictor of attachment security at 36 months. *Development and Psychopathology, 16*, 231–252. https://doi.org/10.1017/S0954579404044499

Clatworthy, J. (2012). The effectiveness of antenatal interventions to prevent postnatal depression in high-risk women. *Journal of Affective Disorders, 137*(1–3), 25–34. https://doi.org/10.1016/j.jad.2011.02.029

Cuijpers, P., Brännmark, J. G., & van Straten, A. (2007). Psychological treatment of postpartum depression: A meta-analysis. *Journal of Clinical Psychology, 64*(1), 103–118. https://doi.org/10.1002/jclp.20432

Cuijpers, P., Franco, P., Ciharova, M., Miguel, C., Segre, L., Quero, S., & Karyotaki, E. (2021). Psychological treatment of perinatal depression: A meta-analysis. *Psychological Medicine*, 1–13. https://doi.org/10.1017/S0033291721004529

Cuijpers, P., Noma, H., Karyotaki, E., Cipriani, A., & Furukawa, T. A. (2019). Effectiveness and acceptability of cognitive behavior therapy delivery formats in adults with depression: A network meta-analysis. *JAMA Psychiatry, 76*(7), 700–707. https://doi.org/10.1001/jamapsychiatry.2019.0268

Danaher, B. G., Milgrom, J., Seeley, J. R., Stuart, S., Schembri, C., Tyler, M. S., Ericksen, J., Lester, W., Gemmill, A. W., & Lewinsohn, P. (2012). Web-based intervention for postpartum depression: Formative research and design of the MomMoodBooster program. *JMIR Research Protocols, 1*(2), e2329. https://doi.org/10.2196/resprot.2329

Deave, T., Heron, J., Evans, J., & Emond, A. (2008). The impact of maternal depression in pregnancy on early child development. *BJOG an International Journal of Obstetrics and Gynecology, 115*, 1043–1051. https://doi.org/10.1111/j.1471-0528.2008.01752.x

Dekker, R. L., King, S., & Lester, K. (2016). Social media and evidence-based maternity care: A cross-sectional survey study. *The Journal of Perinatal Education, 25*(2), 105–115. https://doi.org/10.1891/1058-1243.25.2.105

Dennis, C. L., & Chung-Lee, L. (2006). Postpartum depression help-seeking barriers and maternal treatment preferences: A qualitative systematic review. *Birth, 33*(4), 323–331. https://doi.org/10.1111/j.1523-536X.2006.00130.x

Diego, M., Field, T., Hernandez-Reif, M., Schanberg, S., Kuhn, C., & Gonzalez-Quintero, V. H. (2009). Prenatal depression restricts fetal growth. *Early Human Development, 85*, 65–70. https://doi.org/10.1016/j.earlhumdev.2008.07.002

Ebert, D. D., Buntrock, C., Lehr, D., Smit, F., Riper, H., Baumeister, H., Cuijpers, P., & Berking, M. (2018). Effectiveness of web- and mobile-based treatment of subthreshold depression with adherence-focused guidance: A single-blind randomized controlled trial. *Behavior Therapy, 49*(1), 71–83. https://doi.org/10.1016/j.beth.2017.05.004

Emory, E. K., & Dieter, J. N. (2006). Maternal depression and psychotropic medication effects on the human fetus. *Annals of the NY Academy of Sciences, 1094*, 287–291. https://doi.org/10.1196/annals.1376.036

Erbe, D., Eichert, H. C., Riper, H., & Ebert, D. D. (2017). Blending face-to-face and internet-based interventions for the treatment of mental disorders in adults: Systematic review. *Journal of Medical Internet Research, 19*(9), e306. https://doi.org/10.2196/jmir.6588

Faisal-Cury, A., & Rossi Menezes, P. (2007). Prevalence of anxiety and depression during pregnancy in a private setting sample. *Archives of Women's Mental Health, 10*(1), 25–32. https://doi.org/10.1007/s00737-006-0164-6

Fekadu Dadi, A., Miller, E. R., & Mwanri, L. (2020). Antenatal depression and its association with adverse birth outcomes in low and middle-income countries: A systematic review and meta-analysis. *PLoS One, 15*(1), e0227323. https://doi.org/10.1371/journal.pone.0227323

Ferrari, A. J., Charlson, F. J., Norman, R. E., Patten, S. B., Murray, C. J. L., Vos, T., & Whiteford, H. A. (2013). Burden of depressive disorders by country, sex, age, and year: Findings from the global burden of disease study 2010. *PLoS Medicine, 10*, e1001547. https://doi.org/10.1371/journal.pmed.1001547

Field, T. (2011). Prenatal depression effects on development. *Infant Behavior and Development, 34*, 1–14. https://doi.org/10.1016/j.infbeh.2010.09.008

Field, T. (2017a). Prenatal depression risk factors, developmental effects and interventions: A review. *Journal of Pregnancy and Child Health, 4*(1), 301. https://doi.org/10.4172/2376-127X.1000301

Field, T. (2017b). Postpartum depression effects, risk factors and interventions: A review. *Clinical Depression, 3*(1), 122. https://doi.org/10.4172/2572-0791.1000122

Figueiredo, B., & Conde, A. (2011). Anxiety and depression symptoms in women and men from early pregnancy to 3-months postpartum: Parity differences and effects. *Journal of Affective Disorders, 132*, 146–157. https://doi.org/10.1016/j.jad.2011.02.007

Fisher, J., Cabral de Mello, M., Patel, V., Rahman, A., Tran, T., Holton, S., & Holmes, W. (2012). Prevalence and determinants of common perinatal mental disorders in women in low- and lower-middle-income countries: A systematic review. *Bulletin of the World Health Organization, 90*, 139–149. https://doi.org/10.2471/BLT.11.091850

Fitelson, E., Kim, S., Baker, A. S., & Leight, K. (2010). Treatment of postpartum depression: Clinical, psychological and pharmacological options. *International Journal of Women's Health, 3*, 1–14. https://doi.org/10.2147/IJWH.S6938

Fonseca, A., Alves, S., Monteiro, F., Gorayeb, R., & Canavarro, M. C. (2020). Be a Mom, a web-based intervention to prevent postpartum depression: Results from a pilot randomized controlled trial. *Behavior Therapy, 51*(4), 616–633. https://doi.org/10.1016/j.beth.2019.09.007

Fonseca, A., Gorayeb, R., & Canavarro, M. C. (2016). Women's use of online resources and acceptance of e-mental health tools during the perinatal period. *International Journal of Medical Informatics, 94*, 228–236. https://doi.org/10.1016/j.ijmedinf.2016.07.016

Forsell, E., Bendix, M., Holländare, F., Szymanska von Schutz, B., Nasiell, J., Blomdadahl-Wetterholm, M., Ericksson, C., Kvarned, S., Lindau van der Linden, J., Södeberg, E., Jokinen, J., Wide, K., & Kaldo, V. (2017). Internet delivered cognitive behavior therapy for antenatal depression: A randomised controlled trial. *Journal of Affective Disorders, 221*, 56–64. https://doi.org/10.1016/j.jad.2017.06.013

Fox, M., & Borelli, J. (2015). Attachment moderates the association between mother and child depressive symptoms. *Psi Chi Journal of Psychological Research, 20*(1), 29–36. https://doi.org/10.24839/2164-8204.JN20.1.29

Furukawa, T. A., Suganuma, A., Ostinelli, E. G., Andersson, G., Beevers, C. G., Shumake, J., Berger, T., Boele, F. W., Buntrock, C., Carlbring, P., Choi, I., Christensen, H., Mackinnon, A., Dahne, J., Huibers, M. J. H., Ebert, D. D., Farrer, L., Forand, N. R., Strunk, D. R., et al. (2021). Dismantling, optimising and personalising internet cognitive-behavioural therapy for depression: A systematic review and individual participant data component network meta-analysis. *Lancet Psychiatry, 8*, 500–511. https://doi.org/10.1016/S2215-0366(21)00077-8

Gelaye, B., Rondon, M. B., Araya, R., & Williams, M. A. (2016). Epidemiology of maternal depression, risk factors, and child outcomes in low-income and middle-income countries. *The Lancet Psychiatry, 3*(10), 973–982. https://doi.org/10.1016/S2215-0366(16)30284-X

Goetz, M., Müller, M., Matthies, L. M., Hansen, J., Doster, A., Szabo, A., Pauluschke-Fröhlich, J., Abele, H., Sohn, C., Wallwiener, M., & Wallwiener, S. (2017). Perceptions of patient engagement applications during pregnancy: A qualitative assessment of the patient's perspective. *JMIR mHealth and uHealth, 5*(5), e73. https://doi.org/10.2196/mhealth.7040

Goodman, J. H. (2009). Women's attitudes, preferences, and perceived barriers to treatment for perinatal depression. *Birth, 36*(1), 60–69. https://doi.org/10.1111/j.1523-536X.2008.00296.x

Grace, S. L., Evindar, A., & Stewart, D. (2003). The effect of postpartum depression on child cognitive development and behavior: A review and critical analysis of the literature. *Archives of Women's Mental Health, 6*, 263–274. https://doi.org/10.1007/s00737-003-0024-6

Guerra-Reyes, L., Christie, V. M., Prabhakar, A., Harris, A. L., & Siek, K. A. (2016). Postpartum health information seeking using mobile phones: Experiences of low-income mothers. *Maternal and Child Health Journal, 20*(1), 13–21. https://doi.org/10.1007/s10995-016-2185-8

Haga, S. M., Drozd, F., Lisoy, C., Wentzel-Lrsen, T., & Slinning, K. (2018). Mamma Mia – A randomized controlled trial of internet-based intervention for perinatal depression. *Psychological Medicine, 48*, 1850–1857. https://doi.org/10.1017/S0033291718002544

Hahn-Holbrook, J., Cornwell-Hinrichs, T., & Anaya, I. (2018). Economic and health predictors of national postpartum depression prevalence: A systematic review, meta-analysis, and meta-regression of 291 studies from 56 countries. *Frontiers in Psychiatry, 8*(248), 1–23. https://doi.org/10.3389/fpsyt.2017.00248

Halbreich, U., & Karkun, S. (2006). Cross-cultural and social diversity of prevalence of postpartum depression and depressive symptoms. *Journal of Affective Disorders, 91*, 97–111. https://doi.org/10.1016/j.jad.2005.12.051

Hall, G. C. N., Ibaraki, A. Y., Huang, E. R., Marti, C. N., & Stice, E. (2016). A meta-analysis of cultural adaptations of psychological interventions. *Behavior Therapy, 47*(6), 993–1014. https://doi.org/10.1016/j.beth.2016.09.005

Hawes, C. G. (2020). The role of social isolation as a predetermining factor for postpartum depression development: A literature review. https://doi.org/10.17615/wy71-h444

Hayes, L. J., Goodman, S. H., & Carlson, E. (2013). Maternal antenatal depression and infant disorganized attachment at 12 months. *Attachment & Human Development, 15*(2), 133–153. https://doi.org/10.1080/14616734.2013.743256

Heller, H. M., Hoogendoorn, A. W., Honig, A., Broekman, B. F., & van Straten, A. (2020). The effectiveness of a guided internet-based tool for the treatment of depression and anxiety in pregnancy (MamaKits online): Randomized controlled trial. *Journal of Medical Internet Research, 22*(3), e15172. https://doi.org/10.2196/15172

Hoddinott, P. (2015). A new era for intervention development studies. *Pilot and Feasibility Studies, 1*(36), 1–4. https://doi.org/10.1186/s40814-015-0032-0

Hompoth, E. A., Pető, Z., Balogh, V. F., & Töreki, A. (2020). Associations between depression symptoms, psychological intervention and perinatal complications. *Journal of Clinical Psychology in Medical Settings, 27*(1), 199–205. https://doi.org/10.1007/s10880-019-09632-4

Huang, R., Yan, C., Tian, Y., Lei, B., Yang, D., Liu, D., & Lei, J. (2020). Effectiveness of peer support intervention on perinatal depression: A systematic review and meta-analysis. *Journal of Affective Disorders, 276*, 788–796. https://doi.org/10.1016/j.jad.2020.06.048

Huynh-Nhu, L., Perry, D., Genovez, M., & Cardeli, E. (2013). In their own voices: Latinas' experiences with a randomized controlled trial. *Qualitative Health Research, 23*, 834–846. https://doi.org/10.1177/1049732313482591

Jannati, N., Mazhari, S., Ahmadian, L., & Mirzaee, M. (2020). Effectiveness of an app-based cognitive behavioral therapy program for postpartum depression in primary care: A randomized controlled trial. *International Journal of Medical Informatics, 141*, 104145. https://doi.org/10.1016/j.ijmedinf.2020.104145

Jiménez-Molina, Á., Franco, P., Martínez, V., Martínez, P., Rojas, G., & Araya, R. (2019). Internet-based interventions for the prevention and treatment of mental disorders in Latin America: A scoping review. *Frontiers in Psychiatry, 10*, 1–9. https://doi.org/10.3389/fpsyt.2019.00664

Karyotaki, E., Efthimiou, O., Miguel, C., Bermpohl, F. M. G., Furukawa, T. A., Cuijpers, P., Individual Patient Data Meta-Analyses for Depression (IPDMA-DE) Collaboration, Riper, H., Patel, V., Mira, A., Gemmil, A. W., Yeung, A. S., Lange, A., Williams, A. D., Mackinnon, A., Geraedts, A., van Straten, A., Meyer, B., Björkelund, C., Knaevelsrud, C., Beevers, C. G., Botella, C., Strunk, D. R., Mohr, D. C., Ebert, D. D., Kessler, D., et al. (2021). Internet-based cognitive behavioral therapy for depression: A systematic review and individual patient data network meta-analysis. *JAMA Psychiatry, 78*(4), 361–371. https://doi.org/10.1001/jamapsychiatry.2020.4364

Kersten-Alvarez, L. E., Hosman, C. M., Riksen-Walraven, J. M., Van Doesum, K. T., & Hoefnagels, C. (2011). Which preventive interventions effectively enhance depressed mothers' sensitivity? A meta-analysis. *Infant Mental Health Journal, 32*(3), 362–376. https://doi.org/10.1002/imhj.20301

Knight, M., Bunch, K., Tuffnell, D., Shakespeare, J., Kotnis, R., Kenyon, S. & Kurinczuk, J.J. (Eds.) (2019) on behalf of MBRRACE-UK. Saving Lives, Improving Mothers' Care – Lessons learned to inform maternity care from the UK and Ireland Confidential Enquiries into Maternal Deaths and Morbidity 2015-17. : National Perinatal Epidemiology Unit, University of Oxford.

Koutra, K., Vassilaki, M., Georgiou, V., Koutis, A., Bitsios, P., Chatzi, L., & Kogevinas, M. (2014). Antenatal maternal mental health as determinant of postpartum depression in a population-based mother-child cohort (Rhea Study) in Crete, Greece. *Social Psychiatry and Psychiatric Epidemiology, 49*(5), 711–721. https://doi.org/10.1007/s00127-013-0758-z

Kozinsky, Z., Dudas, R., Devosa, I., Csatordai, S., Tóth, E., Szabó, D., Sikovanyecz, J., Barabás, K., & Pal, A. (2012). Can a brief antepartum preventive group intervention help reduce postpartum depressive symptomatology? *Psychotherapy and Psychosomatics, 81*, 98–107. https://doi.org/10.1159/000330035

Krausz, R. M., Ramsey, D., Wetterlin, F., Tabiova, K., & Thapliyal, A. (2019). Accessible and cost-effective mental health care using E-Mental Health (EMH). In A. Javed & K. N. Fountoulakis (Eds.), *Advances in Psychiatry*. Springer. https://doi.org/10.1007/978-3-319-70554-5_8

Ladyman, C., Signal, T. L., Sweeney, B., Gander, P., Paine, S. J., & Huthwaite, M. (2020). A pilot longitudinal sleep education intervention from early pregnancy and its effect on optimizing sleep and minimizing depressive symptoms. *Sleep Health, 6*(6), 778–786. https://doi.org/10.1016/j.sleh.2020.05.001

Lagan, B. M., Sinclair, M., & George Kernohan, W. (2010). Internet use in pregnancy informs women's decision making: A web-based survey. *Birth, 37*(2), 106–115. https://doi.org/10.1111/j.1523-536X.2010.00390.x

Lal, S. (2019). E-mental health: Promising advancements in policy, research, and practice. *Healthcare Management Forum, 32*(2), 56–62. https://doi.org/10.1177/0840470418818583

Lal, S., & Adair, C. E. (2014). E-mental health: A rapid review of the literature. *Psychiatric Services, 65*(1), 24–32. https://doi.org/10.1176/appi.ps.201300009

Lara, M. A., Navarro, C., & Navarrete, L. (2010). Outcome results of a psycho-educational intervention in pregnancy to prevent PPD: A randomized control trial. *Journal of Affective Disorders, 122*, 109–117. https://doi.org/10.1016/j.jad.2009.06.024

Lau, Y., Htun, T. P., Wong, S. N., Tam, W. S. W., & Klainin-Yobas, P. (2017). Therapist-supported internet-based cognitive behavior therapy for stress, anxiety, and depressive symptoms among postpartum women: A systematic review and meta-analysis. *Journal of Medical Internet Research, 19*(4), e138. https://doi.org/10.2196/jmir.6712

Lee, E. W., Denison, F. C., Hor, K., & Reynolds, R. M. (2016). Web-based interventions for prevention and treatment of perinatal mood disorders: A systematic review. *BMC Pregnancy and Childbirth, 16*(1), 38. https://doi.org/10.1186/s12884-016-0831-1

Lefkovics, E., Rigó, J., Jr., Kovács, I., Talabér, J., Szita, B., Kecskeméti, A., Szabó, L., Somogyvári, Z., & Baji, I. (2018). Effect of maternal depression and anxiety on mother's perception of child and the protective role of social support. *Journal of Reproductive and Infant Psychology, 36*(4), 434–448. https://doi.org/10.1080/02646838.2018.1475726

Letourneau, N. L., Dennis, C. L., Cosic, N., & Linder, J. (2017). The effect of perinatal depression treatment for mothers on parenting and child development: A systematic review. *Depression and Anxiety, 34*(10), 928–966. https://doi.org/10.1002/da.22687

Loughnan, S. A., Butler, C., Sie, A. A., Grierson, A. B., Chen, A. Z., Hobbs, M. J., Joubert, A., Haskelberg, H., Mahoney, A., Holt, C., Gennill, A. W., Milgrom, J., Austin, M. P., Andrews, G., & Newby, J. M. (2019). A randomised controlled trial of 'MUMentum postnatal': Internet-delivered cognitive behavioural therapy for anxiety and depression in postpartum women. *Behaviour Research and Therapy, 116*, 94–103. https://doi.org/10.1016/j.brat.2019.03.001

Loughnan, S. A., Joubert, A. E., Grierson, A., Andrews, G., & Newby, J. M. (2019). Internet-Delivered psychological interventions for clinical anxiety and depression in perinatal women:

A systematic review and meta-analysis. *Archives of Women's Mental Health, 22*(6), 737–750. https://doi.org/10.1007/s00737-019-00961-9

Loughnan, S. A., Sie, A., Hobbs, M. J., Joubert, A. E., Smith, J., Haskelberg, H., Mahoney, A. E. J., Kladnitski, N., Holt, C. J., Milgrom, J., Austin, M., Andrews, G., & Newby, J. M. (2019). A randomized controlled trial of 'MUMentum Pregnancy': Internet-delivered cognitive behavioral therapy program for antenatal anxiety and depression. *Journal of Affective Disorders, 243*, 381–390. https://doi.org/10.1016/j.jad.2018.09.057

Lucena, L., Frange, C., Pinto, A. C. A., Andersen, M. L., Tufik, S., & Hachul, H. (2020). Mindfulness interventions during pregnancy: A narrative review. *Journal of Integrative Medicine, 18*(6), 470–477. https://doi.org/10.1016/j.joim.2020.07.007

Ludden, G. D., Van Rompay, T. J., Kelders, S. M., & van Gemert-Pijnen, J. E. (2015). How to increase reach and adherence of web-based interventions: A design research viewpoint. *Journal of Medical Internet Research, 17*(7), e4201. https://doi.org/10.2196/jmir.4201

Lupton, D., & Pedersen, S. (2016). An Australian survey of women's use of pregnancy and parenting apps. *Women and Birth, 29*(4), 368–375. https://doi.org/10.1016/j.wombi.2016.01.008

Maloni, J. A., Przeworski, A., & Damato, E. G. (2013). Web recruitment and Internet use and preferences reported by women with postpartum depression after pregnancy complications. *Archives of Psychiatric Nursing, 27*(2), 90–95. https://doi.org/10.1016/j.apnu.2012.12.001

Martínez, P., Rojas, G., Martínez, V., Lara, M. A., & Pérez, J. C. (2018). Internet-based interventions for the prevention and treatment of depression in people living in developing countries: A systematic review. *Journal of Affective Disorders, 234*, 193–200. https://doi.org/10.1016/j.jad.2018.02.079

Martins, C., & Gaffan, E. (2000). Effects of early maternal depression on patterns of infant-mother attachment: A meta-analytic investigation. *Journal of Child Psychology and Psychiatry, 41*, 737–746. https://doi.org/10.1111/1469-7610.00661

McMahon, C. A., Barnett, B., Kowalenko, N. M., & Tennant, C. C. (2006). Maternal attachment state of mind moderates the impact of postnatal depression on infant attachment. *The Journal of Child Psychology and Psychiatry and Allied Disciplines, 47*, 660–669. https://doi.org/10.1111/j.1469-7610.2005.01547.x

Mental Health Commission of Canada. (2014). *E-mental health in Canada: Transforming the mental health system using technology*. Mental Health Commission of Canada website: https://www.mentalhealthcommission.ca/

Milgrom, J., Danaher, B. G., Gemmill, A. W., Holt, C., Holt, C. J., Seeley, J. R., Tyler, M. S., Ross, J., & Ericksen, J. (2016). Internet cognitive behavioral therapy for women with postnatal depression: A randomized controlled trial of MumMoodBooster. *Journal of Medical Internet Research, 18*(3), e54. https://doi.org/10.2196/jmir.4993

Milgrom, J., Gemmill, A., & Bilszt, J. (2008). Antenatal risk factors for postnatal depression: A large prospective study. *Journal of Affective Disorders, 108*, 147–157. https://doi.org/10.1016/j.jad.2007.10.014

Milgrom, J., Schembri, C., Ericksen, J., Ross, J., & Gemmill, A. (2011). Towards parenthood: An antenatal intervention to reduce depression, anxiety and parenting difficulties. *Journal of Affective Disorders, 130*, 385–394. https://doi.org/10.1016/j.jad.2010.10.045

Ministerio de Salud. (2014). *Protocolo de detección de la depresión durante el embarazo y posparto y apoyo al tratamiento*. MINSAL. Minsal website: https://www.minsal.cl/sites/default/files/files/ProtocoloProgramaEmbarazoypospartofinal12032014.pdf

Molenaar, N. M., Kamperman, A. M., Boyce, P., & Bergink, V. (2018). Guidelines on treatment of perinatal depression with antidepressants: An international review. *The Australian and New Zealand Journal of Psychiatry, 52*(4), 320–327. https://doi.org/10.1177/0004867418762057

Moore, D., & Ayers, S. (2011). A review of postnatal mental health websites: Help for healthcare professionals and patients. *Archives of Women's Mental Health, 14*(6), 443–452. https://doi.org/10.1007/s00737-011-0245-z

Moore, D., Drey, N., & Ayers, S. (2017). Use of online forums for perinatal mental illness, stigma, and disclosure: An exploratory model. *JMIR Mental Health, 4*(1). https://doi.org/10.2196/mental.5926

Morris, M. R. (2014). Social networking site use by mothers of young children. In *Proceedings of the 17th ACM conference on Computer supported cooperative work & social computing* (pp. 1272–1282). https://doi.org/10.1145/2531602.2531603

Moshe, I., Terhorst, Y., Cuijpers, P., Cristea, I., Pulkki-Råback, L., & Sander, L. (2020). Three decades of Internet-and computer-based interventions for the treatment of depression: Protocol for a systematic review and meta-analysis. *JMIR Research Protocols, 9*(3), e14860. https://doi.org/10.2196/14860

Moshe, I., Terhorst, Y., Philippi, P., Domhardt, M., Cuijpers, P., Cristea, I., Pulkki-Råback, L., Baumeister, H., & Sander, L. B. (2021). Digital interventions for the treatment of depression: A meta-analytic review. *Psychological Bulletin, 147*(8), 749–786. https://doi.org/10.1037/bul0000334

Mu, T. Y., Li, Y. H., Xu, R. X., Chen, J., Wang, Y. Y., & Shen, C. Z. (2021). Internet-based interventions for postpartum depression: A systematic review and meta-analysis. *Nursing Open, 8*(3), 1125–1134. https://doi.org/10.1002/nop2.724

Muñoz, R. F. (2019). Prevent depression in pregnancy to boost all mental health. https://doi.org/10.1038/d41586-019-03226-8

Muñoz, R. F., Bunge, E. L., Chen, K., Schueller, S. M., Bravin, J. I., Shaughnessy, E. A., & Pérez-Stable, E. J. (2016). Massive open online interventions: A novel model for delivering behavioral-health services worldwide. *Clinical Psychological Science, 4*(2), 194–205. https://doi.org/10.1177/2167702615583840

Muñoz, R. F., Le, H. N., Barrera, A. Z., & Pineda, B. S. (2021). Leading the charge toward a world without depression: Perinatal depression can be prevented. *Archives of Women's Mental Health, 24*(5), 807–815. https://doi.org/10.1007/s00737-021-01160-1

Muñoz, R. F., Pineda, B. S., Barrera, A. Z., Bunge, E., & Leykin, Y. (2021). Digital tools for prevention and treatment of depression: Lessons from the Institute for International Internet Interventions for Health. *Clinical and Health, 32*(1), 37–40. https://doi.org/10.5093/clysa2021a2

Murray, L., Cooper, P., & Fearon, P. (2014). Parenting difficulties and postnatal depression: Implications for primary healthcare assessment and intervention. *Community Practitioner, 87*(11), 34–38. PMID: 25612413.

Murray, L., Cooper, P., Wilson, A., & Romaniuk, H. (2003). Controlled trial of the short and long-term effect of psychological treatment of postpartum depression. Impact on the mother–child relationship and child outcome. *British Journal of Psychiatry, 182*, 420–427. https://doi.org/10.1192/bjp.182.5.420

Nelson, E. C., Heath, A. C., Madden, P. A., Cooper, M. L., Dinwiddie, S. H., Bucholz, K. K., Glowinski, A., McLaughlin, T., Dunne, M. P., Statham, D. J., & Martin, N. G. (2002). Association between self-reported childhood sexual abuse and adverse psychosocial outcomes: Results from a twin study. *Archives of General Psychiatry, 59*(2), 139–145. https://doi.org/10.1001/archpsyc.59.2.139

Newby, J., Mason, E., Kladnistki, N., Murphy, M., Millard, M., Haskelberg, H., et al. (2021). Integrating internet CBT into clinical practice: A practical guide for clinicians. *Clinical Psychologist, 25*(2), 164–178. https://doi.org/10.1080/13284207.2020.1843968

Nicholas, J., Huckvale, K., Larsen, M. E., Basu, A., Batterham, P. J., Shaw, F., & Sendi, S. (2017). Issues for eHealth in psychiatry: Results of an expert survey. *Journal of Medical Internet Research, 19*(2), e55. https://doi.org/10.2196/jmir.6957

O'Connor, E., Rossom, R. C., Henninger, M., Groom, H. C., & Burda, B. U. (2016). Primary care screening for and treatment of depression in pregnant and postpartum women: Evidence report and systematic review for the US Preventive Services Task Force. *JAMA, 315*(4), 388–406. https://doi.org/10.1001/jama.2015.18948

O'Hara, M. W., & McCabe, J. E. (2013). Postpartum depression: Current status and future directions. *Annual Review of Clinical Psychology, 9*(1), 379–407. https://doi.org/10.1146/annurev-clinpsy-050212-185612

O'Mahen, H., Fedock, G., Henshaw, E., Himle, J. A., Forman, J., & Flynn, H. A. (2012). Modifying CBT for perinatal depression: What do women want?: A qualitative study. *Cognitive and Behavioral Practice, 19*(2), 359–371. https://doi.org/10.1016/j.cbpra.2011.05.005

O'Mahen, H. A., Grieve, H., Jones, J., McGinley, J., Woodford, J., & Wilkinson, E. L. (2015). Women's experiences of factors affecting treatment engagement and adherence in internet delivered behavioural activation for postnatal depression. *Internet Interventions, 2*(1), 84–90. https://doi.org/10.1016/j.invent.2014.11.003

O'Mahen, H. A., Richards, D. A., Woodford, J., Wilkinson, E., McGinley, J., Taylor, R. S., & Warren, F. C. (2013). Netmums: A phase II randomized controlled trial of a guided Internet behavioural activation treatment for postpartum depression. *Psychological Medicine, 44*(8), 1675–1689. https://doi.org/10.1017/S0033291713002092

O'Mahen, H. A., Woodford, J., McGinley, J., Warren, F. C., Richardson, D. A., Lynch, T. R., & Tylor, R. S. (2013). Internet-based behavioral activation-Treatment for postnatal depression (Netmums): A randomized controlled trial. *Journal of Affective Disorders, 150*, 814–822. https://doi.org/10.1016/j.jad.2013.03.005

Oinas-Kukkonen, H., & Harjumaa, M. (2009). Persuasive systems design: Key issues, process model, and system features. *Communications of the Association for Information Systems, 24*(1), 28. https://doi.org/10.17705/1CAIS.02428

Olhaberry, M., Escobar, M., Mena, C., Santelices, P., Morales-Reyes, I., Rojas, G., & Martínez, V. (2015). Intervención grupal para reducir la sintomatología depresiva y promover la sensibilidad materna en embarazadas chilenas. *Revista SUMA Psicológica, Konrad Lorenz, 22*, 93–101. https://doi.org/10.1016/j.sumpsi.2015.08.002

Olhaberry, M., Escobar, M., San Cristobal, P., Santelices, P., Farkas, C., Rojas, G., & Martínez, V. (2013). Intervenciones psicológicas perinatales en depresión materna y vínculo madre-bebé: Una revisión sistemática. *Terapia Psicológica, 31*(2), 249–261. https://doi.org/10.4067/S0718-48082013000200011

Olhaberry, M., León, M. J., Seguel, M., & Mena, C. (2015). Video-feedback intervention in mother-baby dyads with depressive symptomatology and relationship difficulties. *Research in Psychotherapy: Psychopathology, Process and Outcome, 18*(2), 82–92. https://doi.org/10.4081/ripppo.2015.177

Olhaberry, M., Zapata, J., Escobar, M., Mena, C., Farkas, C., Santelices, P., & Krause, M. (2014). Antenatal depression and its relationship with problem-solving strategies, childhood abuse, social support, and attachment styles in a low-income Chilean sample. *Mental Health & Prevention, 2*(3-4), 86–97. https://doi.org/10.1016/j.mhp.2014.09.001

Osma, J., Barrera, A. Z., & Ramphos, E. (2016). Are pregnant and postpartum women interested in health-related apps? Implications for the prevention of perinatal depression. *Cyberpsychology, Behavior and Social Networking, 19*(6), 412–415. https://doi.org/10.1089/cyber.2015.0549

Paganini, S., Teigelkoetter, W., Buntrock, C., & Baumeister, H. (2018). Economic evaluations of internet-and mobile-based interventions for the treatment and prevention of depression: A systematic review. *Journal of Affective Disorders, 225*, 733–755. https://doi.org/10.1016/j.jad.2017.07.018

Pawlby, S., Hay, D., Sharp, D., Waters, C., & O'Keane, V. (2009). Antenatal depression predicts depression in adolescent offspring: Prospective longitudinal community-based study. *Journal of Affective Disorders, 113*, 236–243. https://doi.org/10.1016/j.jad.2008.05.018

Pearlstein, T., Howard, M., Salisbury, A., & Zlotnick, C. (2009). Postpartum depression. *American Journal of Obstetrics and Gynecology, 200*(4), 357–364. https://doi.org/10.1016/j.ajog.2008.11.033

Pearson, R. M., Melotti, R., Heron, J., Joinson, C., Stein, A., Ramchandani, P. G., & Evans, J. (2012). Disruption to the development of maternal responsiveness? The impact of prenatal depression on mother-infant interactions. *Infant Behavior and Development, 35*, 613–626. https://doi.org/10.1016/j.infbeh.2012.07.020

Peragallo Urrutia, R. P., Berger, A. A., Ivins, A. A., Urrutia, E. G., Beckham, A. J., Thorp, J. M., Jr., & Nicholson, W. K. (2015). Internet use and access among pregnant women via computer and mobile phone: Implications for delivery of perinatal care. *JMIR mHealth and uHealth, 3*(1), e25. https://doi.org/10.2196/mhealth.3347

PMMRC. (2016). *Tenth annual report of the Perinatal and Maternal Mortality Review Committee: Reporting mortality 2014.* Health Quality & Safety Commission.

Pugh, N. E., Hadjistavropoulos, H. D., & Dirkse, D. (2016). A randomised controlled trial of therapist-assisted, internet-delivered cognitive behavior therapy for women with maternal depression. *PLoS One, 11*(3), e0149186. https://doi.org/10.1371/journal.pone.0149186

Ramphos, E. S., Kelman, A. R., Stanley, M. L., & Barrera, A. Z. (2019). Responding to women's needs and preferences in an online program to prevent postpartum depression. *Internet Interventions, 18*, 100275. https://doi.org/10.1016/j.invent.2019.100275

Raskin, M., Easterbrooks, M. A., Lamoreau, R. N., Chie Kotake, B. A., & Goldberg, J. (2016). Depression Trajectories of Antenatally Depressed and Non-depressed Young Mothers: Implications for Child Socioemotional Development. *Women's Health Issues, 26*, 344–350. https://doi.org/10.1016/j.whi.2016.02.002

Richards, D., & Richardson, T. (2012). Computer-based psychological treatments for depression: A systematic review and meta-analysis. *Clinical Psychology Review, 32*(4), 329–342. https://doi.org/10.1016/j.cpr.2012.02.004

Rigabert, A., Motrico, E., Moreno-Peral, P., Resurrección, D. M., Conejo-Cerón, S., Cuijpers, P., Martín-Gómez, C., López-Del-Hoyo, Y., & Bellón, J. Á. (2020). Effectiveness of online psychological and psychoeducational interventions to prevent depression: Systematic review and meta-analysis of randomized controlled trials. *Clinical Psychology Review, 82*, 101931. https://doi.org/10.1016/j.cpr.2020.101931

Riper, H., Andersson, G., Christensen, H., Cuijpers, P., Lange, A., & Eysenbach, G. (2010). Theme issue on e-Mental health: A growing field in internet research: Editorial. *Journal of Medical Internet Research, 12*(5), e74. https://doi.org/10.2196/jmir.1713

Rojas, G., Guajardo, V., Martínez, P., & Fritsch, R. (2018). Depresión posparto: Tamizaje, uso de servicios y barreras para su tratamiento en centros de atención primaria. *Revista Médica de Chile, 146*(9), 1001–1007. https://doi.org/10.4067/s0034-98872018000901001

Rojas, G., Santelices, M. P., Martínez, P., Tomicic, A., Reinel, M., Olhaberry, M., & Krause, M. (2015). Barreras de acceso a tratamiento de la depresión posparto en Centros de Atención Primaria de la Región Metropolitana: Un estudio cualitativo. *Revista Médica de Chile, 143*(4), 424–432. https://doi.org/10.4067/S0034-98872015000400002

Rollè, L., Prino, L. E., Sechi, C., Vismara, L., Neri, E., Polizzi, C., Trovato, A., Volpi, B., Molgora, S., Fenaroli, V., Lerardi, E., Ferro, V., Lucarelli, L., Agostini, F., Tambelli, R., Saita, E., Riva Crugnola, C., & Brustia, P. (2017). Parenting stress, mental health, dyadic adjustment: A structural equation model. *Frontiers in Psychology, 8*, 1–10. https://doi.org/10.3389/fpsyg.2017.00839

Santelices, M., Guzmán, M., Aracena, M., Farkas, C., Armijo, I., Pérez-Salas, C., & Borghini, A. (2010). Promoting secure attachment: Evaluation of the effectiveness of an early intervention pilot programme with mother-infant dyads in Santiago, Chile. *Child: Care, Health and Development, 37*(2), 203–2010. https://doi.org/10.1111/j.1365-2214.2010.01161.x

Sawyer, A., Kaim, A., Le, H. N., McDonald, D., Mittinty, M., Lynch, J., & Sawyer, M. (2019). The effectiveness of an app-based nurse-moderated program for new mothers with depression and parenting problems (eMums Plus): Pragmatic randomized controlled trial. *Journal of Medical Internet Research, 21*(6), e13689. https://doi.org/10.2196/13689

Schröder, J., Berger, T., Westermann, S., Klein, J. P., & Moritz, S. (2016). Internet interventions for depression: New developments. *Dialogues in Clinical Neuroscience, 18*(2), 203. https://doi.org/10.31887/DCNS.2016.18.2/jschroeder

Schueller, S. M. (2018). Mental health and eHealth technology. In L. van Gemert-Pijnen, S. M. Kelders, H. Kip, & R. Sanderman (Eds.), *eHealth research theory and development: A multidisciplinary approach.* Routledge. https://doi.org/10.4324/9781315385907

Shen, N., Levitan, M. J., Johnson, A., Bender, J. L., Hamilton-Page, M., Jadad, A. A. R., & Wiljer, D. (2015). Finding a depression app: A review and content analysis of the depression app marketplace. *JMIR mHealth and uHealth, 3*(1), e16. https://doi.org/10.2196/mhealth.3713

Shieh, C., Mays, R., McDaniel, A., & Yu, J. (2009). Health literacy and its association with the use of information sources and with barriers to information seeking in clinic-based pregnant women. *Health Care for Women International, 30*(11), 971–988. https://doi.org/10.1080/07399330903052152

Shim, M., Mahaffey, B., Bleidistel, M., & Gonzalez, A. (2017). A scoping review of human-support factors in the context of Internet-based psychological interventions (IPIs) for depression and anxiety disorders. *Clinical Psychology Review, 57*, 129–140. https://doi.org/10.1016/j.cpr.2017.09.003

Shorey, S., Chee, C., Ng, E. D., Lau, Y., Dennis, C. L., & Chan, Y. H. (2019). Evaluation of a Technology-Based Peer-Support Intervention Program for Preventing Postnatal Depression (Part 1): Randomized Controlled Trial. *Journal of Medical Internet Research, 21*(8), e12410. https://doi.org/10.2196/12410

Slomian, J., Bruyère, O., Reginster, J. Y., & Emonts, P. (2017). The internet as a source of information used by women after childbirth to meet their need for information: A web-based survey. *Midwifery, 48*, 46–52. https://doi.org/10.1016/j.midw.2017.03.005

Slomian, J., Honvo, G., Emonts, P., Reginster, J. Y., & Bruyère, O. (2019). Consequences of maternal postpartum depression: A systematic review of maternal and infant outcomes. *Women's Health, 15*, 1–55. https://doi.org/10.1177/1745506519844044

Sockol, L. E., Epperson, C. N., & Barber, J. P. (2011). A meta-analysis of treatments for perinatal depression. *Clinical Psychology Review, 31*(5), 839–849. https://doi.org/10.1016/j.cpr.2011.03.009

Sockol, L. E., Eppersond, N., & Barbere, J. P. (2013). Preventing postpartum depression: A meta-analytic review. *Clinical Psychology Review, 33*(8), 1205–1217. https://doi.org/10.1016/j.cpr.2013.10.004

Soto, A., Smith, T. B., Griner, D., Domenech Rodríguez, M., & Bernal, G. (2018). Cultural adaptations and therapist multicultural competence: Two meta-analytic reviews. *Journal of Clinical Psychology, 74*(11), 1907–1923. https://doi.org/10.1002/jclp.22679

Spanhel, K., Balci, S., Feldhahn, F., Bengel, J., Baumeister, H., & Sander, L. B. (2021). Cultural adaptation of internet-and mobile-based interventions for mental disorders: A systematic review. *NPJ Digital Medicine, 4*(1), 1–18. https://10.1038/s41746-021-00498-1.

Stein, A., Pearson, R. M., Goodman, S. H., Rapa, E., Rahman, A., McCallum, M., Howard, L. M., & Pariante, C. M. (2014). Effects of perinatal mental disorders on the fetus and child. *The Lancet, 384*(9956), 1800–1819. https://doi.org/10.1016/S0140-6736(14)61277-0

Summers, A. L., & Logsdon, M. C. (2005). Web sites for postpartum depression: Convenient, frustrating, incomplete, and misleading. *MCN: The American Journal of Maternal/Child Nursing, 30*(2), 88–94. https://doi.org/10.1097/00005721-200503000-00004

Sun, Y., Li, Y., Wang, J., Chen, Q., Bazzano, A. N., & Cao, F. (2021). Effectiveness of smartphone-based mindfulness training on maternal perinatal depression: randomized controlled trial. *Journal of medical Internet Research, 23*(1), e23410. https://doi.org/10.2196/23410

Svanberg, P., Mennet, L., & Spieker, S. (2010). Promoting a secure attachment: A primary prevention practice model. *Clinical Child Psychology and Psychiatry, 15*, 363–378. https://doi.org/10.1177/1359104510367584

Sword, W., Busser, D., Ganann, R., McMillan, T., & Swinton, M. (2008). Women's care-seeking experiences after referral for postpartum depression. *Qualitative Health Research, 18*(9), 1161–1173. https://doi.org/10.1177/1049732308321736

Toohey, J. (2012). Depression during pregnancy and postpartum. *Clinical Obstetrics and Gynecology, 55*(3), 788–797. https://doi.org/10.1097/GRF.0b013e318253b2b4

Tronick, E., & Reck, C. (2009). Infants of depressed mothers: A review of longitudinal studies on antenatal and postnatal depression. *Harvard Review of Psychiatry, 17*(2), 147–156. https://doi.org/10.1080/10673220902899714

Tsivos, Z. L., Calam, R., Sanders, M. R., & Wittkowski, A. (2015). Interventions for postnatal depression assessing the mother–infant relationship and child developmental outcomes: A systematic review. *International Journal of Women's Health, 7*, 429. https://doi.org/10.2147/IJWH.S75311

van Gemert-Pijnen, J. E., Nijland, N., van Limburg, M., Ossebaard, H. C., Kelders, S. M., Eysenbach, G., & Seydel, E. R. (2011). A holistic framework to improve the uptake and impact of eHealth technologies. *Journal of Medical Internet Research, 13*(4), e111. https://doi.org/10.2196/jmir.1672

van Gemert-Pijnen, L., Kip, H., Kelders, S. M., & Sanderman, R. (2018). Introducing eHealth. In L. van Gemert-Pijnen, S. M. Kelders, H. Kip, & R. Sanderman (Eds.), *eHealth research theory and development: A multidisciplinary approach*. Routledge. https://doi.org/10.4324/9781315385907

Vismara, L., Rollè, L., Agostini, F., Sechi, C., Fenaroli, V., Molgora, S., Neri, E., Prino, L. E., Odorisio, F., Trovato, A., Polizzi, C., Brustia, P., Lucarelli, L., Monti, F., Saita, E., & Tambelli, R. (2016). Perinatal parenting stress, anxiety, and depression outcomes in first-time mothers and fathers: A 3- to 6-months postpartum follow-up study. *Frontiers in Psychology, 7*, 1–10. https://doi.org/10.3389/fpsyg.2016.00938

Walker, L. O., Mackert, M. S., Ahn, J., Vaughan, M. W., Sterling, B. S., Guy, S., & Hendrickson, S. (2017). e-Health and new moms: Contextual factors associated with sources of health information. *Public Health Nursing, 34*(6), 561–568. https://doi.org/10.1111/phn.12347

Webb, C. A., Rosso, I. M., & Rauch, S. L. (2017). Internet-based cognitive behavioral therapy for depression: Current progress & future directions. *Harvard Review of Psychiatry, 25*(3), 114–122. https://doi.org/10.1097/HRP.0000000000000139

Werner, E., Miller, M., Osborne, L. M., Kuzava, S., & Monk, C. (2015). Preventing postpartum depression: Review and recommendations. *Archives of Women's Mental Health, 18*(1), 41–60. https://doi.org/10.1007/s00737-014-0475-y

Wildeboer, G., Kelders, S. M., & van Gemert-Pijnen, J. E. (2016). The relationship between persuasive technology principles, adherence and effect of web-Based interventions for mental health: A meta-analysis. *International Journal of Medical Informatics, 96*, 71–85. https://doi.org/10.1016/j.ijmedinf.2016.04.005

Wisner, K. L., Sit, D. K., McShea, M. C., Rizzo, D. M., Zoretich, R. A., Hughes, C. L., Eng, H. F., Luther, J. F., Wsisniewski, S. R., Constantino, M. L., Confer, A. L., Moses-Kolko, E. L., Farmy, C. S., & Hanusa, B. H. (2013). Onset timing, thoughts of self-harm, and diagnoses in postpartum women with screen-positive depression findings. *JAMA Psychiatry, 70*(5), 490–498. https://doi.org/10.1001/jamapsychiatry.2013.87

Woody, C. A., Ferrari, A. J., Siskind, D. J., Whiteford, H. A., & Harris, M. G. (2017). A systematic review and meta-regression of the prevalence and incidence of perinatal depression. *Journal of Affective Disorders, 219*, 86–92. https://doi.org/10.1016/j.jad.2017.05.003

Yang, M., Jia, G., Sun, S., Ye, C., Zhang, R., & Yu, X. (2019). Effects of an online mindfulness intervention focusing on attention monitoring and acceptance in pregnant women: A randomized controlled trial. *Journal of Midwifery & Women's Health, 64*(1), 68–77. https://doi.org/10.1111/jmwh.12944

Zale, A., Lasecke, M., Baeza-Hernandez, K., Testerman, A., Aghakhani, S., Muñoz, R. F., & Bunge, E. L. (2021). Technology and psychotherapeutic interventions: Bibliometric analysis of the past four decades. *Internet Interventions, 25*, 100425. https://doi.org/10.1016/j.invent.2021.100425

Zhang, P., Dong, L., Chen, H., Chai, Y., & Liu, J. (2018). The rise and need for mobile apps for maternal and child health care in China: Survey based on app markets. *JMIR mHealth and uHealth, 6*(6), e140. https://doi.org/10.2196/mhealth.9302

Zhou, C., Hu, H., Wang, C., Zhu, Z., Feng, G., Xue, J., & Yang, Z. (2020). The effectiveness of mHealth interventions on postpartum depression: A systematic review and meta-analysis. *Journal of Telemedicine and Telecare, 28*(2), 83–95. https://doi.org/10.1177/1357633X20917816

Chapter 9
Preventive and Early Treatment of Depression in Older Adults

Sandra Saldivia, Félix Cova, Carolina Inostroza, Joseph Aslan, and Maryam Farhang

9.1 Background

The aging population is a visible trend across the world, more accelerated in higher-income countries but with notable manifestations in the entire world. In Latin America and the Caribbean, people over 60 currently represent 12% of the total population, and it is estimated that, by 2037, the proportion of older people will surpass the proportion of children under 15 (20%) (Huenchuan, 2018). In this context, the promotion and protection of the well-being and mental health of older adults is an increasingly relevant challenge.

S. Saldivia (✉)
Departamento de Psiquiatría y Salud Mental, Facultad de Medicina, Universidad de Concepción, Concepción, Chile
e-mail: ssaldivi@udec.cl

F. Cova · C. Inostroza
Departamento de Psicología, Facultad de Ciencias Sociales, Universidad de Concepción, Concepción, Chile

J. Aslan
Programa de Doctorado en Psicología, Facultad de Ciencias Sociales, Universidad de Concepción, Concepción, Chile

M. Farhang
Escuela de Enfermería, Facultad de Salud y Ciencias Sociales, Universidad de Las Américas, Santiago, Chile

Millennium Institute for Research in Depression and Personality (MIDAP), Santiago, Chile

Millennium Institute for Care Research (MICARE), Santiago, Chile

Departamento de Psiquiatría y Salud Mental, Hospital Clínico Universidad de Chile, Santiago, Chile

V. Martínez, C. Miranda-Castillo (eds.), *Prevention and Early Treatment of Depression Through the Life Course*, Depression and Personality,
https://doi.org/10.1007/978-3-031-13029-8_9

The age of onset of what is classified as "older" is relative, with important local variations according to variables like general health of the population, income status, and medical facilities to reduce the burden of old age. The increase in life expectancy and improved population health have postponed the start of this life stage to later years. Many older adults have relatively normal health up to advanced age and have shown the trend towards a more generalized physical and mental decline after the age of 80, in what is called the "fourth age" (Broderick & Blewitt, 2015).

Contradicting certain social stereotypes, many older adults experience "successful aging" and positive emotional well-being (Bar-Tur & Malkinson, 2014). However, mental problems and disorders that can significantly affect the well-being and quality of life of older adults are not uncommon. Using current diagnostic criteria, the annual prevalence rates of mental disorders, as per the limited Latin American studies (Andrade et al., 2002; Kohn et al., 2008; Torres de Galvis & Montoya, 1997), vary from 8.0% to 26.0%, analogous to studies in high-income countries (Kirchberger et al., 2012; Baladón et al., 2015).

9.2 Depression in Later Years of Life

Depression in late life is the term used to refer to depressive episodes that occur in the later years. The term includes both people who have already had episodes of depression (early-onset depression) and those who these episodes appear for the first time in late adulthood (late-onset depression).

Late-life depression is frequently under-recognized for various reasons. One of them is that it presents characteristics that are slightly different from depression in other stages of life, such as a greater prevalence of somatic symptoms (e.g., fatigue, sleep disturbance, chronic pain, appetite loss, etc.) or concerns about physical health, social relationships, or economic burdens. It is also frequently observed that manifestations of late depression such as hopelessness, sadness, tiredness, anhedonia, sleep disturbances, hypochondriasis, and subjective cognitive complaints (e.g., poor concentration and memory) are confused with aspects of aging processes (Hegeman et al., 2012). The presence of "subclinical" depression in older adults, that is, a universe of depressive symptoms that do not completely fit the set of typical diagnostic criteria, is often associated with the same negative consequences as the depressive episodes that do satisfy these diagnostic criteria, including a reduction of well-being and quality of life, a worsening of the state of health, greater disability, morbidity, and mortality (Cherubini et al., 2012), which is why "subclinical" depression must not be written off a priori.

Late-life depression can be influenced by a broad and interdependent set of factors (Fiske et al., 2009). Blazer (2010) proposes an etiological model that highlights the following factors: (1) biological (genetic predisposition, comorbid diseases), (2) psychological (loss of interest in pleasurable activities, maladaptive cognitions, comorbid psychiatric disorders), and (3) social (daily stressors and negative life events, poor social support). In late depression, the general health of the person may be particularly important. Some diseases may share some etiological elements with late depression or may favor it by affecting the person's daily life and physical or mental abilities. Many older adults are deprived of the ability to live independently due to mobility issues, chronic pain, frailty, or other mental or physical problems. It has been suggested that the reduction of daily activities would be a common final pathway predisposing to late-life depression (Fiske et al., 2009).

The decline in socioeconomic status and social integration due to retirement can be another important factor as well as the exposure to painful experiences, such as the loss of closely related friends or family (Cole & Dendukuri, 2003). Isolation, poor living conditions, and the loss of social roles are sociocultural factors that can significantly affect the mental health of older adults, as well as the exposure to forms of abandonment, mistreatment, violence, and abuse (Dong et al., 2013).

Having wide-reaching and diverse social networks and experiencing higher levels of perceived social support both instrumental and social are important protective factors against depression (Jacobson et al., 2017; Santini et al., 2015). It has been seen that the relationship between functional disability and the presence of symptoms of anxiety and depression in adults over the age of 75 is mediated by perceived social support (Feng et al., 2014). Low levels of social support and a higher need for affiliation are associated with greater depression in older adults, with an increased vulnerability seen in men (Sonnenberg et al., 2013). The recovery of older adults from depressive episodes is also affected by the social support perceived. It has particularly been seen that having a partner, and the amount of time they share with others, is linked to the recovery from depressive episodes in hospitalized older people (Li et al., 2013).

Loneliness is defined as feelings of sadness, frustration, anxiety, or anguish that accompany the perception that the social needs of the person are not satisfied by the amount, and especially, the quality of their social relationships. Unlike isolation, which is an objective measurement of poor social integration, loneliness is an experience and a complex construct that includes three dimensions: (a) intimate loneliness, (b) relational loneliness, and (c) collective loneliness (Hawkley & Cacioppo, 2010). This experience of loneliness is particularly intense in subgroups of older people, although there are differences highlighted among countries and cultural contexts (Yang & Victor, 2011). Knowledge about how social and environmental experiences affect the experience of loneliness at advanced ages is limited. A systematic revision of the experiences and predictors of loneliness in older people found an association with women, being unmarried, being older, low-income level, low qualification, living alone, low-quality social relationships, poor self-reporting of health, lack of belief in self-efficacy, negative life events, and cognitive shortcomings (Cohen-Mansfield et al., 2016). Loneliness is positively associated with depression in older adults. Individuals with higher levels of loneliness show a lower satisfaction with life, more negative emotions, and depressive symptoms (Hansen et al., 2013; Hawkley & Cacioppo, 2010). Cross-sectional and longitudinal studies show reciprocal influences over time between loneliness and symptoms of depression, often co-occurring but loneliness is considered a consistent and strong risk factor for depression (Luanaigh & Lawlor, 2008).

Many of the studies on risk factors for depression are not longitudinal, raising questions as to whether some of the factors reported are mere correlates of depression or whether they are true risk factors (Kraemer et al., 1997). A recent systematic review of risk and protective factors in older adults found that the most consistent predictors were physical activity, the presence of chronic diseases, difficulties in initiating sleep, motor impairment, visual impairment, and disabilities in daily activities (Maier et al., 2021). Depression in later years of life has been associated with poorer physical health, impaired cognitive functioning, decreased quality of life, limited social functioning, increased suicide risk, and high overall mortality (Corrêa et al., 2021; Power et al., 2017). Late-life depression has been also associated with other mental health problems and disorders, such as anxiety disorders, substance and medication abuse, and cognitive functioning impairment. Suicidal ideation and attempts in depressed older adults are relatively less than in depressed people in other stages of life. However, the increment in the age in older adults is associated with an increased suicidal risk and, compared to younger adults, suicidal behavior is more related to health problems than alcohol use and is more likely to be lethal (Kim et al., 2018; Power et al., 2017).

9.3 Prevention of Depression in Older Adults

Efforts focused on preventing late depression are a relevant line of action to favor the well-being and mental health of the older adult population (Norton et al., 2014). However, depression prevention must not be conceived as an isolated goal. Preventive actions for depression in older people make sense in a broader context that addresses the care and promotion of the quality of life and mental health of this group (Petersen et al., 2014; Norton et al., 2014). Conditions that allow older adults to conserve and strengthen their social integration, have an active and meaningful life, keep the highest possible degree of control over their decisions, and preserve and develop valuable ties with others are core lines of care and protection for mental health in this population (Forsman et al., 2011a). For this reason, mental health promotion actions along these lines may also have a preventive effect on depression in older adults.

The mental health of older adults is greatly affected by their prior biographical path and its determining factors: the social conditions throughout their life, the experiences they have lived, and the habits and behaviors they have had for years, all have effects that are ingrained throughout life (Beard & Bloom, 2015). Thus, there is a need to plan ahead of time when it comes to older people's mental health. Improving living conditions, promoting health throughout the life cycle, suitable prevention and handling of chronic diseases, and access to health and mental healthcare in earlier stages of life are the determining actions for the later mental health of older adults (Patel et al., 2008; Mangialasche et al., 2012).

The interaction between physical and mental health is especially accentuated in older adults (Wang & Kim, 2020). Prompt and effective care for the overall health of older adults can prevent harmful cycles of a loop between poorly treated health conditions, progressive isolation, loss of autonomy, sense of handicap, and progressive deterioration of mental health. The regular control of risk factors for cardiovascular and chronic diseases is essential for the physical and mental well-being of the older population (Mangialasche et al., 2012).

Preventive programs, depending on their nature and goals, can be categorized differently. It is usual to distinguish universal programs, namely, those directed at the entire population that has a condition, in this case, older people in general, or focused ones. Focused programs can be broken down into selective programs, aimed at people who have one or several risky health conditions, or indicated programs, where the risk factor considered is the subthreshold presence of the condition to be prevented. The so-called early interventions comprise indicated programs and programs that aim at the early treatment of people who already have the target condition. Preventive programs also have a promotion dimension, especially those of universal prevention (Cova et al., 2006).

Although it is expected that focused programs show more measurable effects than the universal ones do, as they are specifically aimed at the high-risk population, no clear differences in the effectiveness have been observed between both types of preventive programs in the field of depression in older people. In general, depression prevention programs at different ages have shown positive effects, though small, without clarity as to what would be the core aspects of the most successful interventions (van Zoonen et al., 2014). The same has been observed in depression prevention programs in older adults (Cole, 2012; Forsman et al., 2011a, b).

In recent decades, special attention has been paid to selective and indicated prevention programs. Lee et al. (2012) summarize the findings of five studies, which included an older adult population with sub-syndromic depressive symptoms. These include psychotherapeutic interventions as a core component, or complemented with other actions, with the different psychotherapeutic strategies showing benefits, including the revision of their own life, behavioral activation, problem-solving, and broader cognitive behavioral strategies. In general, and consistent with the observations by Lee et al. (2012), the typical components of depression prevention programs for older adults are encouraging physical exercise, cognitive and skill training, group support, evoking memories, and developing social activities (Forsman et al., 2011a).

From a public health perspective, a relevant preventive strategy would be that professionals identify people who are at risk of major depression, as well as people with subsyndromal symptoms to prevent or mitigate those disorders. For example, people with functional limitations resulting from strokes, with limited social support, and with subsyndromal symptoms could be the best targets for preventive interventions. This also may prove to be the case with other conditions that limit physical functioning (e.g., chronic obstructive pulmonary disease, macular degeneration, hip fracture) (Hindi et al., 2011). An intervention format of particular interest that integrates prevention and early intervention actions is multistage or multicomponent intervention, which includes different and successive support activities depending on the level of risk and the difficulties of the older adults whom these activities target and considering the evolution they start having. Currently, there are some previous studies with interesting results along this line (van't Veer-Tazelaar et al., 2011; van der Aa et al., 2017).

9.4 Psychosocial Preventive Programs for Depression

In recent decades, several preventive programs for depressive symptoms or disorders have been developed and evaluated in people aged 55 or older using randomized controlled trials (RCT) or quasi-experimental designs. In these studies, four main types of programs can be identified according to their dominant components: exercise-based, mind-body-based, psychology-based, and multicomponent interventions.

9.4.1 Exercise-Based Interventions

The World Health Organization defines physical activity as any bodily movement produced by skeletal muscles that require energy expenditure. Components of exercise-based preventive interventions in the older people include resistance, strength, aerobic, and combinations, ranging from moderate to vigorous physical activity. RCT studies support its usefulness in preventing depression. One study applied a 9-month resistance training program whose focus was specific muscular endurance in the first 3 months, and for the remaining 6 months, the training groups were split into different training frequencies ranging from reduced to increased. This program found a decrease in depressive symptoms in the initial 3 months, findings that were maintained until the end of the intervention (Kekäläinen et al., 2018). Resnick et al. (2008) developed a training program comprised of stretching, resistance, and aerobic exercise activities with a self-efficacy component, with statistically significant improvements in depressive symptoms (Resnick et al., 2008), while Huang et al. (2015) designed a physical approach intervention including warm-up, cardiovascular exercises, muscle strength, and a cooldown period, showing decreased depressive symptoms. A similar study trialed a DVD-delivered, home-based, physical activity intervention focused on flexibility, muscle strength, and balance, finding a marginally significant effect in the total sample. However, in the participants who reported elevated depression, the intervention demonstrated effects that were two to four times greater than the control group (Aguiñaga et al., 2018). Other studies focus on aerobic training, such as Underwood et al. (2013) and Bouaziz et al. (2019), with the former using 45-min physiotherapist-led group exercise sessions with no effect on depressive symptoms, and the latter, an interval aerobic training program with active recovery bouts to improve functional, cognitive performances and mental health, which had significant improvements in depression scores.

One study randomized participation to three different exercise training programs: dancing, walking, and strengthening/stretching/stability, where each group increased intensity as sessions progressed and the findings suggest that physical activity can be effective in reducing depressive symptoms (Awick et al., 2017). A more recent study used a multisystem physical training program consisting of three levels (beginner, intermediate, and advanced) of proprioception training, muscle strength training, reaction time exercise training with auditory cues, and postural balance training, with a significant decrease in depression symptoms at 12 weeks post-intervention (Chittrakul et al., 2020).

9.4.2 *Mind-Body-Based Interventions*

Mind-body interventions that focus on interactions among the brain, body, mind, and behavior by including different combinations of breathing exercises (Lavretsky, 2009), meditation, and structured movements (Bo et al., 2017) are one of the potential approaches to prevention programs that address not only physical but also psychological health.

Yoga is an ancient mind-body practice rooted in India, which focuses on the present moment by using mediation techniques consisting of physical postures (*asanas*), breathing control (*pranayama*), and the use of meditation (*dhyana*) (Büssing et al., 2012). The influence of yoga in the reduction of depression scores in older subjects is evident in some studies (Noradechanunt et al., 2017; Ramanathan et al., 2017). However, it is not recommended as a first-line intervention but rather as a complementary one if the older person presents depressive symptoms since it could provide a healthy and positive alternative to depressing negative thoughts (Ramanathan et al., 2017) where they are more likely to benefit from the intervention.

Mindfulness therapy is a well-accepted mind-body intervention that involves developing awareness in the present moment in a nonjudgmental way and with acceptance (Kabat-Zinn, 2003). A common type of mindfulness-based intervention (MBI) is the mindfulness-based stress reduction (MBSR) program, which teaches mindfulness meditation and yoga (Kabat-Zinn, 1990). Mindfulness-based cognitive therapy (MBCT) integrates elements of cognitive behavioral therapy (Beck, 1976) with systematic training in mindfulness meditation (Kabat-Zinn, 1990). In a quasi-experimental study conducted by O'Connor et al. (2014), they found a significant interaction effect of MBCT on depressive symptoms at follow-up between the intervention and the waiting list group, which reflected a significant decrease in depressive symptoms in the intervention group, but not in the waiting list group. The frequency of elevated depressive symptoms went from 50% post-intervention to 0% at follow-up in those who completed their participation in the intervention group, while the frequency of elevated depressive symptoms remained stable at 29% in the waiting list group. MBCT may be an effective way of reducing depressive symptoms in older bereaved people, especially those with clinically relevant depressive symptoms. The result of another study with a quasi-experimental design revealed a significant reduction in depression among the older people in the experimental group, who were subjected to the MBSR program (Kumar et al., 2014). The results suggest that the MBSR program improves depressive symptoms in older adults (over 75 years of age) with chronic insomnia (Zhang et al., 2015). Similarly, the results of an RCT study regarding the effect of flow meditation revealed a significant decrease in geriatric depression in older adults in the experimental group compared to the control group, confirming the effectiveness of mindfulness techniques in reducing this condition (Franco et al., 2017).

Qigong intervention is a form of mind-body approach involving meditative movement, breathing, meditation, and relaxation (Ladawan et al., 2017). Two Qigong intervention studies with an RCT design have been conducted (Phansuea et al., 2020; Tsang et al., 2013). The findings of the study performed by Phansuea et al. (2020) support that the Qigong program was effective in reducing the depression scores both in mild and moderate depression community-dwelling older adults. Also, Tsang et al. (2013) found that Qigong significantly reduced depressive symptoms compared to a control group. However, the available reviews focused on Qigong and Yoga for older adults, are limited and do not provide strong evidence about their effects on quality of life and depression (Gouw et al., 2019).

A systematic review examining the efficacy of mind-body interventions designed to reduce depressive symptoms among older adults (Bo et al., 2017), showed that mind-body interventions had short-term effects in reducing depressive symptoms in older adults with depressive symptoms. Subsequently, the findings may suggest the capacity of mind-body interventions to impact a range of symptom expressions from the most severe to less severe or subsyndromal symptom expressions (Bo et al., 2017). Nonetheless, mind-body interventions have not yet confirmed their long-term effect in alleviating depressive symptoms among older adults.

9.4.3 Psychology-Based Interventions

Psychological interventions cover a broad group that includes diverse non-pharmacological interventions focused on psychological or social factors. Lee et al. (2012) summarize the findings of five studies conducted with an older adult population with sub-syndromic depressive symptoms. These include psychotherapeutic interventions as a core component or complemented with other actions, showing the usefulness of the different psychotherapeutic strategies including life review, reminiscence therapy, cognitive behavioral therapy (CBT), problem-solving treatment (PST), psychosocial programs, and behavioral activation. Some of these are not only preventive but rather early intervention programs.

Reminiscence group therapy refers to a group activity, where the participants are encouraged to recall personal past events with one another. This group therapy differs from life review interventions, which is a more structured activity that can be done individually or in a group. Life review interventions are based on Erik Erikson's theory of human development to make the participant reflect and tell stories about their entire lifespan. Two RCT studies in the Netherlands found a significant decrease in depressive symptoms, with programs where the effect lasted 9 months after the intervention: The first study used three core elements – integration of difficult life events from the past, development of agentic life stories, and the retrieval of specific positive memories (Korte et al., 2012). The second developed an intervention for older adults called "Looking for Meaning" including sensory recall exercises, creative activity, and verbal exchange of experiences related to the course of life, linking the past and the present of the participants (Pot et al., 2010).

Behavioral activation (BA) interventions use the concepts of operant conditioning and scheduling to help people reconnect with positive reinforcement in their surroundings. Dozeman et al. (2011) did an RCT study with a self-help activity scheduling program that consisted of four steps, where participants learned to monitor their mood and daily activities and designed a pleasurable activity plan. Two similar RCT studies aimed at preventing depression in older people samples, using BA interventions to enhance daily routine activities, reduce avoidance behaviors and increase pleasurable, meaningful, or important activities (Almeida et al., 2021; Gilbody et al., 2021); overall, these studies found positive improvements in depression symptoms, but none were statistically significant.

Regarding cognitive behavioral therapy (CBT) interventions for the prevention and treatment of depression in older adults, the main aim is to restructure misconceptions and promote positive thinking and behavior. RCT evidence favors this type of intervention: Some studies have used a CBT-developed plan for depression consisting of three phases, the first one being behavioral activation (scheduling), the second cognitive assessment and restructuring, and the third, altering core beliefs that trigger negative thoughts, as well as behavioral analysis of dysfunctional coping mechanisms and problem-solving strategies (Huang et al., 2015). Another study developed an intervention consisting of receiving a CBT manual, psychoeducation, case reformulation, identifying, evaluating, and responding to automatic negative thoughts, homework assignments, evaluation, and feedback (Longchoopol et al., 2018). Other studies have also presented Internet-delivered CBT interventions (Read et al., 2020; Titov et al., 2015), consisting of five lessons in the form of a slideshow format over 8 weeks. The first lesson is psychoeducation; the second is the basics of CBT; the third is controlling physical symptoms of depression and anxiety; the fourth is education and guidelines about behavioral activation and graded exposure; and the last is information about relapse prevention and plans. Overall, these CBT studies found significantly fewer symptoms of depression in the intervention groups.

A variant of CBT intervention is problem-solving therapy. These interventions aim to break down problems into manageable components, generate strategies to find solutions, to later implement and evaluate their results. RCT studies carried out with older samples aim at teaching participants a positive problem orientation and active problem-solving skills instead of avoidant coping, where the most common problems are interpersonal issues and practical problems related to service needs

(Albert et al., 2019; Dias et al., 2019). In their study, Albert et al. (2019) found a small, yet significant decrease over time in depression scores, and Dias et al. (2019) reported that the intervention led to a reduced incidence of major depressive episodes.

A recent RCT study developed an active learning program consisting of 24-week 90-min sessions that addressed health promotion in old age, including group discussions, generation of individual ideas, and self-reflection as key components. This program was effective on improving depressive symptoms, communicative health literacy, and lifestyle behaviors among older adults (Uemura et al., 2021).

A quasi-experimental study conducted by Winocur et al. (2007) focused on cognitive aspects and developed a cognitive rehabilitation program for the older people consisting of three modules – memory skills training, modified goal management training, and psychosocial training; another study with the same design, aimed at reducing depressive symptoms in older adults through a humor intervention which consisted of a series of warm-up practices, watching humorous videos, game time, and humor sharing components (Zhao et al., 2020); both of these studies reported a significant improvement in depressive symptoms after the intervention.

9.4.4 Multicomponent Program-Based Interventions

Multicomponent interventions refer to combinations of educational interventions, support, psychotherapy, or group psychoeducation and therapeutic-psychosocial activities, physical exercise, and skill training (Forsman et al., 2011a). In this regard, there are several multicomponent intervention studies that used an RCT design (Uemura et al., 2021; Stahl et al., 2020; van der Aa et al., 2017; Dozeman et al., 2012; van't Veer-Tazelaar et al., 2011, 2010) as well as a quasi-experimental design (Hong et al., 2020; Greenawalt et al., 2019).

Life-Love program therapeutic activities and strategies involve providing education about depression and suicide, managing negative emotions, and promoting a more accurate and positive self-image among the older people, challenging their distorted, negative self-conception through group psychoeducation and therapeutic-psychosocial activities (Hong et al., 2020). The program showed effects in reducing the perception of being a burden and in reducing suicidal ideation among the participants.

Music and Tai Chi combined intervention is a variant of multicomponent programs. Tai Chi is a traditional Chinese martial art and is commonly believed to increase physical activity and lower depression among older persons (Sherman, 2012), by combining mind management with body movement, as well as increasing social participation (Chan et al., 2013). Combined music and Tai Chi reduced depressive symptoms among community-dwelling older people. This may represent an economically viable solution to manage depression in highly populous and developing nations. The potential synergistic effect of exercise and music as well as the long-term effects of the intervention will need to be explored in future studies (Uemura et al., 2021).

A positive psychology intervention program, called the Art of Happiness, based on key concepts including defining happiness, stress management, reflecting on happiness, compassion, and human connection, forgiveness, transforming suffering, mindfulness, and humor, has been incorporated into 8 weekly 90-min classes, which were specifically tailored to older adults to promote positive aging and overall mental well-being among this population (Greenawalt et al., 2019). Results showed that the intervention participants were significantly less stressed at the end of the program and there were significant improvements in both subjective happiness and depression. Such positive psychological states are closely intertwined with enhanced physical and mental health outcomes (Chida & Steptoe, 2008; Greenawalt et al., 2019).

In a digital monitoring (DM) study conducted by Stahl et al. (2020), participants randomized to DM recorded the times of sleep, meals, and physical activity behaviors twice daily using a diary-like app on a tablet for 12 weeks. The app also provided real-time feedback about the participants' sleep, meals, and physical activity. In addition to DM, participants received weekly calls from a health coach who used motivational interviewing (MI) techniques to strengthen participants' intrinsic motivation to engage in a regular behavioral routine. The results revealed that depression symptoms significantly decreased but the interaction between time and intervention was not significant. However, it was concluded that behavioral intervention that uses both digital monitoring and motivational health coaching is feasible and acceptable to older bereaved adults.

Another type of multicomponent depression prevention program is the stepped-care program. Prevention studies by Dozeman et al. (2012) and van't Veer-Tazelaar et al. (2011, 2010) have shown considerable promise. These authors have demonstrated that stepped-care prevention programs are effective in reducing the cumulative incidence of depression among older adults who were considered at risk of depression based on subsyndromal depressive symptoms. The intervention decreased the 12-month incidence of depressive disorders, from 0.24 (20 of 84) in the usual care group to 0.12 (10 of 86) in the stepped-care group (RR, 0.49; 95% CI, 0.24–0.98) (van't Veer-Tazelaar et al., 2011). Briefly, the four steps of the program, each lasting 3 months, include watchful waiting (step one), cognitive behavioral therapy (CBT) (step two), problem-solving therapy (PST) (step three), and referral to a primary care physician (step four). The stepped-care program is consistent with the suggestions of Reynolds III et al. (2012), who encouraged the use of brief, learning-based approaches that have proven to be effective with affective disorders and insomnia.

In another study, van der Aa et al. (2017) applied a stepped-care program consisting of four steps including watchful waiting, a guided self-help course based on cognitive behavioral therapy (CBT), problem-solving treatment (PST), and a referral to the general practitioner (GP) to discuss other treatments and the use of medication. The total intervention period lasted 12 months, and significant differences were found in the incidence of depressive disorders, but no significant difference was found for the symptoms of depression, although the stepped-care program was effective in preventing major depressive disorder when compared to usual care. Stepped-care programs allow limited resources to be used efficiently and, thus, help a larger portion of the population (van der Aa et al., 2017).

9.5 Discussion

Population aging demands that society generate responses to support this age group's well-being and mental health, both at a level of public policies, programs, and resources specifically designed for this population.

Care for the well-being and mental health among older adults must start several decades before this vital stage begins. Alongside this, it is necessary to develop promotional and preventive mental healthcare models for the current old population that are sensitive to their main difficulties and needs. This includes actions at very different levels to reduce risk factors and strengthen protective and promoting factors. At a macro level, the care of living conditions, the alignment of the health systems with the needs and human rights of older people, the development of friendly environments, increased opportunities for education, recreation, and playing sports, and the strengthening of the quality of long-term care are important (Patel et al., 2008). The actions that foster joining social networks that benefit social interaction and affective support require special attention; peer groups, volunteer, and intergenerational projects are some examples of interest along this line (Petersen et al., 2014). Evidence of the cost-effectiveness of psychosocial interventions to reduce social isolation and loneliness is emerging. One study in the United Kingdom (Coulton et al., 2015) evaluated the impact of participating in a community choir group on well-being, with promising results benefiting the intervention group, which reported better mental health indicators at a low cost. It is necessary to develop more group and volunteer programs.

The growing interest in depression prevention in older adults is leading to different initiatives, both at a level of broader social policies and in specific programs, although valuing the effectiveness of these initiatives from an empirical point of view has a series of complexities. One of the reasons behind this complexity is the broad age range this target population considers, which is even broader with the progressively longer life expectancy. In addition, older adults of similar ages have an accentuated heterogeneity of conditions and health statuses (Kessler et al., 2014). The evaluation of programs must consider this double source of diversity.

Effective studies of preventive interventions in mental health require long follow-up times and very large samples, even more so if the goal is the reduction of the incidence of certain mental disorders (Cuijpers, 2003). This complexity is even greater in universal programs, where many of the beneficiaries do not present difficulties when they start taking part in a program. Some authors opt for the development of highly focused programs to facilitate the detection of effects (Cuijpers et al., 2015). However, more universal programs have the potential of reaching more people that can benefit from them than focused programs do. At a population level, intervening with many people with moderate risk leads to a more effective frequency than doing so with fewer people with an elevated risk (Hotopf et al., 2015). In the prevention of depression in older adults, it is still premature to assert the superiority of universal programs over the focused ones. Furthermore, it does not seem to be appropriate to use the same indicators to evaluate both types of programs. The first tends to have a much more relevant promotional component and is a challenge that transcends the strict healthcare area. Care and promotion of mental health in older adults must be, by nature, an intersectoral effort.

On the other hand, it is debatable whether the evaluation of mental health prevention programs must be focused on the reduction of the incidence of particular disorders, identified with the standardized diagnostic criteria used for this. The presence/absence of a depressive disorder according to these criteria can underestimate the limitations of people who do not fully satisfy the criteria and overestimate the durability and seriousness of the condition in those that do satisfy them (Spitzer & Wakefield, 1999). The dichotomic nature of these analyses and the exclusion of other possible relevant outcomes also relativize its importance.

Although evidence is insufficient, the available reviews of psychosocial or psychological interventions show interesting efforts of implemented preventive programs, without being possible to state which are the most effective or what their essential components are (Cole, 2012; Forsman et al., 2011a; Hall & Reynolds III, 2014; Lee et al., 2012; van Zoonen et al., 2014). It should also be noted that most studies compare changes in depressive symptoms or quality of life indicators between experimental and control groups and not the reduction of depression incidence.

Preventive interventions based on physical exercise are very interesting for the older population since they improve psychological well-being and, at the same time, prevent the deterioration of physical health, which is a paramount aspect in older adulthood. While the results to date are promising, more follow-up studies are needed. Mind and body interventions contain varied interventions that could facilitate acceptance in large population groups of both Eastern and Western cultures. Despite their large increase, it should be noted that mind-body interventions have no evidence of long-term effectiveness in reducing depressive symptoms in older adults, except for mindfulness-based cognitive therapy (MBCT) interventions, which have proved their efficacy in adults and begun to accumulate evidence in older people. There are numerous programs for the prevention and treatment of depression based on psychotherapeutic interventions. Several of them have favorable, although still preliminary, evidence for older adults, especially compared to those available for the adult population. As noticed by van der Aa et al. (2017), stepped-care programs allow for the efficient use of resources that are always limited and, therefore, reach a greater proportion of the population.

Reynolds III et al. (2012) argued that, regarding indicated and early intervention programs, psychological interventions are preferable to antidepressants because antidepressants have demonstrated little efficacy with mild depression, and they have several potential adverse effects, particularly, when used with older adults.

9.6 Conclusion

Generating conditions for older adults to maintain the highest possible degree of control of their lives, participation in significant activities, and social ties, are crucial for promoting well-being and helping to prevent depressive disorders in this population. Even when there is a sustained accumulation of evidence of the efficacy, effectiveness, and cost-effectiveness of different programs, some challenges remain. Programs' capacity to generate significant clinical changes needs to be improved, and a more accurate understanding of the risk factors and processes involved, and the protection and promotion implied in the well-being and mental health of older adults, is required (Greenberg & Riggs, 2015; Toth et al., 2016). This need is amplified if the preeminence of evidence comes from high-income countries, with a gap in knowledge and experience from low- and middle-income ones, which becomes a relevant problem because factors that affect mental health have a strong contextual component (Patel et al., 2008).

Both depression and depressive symptoms are mental health problems that diminish well-being in older people with negative consequences on daily life. The United Nations' sustainable development goals include ensuring healthy lives and promoting mental health and well-being for all at all ages. Public mental health strategies that target screening and early diagnosis and offer preventive interventions are necessary and should increase the coverage in this population by delivering accurate and effective interventions.

Acknowledgments SS, FC, and CI received funding from ANID – FONDECYT – 1201158. JA received funding from the National Agency for Research and Development (ANID)/Scholarship Program/Doctorado Nacional/2018–21181769. MF received funding from ANID – FONDECYT – 3190275 as well as the ANID Millennium Science Initiative Program – ICS13_005 and ICS2019_024.

References

Aguiñaga, S., Ehlers, D. K., Salerno, E. A., Fanning, J., Motl, R. W., & McAuley, E. (2018). Home-based physical activity program improves depression and anxiety in older adults. *Journal of Physical Activity and Health, 15*(9), 692–696. https://doi.org/10.1123/jpah.2017-0390

Albert, S. M., King, J., Anderson, S., Dew, M. A., Zhang, J., Stahl, S. T., Karp, J. F., Gildengers, A. G., Butters, M. A., & Reynolds, C. F., III. (2019). Depression agency-based collaborative: Effect of problem-solving therapy on risk of common mental disorders in older adults with home care needs. *The American Journal of Geriatric Psychiatry, 27*(6), 619–624. https://doi.org/10.1016/j.jagp.2019.01.002

Almeida, O. P., Patel, H., Kelly, R., Ford, A., Flicker, L., Robinson, S., Araya, R., Gilbody, S., & Thompson, S. (2021). Preventing depression among older people living in rural areas: A randomised controlled trial of behavioural activation in collaborative care. *International Journal of Geriatric Psychiatry, 36*(4), 530–539. https://doi.org/10.1002/gps.5449

Andrade, L., Walters, E. E., Gentil, V., & Laurenti, R. (2002). Prevalence of ICD-10 mental disorders in a catchment area in the city of São Paulo, Brazil. *Social Psychiatry and Psychiatric Epidemiology, 37*(7), 316–325. https://doi.org/10.1007/s00127-002-0551-x

Awick, E. A., Ehlers, D. K., Aguiñaga, S., Daugherty, A. M., Kramer, A. F., & McAuley, E. (2017). Effects of a randomized exercise trial on physical activity, psychological distress and quality of life in older adults. *General Hospital Psychiatry, 49*, 44–50. https://doi.org/10.1016/j.genhosppsych.2017.06.005

Baladón, L., Fernández, A., Rubio-Valera, M., Cuevas-Esteban, J., Palao, D., Bellon, J., & Serrano-Blanco, A. (2015). Prevalence of mental disorders in non-demented older people in primary care. *International Psychogeriatrics, 27*, 757–768. https://doi.org/10.1017/S1041610214002841

Bar-Tur, L., & Malkinson, R. (2014). Positive ageing. New horizons for older adults. In N. Pachana & K. Laidlaw (Eds.), *The Oxford handbook of clinical geropsychology* (pp. 927–948). Oxford University Press.

Beard, J. R., & Bloom, D. E. (2015). Towards a comprehensive public health response to population ageing. *Lancet, 385*, 658–661. https://doi.org/10.1016/S0140-6736(14)61461-6

Beck, A. T. (1976). *Cognitive therapy and the emotional disorders*. New American Library.

Blazer, D. G. (2010). The origins of late-life depression. *Psychiatric Annals, 40*(1), 13–18. https://doi.org/10.3928/00485718-20091229-01

Bo, A., Mao, W., & Lindsey, M. A. (2017). Effects of mind-body interventions on depressive symptoms among older Chinese adults: A systematic review and meta-analysis. *International Journal of Geriatric Psychiatry, 32*(5), 509–521. https://doi.org/10.1002/gps.4688

Bouaziz, W., Schmitt, E., Vogel, T., Lefebvre, F., Leprêtre, P.-M., Kaltenbach, G., Geny, B., & Lang, P.-O. (2019). Effects of a short-term Interval Aerobic Training Programme with active Recovery bouts (IATP-R) on cognitive and mental health, functional performance and quality of life: A randomised controlled trial in sedentary seniors. *International Journal of Clinical Practice, 73*(1), e13219. https://doi.org/10.1111/ijcp.13219

Broderick, P., & Blewitt, P. (2015). *The life span*. Pearson.

Büssing, A., Michalsen, A., Khalsa, S. B. S., Telles, S., & Sherman, K. J. (2012). Effects of yoga on mental and physical health: A short summary of reviews. *Evidence-Based Complementary and Alternative Medicine, 2012*, 165410. https://doi.org/10.1155/2012/165412

Chan, A. W. K., Lee, A., Lee, D. T. F., Suen, L. K. P., Tam, W. W. S., Chair, S. Y., & Griffiths, P. (2013). The sustaining effects of Tai chi Qigong on physiological health for COPD patients: A randomized controlled trial. *Complementary Therapies in Medicine, 21*(6), 585–594. https://doi.org/10.1016/j.ctim.2013.09.008

Cherubini, A., Nistico, G., Rozzini, R., Liperoti, R., Di Bari, M., Zampi, E., Ferrannini, L., Aguglia, E., Pani, L., Bernabei, R., Marchionni, N., & Trabucchi, M. (2012). Subthreshold depression in older subjects: An unmet therapeutic need [journal article]. *Journal of Nutrition, Health & Aging, 16*(10), 909–913. https://doi.org/10.1007/s12603-012-0373-9

Chida, Y., & Steptoe, A. (2008). Positive psychological well-being and mortality: A quantitative review of prospective observational studies. *Psychosomatic Medicine, 70*(7), 741–756. https://doi.org/10.1097/PSY.0b013e31818105ba

Chittrakul, J., Siviroj, P., Sungkarat, S., & Sapbamrer, R. (2020). Multi-system physical exercise intervention for fall prevention and quality of life in pre-frail older adults: A randomized controlled trial. *International Journal of Environmental Research and Public Health, 17*(9), 3102. https://www.mdpi.com/1660-4601/17/9/3102

Cohen-Mansfield, J., Hazan, H., Lerman, Y., & Shalom, V. (2016). Correlates and predictors of loneliness in older-adults: A review of quantitative results informed by qualitative insights. *International Psychogeriatrics, 28*(4), 557–576. https://doi.org/10.1017/S1041610215001532

Cole, M. G. (2012). Preventing major depression in older medical inpatients: Innovation or flight of fancy? *International Psychogeriatrics, 24*(8), 1193–1196. https://doi.org/10.1017/S1041610212000671

Corrêa, V. P., Confortin, S. C., d'Orsi, E., de Sá-Junior, A. R., de Oliveira, C., & Schneider, I. J. (2021). Depressive symptoms as an independent risk factor for mortality. *Brazilian Journal of Psychiatry, 43*(3), 247–253. https://doi.org/10.1590/1516-4446-2019-0749

Coulton, S., Clift, S., Skingley, A., & Rodriguez, J. (2015). Effectiveness and cost-effectiveness of community singing on mental health-related quality of life of older people: Randomised controlled trial. *The British Journal of Psychiatry, 207*(3), 250–255. https://doi.org/10.1192/bjp.bp.113.129908

Cole, M. G., & Dendukuri, N. (2003). Risk factors for depression among older people community subjects: A systematic review and meta-analysis. *American Journal of Psychiatry, 160*(6), 1147–1156. https://doi.org/10.1176/appi.ajp.160.6.1147

Cova, F., Aburto, B., Sepúlveda, M. J., & Silva, M. (2006). Potencialidades y obstáculos de la prevención de la depresión en niños y adolescentes. *Psykhe, 15*(1), 57–65. https://doi.org/10.4067/S0718-22282006000100005

Cuijpers, P. (2003). Examining the effects of prevention programs on the incidence of new cases of mental disorders: The lack of statistical power. *American Journal of Psychiatry, 160*(8), 1385–1391. https://doi.org/10.1176/appi.ajp.160.8.1385

Cuijpers, P., Smit, F., Patel, V., Dias, A., Li, J., & Reynolds, C. F., III. (2015). Prevention of depressive disorders in older adults: An overview. *PsyCh Journal, 4*(1), 3–10. https://doi.org/10.1002/pchj.86

Dias, A., Azariah, F., Anderson, S. J., Sequeira, M., Cohen, A., Morse, J. Q., Cuijpers, P., Patel, V., & Reynolds, C. F., III. (2019). Effect of a lay counselor intervention on prevention of major depression in older adults living in low- and middle-income countries: A randomized clinical trial. *JAMA Psychiatry, 76*(1), 13–20. https://doi.org/10.1001/jamapsychiatry.2018.3048

Dong, X., Chen, R., Chang, E. S., & Simon, M. (2013). Elder abuse and psychological well-being: A systematic review and implications for research and policy-A mini review. *Gerontology, 59*(2), 132–142. https://doi.org/10.1159/000341652

Dozeman, E., Van Marwijk, H. W. J., Van Schaik, D. J. F., Smit, F., Stek, M. L., Van Der Horst, E., et al. (2012). Contradictory effects for prevention of depression and anxiety in residents in homes for the older people: A pragmatic randomized controlled trial. *International Psychogeriatric, 24*(8), 1242–1251. https://doi.org/10.1017/S1041610212000178

Dozeman, E., van Schaik, D. J. F., van Marwijk, H. W. J., Stek, M. L., Beekman, A. T. F., & van der Horst, H. E. (2011). Feasibility and effectiveness of activity-scheduling as a guided self-help intervention for the prevention of depression and anxiety in residents in homes for the older people: A pragmatic randomized controlled trial. *International Psychogeriatrics, 23*(6), 969–978. https://doi.org/10.1017/S1041610211000202

Feng, D., Ji, L., & Xu, L. (2014). Mediating effect of social support on the association between functional disability and psychological distress in older adults in rural China: Does age make a difference? *PLoS One, 9*(6), e100945. https://doi.org/10.1371/journal.pone.0100945

Fiske, A., Wetherell, J. L., & Gatz, M. (2009). Depression in older adults. *Annual Review of Clinical Psychology, 5*, 363–389. https://doi.org/10.1146/annurev.clinpsy.032408.153621

Forsman, A. K., Nordmyr, J., & Wahlbeck, K. (2011a). Psychosocial interventions for the promotion of mental health and the prevention of depression among older adults. *Health Promotion International, 26*, 85–107. https://doi.org/10.1093/heapro/dar074

Forsman, A. K., Schierenbeck, I., & Wahlbeck, K. (2011b). Psychosocial interventions for the prevention of depression in older adults: Systematic review and meta-analysis. *Journal of Aging and Health, 23*(3), 387–416. https://doi.org/10.1177/0898264310378041

Franco, C., Amutio, A., Mañas, I., Gázquez, J. J., & Pérez-Fuentes, M. d. C. (2017). Reducing anxiety, geriatric depression and worry in a sample of older adults through a mindfulness training program. *Terapia Psicológica, 35*, 71–79. http://www.scielo.cl/scielo.php?script=sci_arttext&pid=S0718-48082017000100007&nrm=iso

Gilbody, S., Brabyn, S., Mitchell, A., Ekers, D., McMillan, D., Bailey, D., Hems, D., Chew Graham, C. A., Keding, A., & Bosanquet, K. (2021). Can we prevent depression in at-risk older adults using self-help? The UK SHARD trial of Behavioral Activation. *The American Journal of Geriatric Psychiatry, 30*(2), 197–207. https://doi.org/10.1016/j.jagp.2021.06.006

Gouw, V. X. H., Jiang, Y., Seah, B., He, H., Hong, J., & Wang, W. (2019). Effectiveness of internal Qigong on quality of life, depressive symptoms and self-efficacy among community-dwelling older adults with chronic disease: A systematic review and meta-analysis. *International Journal of Nursing Studies, 99*, 103378. https://doi.org/10.1016/j.ijnurstu.2019.06.009

Greenawalt, K. E., Orsega-Smith, E., Turner, J. L., Goodwin, S., & Rathie, E. J. (2019). The impact of "the art of happiness" class on community dwelling older adults: A positive psychology intervention. *Activities, Adaptation & Aging, 43*(2), 118–132. https://doi.org/10.1080/01924788.2018.1493898

Greenberg, M. T., & Riggs, N. R. (2015). Prevention of mental disorders and promotion of competence. In *Rutter's child and adolescent psychiatry* (6th ed., pp. 215–226). John Wiley and Sons Ltd. https://doi.org/10.1002/9781118381953.ch17

Hall, C. A., & Reynolds, C. F., III. (2014). Late-life depression in the primary care setting: Challenges, collaborative care, and prevention. *Maturitas, 79*(2), 147–152. https://doi.org/10.1016/j.maturitas.2014.05.026

Hansen, N. B., Harrison, B., Fambro, S., Bodnar, S., Heckman, T. G., & Sikkema, K. J. (2013). The structure of coping among older adults living with HIV/AIDS and depressive symptoms. *Journal of Health Psychology, 18*(2), 198–211. https://doi.org/10.1177/1359105312440299

Hawkley, L. C., & Cacioppo, J. T. (2010). Loneliness matters: A theoretical and empirical review of consequences and mechanisms. *Annals of Behavioral Medicine, 40*(2), 218–227. https://doi.org/10.1007/s12160-010-9210-8

Hegeman, J. M., Kok, R. M., Van der Mast, R. C., & Giltay, E. J. (2012). Phenomenology of depression in older compared with younger adults: Meta-analysis. *British Journal of Psychiatry, 200*, 275–281. https://doi.org/10.1192/bjp.bp.111.095950

Hindi, F., Dew, M. A., Albert, S. M., Lotrich, F. E., & Reynolds, C. F., III. (2011). Preventing depression in later life: State of the art and science circa 2011. *Psychiatric Clinics of North America, 34*(1), 67. https://doi.org/10.1016/j.psc.2010.11.008

Hong, M., Gang, M., & Lee, J. (2020). Effects of the Life-Love Program on depression, perceived burdensomeness, and suicidal ideation. *Collegian, 27*(1), 102–108. https://doi.org/10.1016/j.colegn.2019.04.003

Hotopf, M., Mehta, N., Henderson, M., & Wessely, S. (2015). Wellbeing interventions: No evidence they prevent mental illness. *Lancet, 386*, 852–853.

Huang, T.-T., Liu, C.-B., Tsai, Y.-H., Chin, Y.-F., & Wong, C.-H. (2015). Physical fitness exercise versus cognitive behavior therapy on reducing the depressive symptoms among community-dwelling older people adults: A randomized controlled trial. *International Journal of Nursing Studies, 52*(10), 1542–1552. https://doi.org/10.1016/j.ijnurstu.2015.05.013

Huenchuan, S. (2018). *Envejecimiento, personas mayores y Agenda 2030 para el Desarrollo Sostenible: Perspectiva regional y de derechos humanos, Libros de la CEPAL, N° 154 (LC/PUB.2018/24-P)*. Comisión Económica para América Latina y el Caribe (CEPAL).

Jacobson, N. C., Lord, K. A., & Newman, M. G. (2017). Perceived emotional social support in bereaved spouses mediates the relationship between anxiety and depression. *Journal of Affective Disorders, 211*(Supplement C), 83–91. https://doi.org/10.1016/j.jad.2017.01.011

Kabat-Zinn, J. (1990). *Full catastrophe living: Using the wisdom of your body and mind to face stress, pain and illness*. Delacorte.

Kabat-Zinn, J. (2003). Mindfulness-based interventions in context: Past, present, and future. *Clinical Psychology: Science and Practice, 10*(2), 144–156. https://doi.org/10.1093/clipsy.bpg016

Kekäläinen, T., Kokko, K., Sipilä, S., & Walker, S. (2018). Effects of a 9-month resistance training intervention on quality of life, sense of coherence, and depressive symptoms in older adults: Randomized controlled trial. *Quality of Life Research, 27*(2), 455–465. https://doi.org/10.1007/s11136-017-1733-z

Kessler, E. M., Kruse, A., & Wahl, H. W. (2014). Clinical gero-psychology: A lifespan perspective. In *The Oxford handbook of clinical geropsychology* (pp. 3–25). https://doi.org/10.1093/oxfordhb/9780199663170.013.001

Kim, H., Ahn, J.-S., Kim, H., Cha, Y. S., Lee, J., Kim, M.-H., & Min, S. (2018). Sociodemographic and clinical characteristics of old-old suicide attempters compared with young-old and middle-aged attempters. *International Journal of Geriatric Psychiatry, 33*(12), 1717–1726. https://doi.org/10.1002/gps.4976

Kirchberger, I., Meisinger, C., Heier, M., Zimmermann, A.-K., Thorand, B., Autenrieth, C. S., Peters, A., Ladwig, K. H., & Doring, A. (2012). Patterns of multimorbidity in the aged population. Results from the KORA-Age study. *PLoS ONE, 7*(1), e30556. https://doi.org/10.1371/journal.pone.0030556

Kohn, R., Vicente, B., Saldivia, S., Rioseco, P., & Torres, S. (2008). Psychiatric epidemiology of the older people population in Chile. *American Journal Geriatric Psychiatry, 16*, 1020–1028. https://doi.org/10.1097/JGP.0b013e31818a0e1c

Korte, J., Bohlmeijer, E. T., Cappeliez, P., Smit, F., & Westerhof, G. J. (2012). Life review therapy for older adults with moderate depressive symptomatology: A pragmatic randomized controlled trial. *Psychological Medicine, 42*(6), 1163–1173. https://doi.org/10.1017/S0033291711002042

Kraemer, H. C., Kazdin, A. E., Offord, D. R., Kessler, R. C., Jensen, P. S., & Kupfer, D. J. (1997). Coming to terms with the terms of risk. *Archives of General Psychiatry, 54*(4), 337–343. https://doi.org/10.1001/archpsyc.1997.01830160065009

Kumar, S., Adiga, K. R., & George, A. (2014). Impact of Mindfulness-based Stress Reduction (MBSR) on depression among older people residing in residential homes. *Nursing Journal of India, 105*(6), 248–251. http://europepmc.org/abstract/MED/26182818

Ladawan, S., Klarod, K., Philippe, M., Menz, V., Versen, I., Gatterer, H., & Burtscher, M. (2017). Effect of Qigong exercise on cognitive function, blood pressure and cardiorespiratory fitness in healthy middle-aged subjects. *Complementary Therapies in Medicine., 33*, 39–45. https://doi.org/10.1016/j.ctim.2017.05.005

Lavretsky, H. (2009). Complementary and alternative medicine use for treatment and prevention of late-life mood and cognitive disorders. *Aging Health, 5*(1), 61–78. https://doi.org/10.2217/1745509X.5.1.61

Lee, S. Y., Franchetti, M. K., Imanbayev, A., Gallo, J. J., Spira, A. P., & Lee, H. B. (2012). Non-pharmacological prevention of major depression among community-dwelling older adults: A systematic review of the efficacy of psychotherapy interventions. *Archives of Gerontology and Geriatrics, 55*(3), 522–529. https://doi.org/10.1016/j.archger.2012.03.003

Li, H., Morrow-Howell, N., Proctor, E., & Rubin, E. (2013). Social support resources and post-acute recovery for older adults with major depression. *Community Mental Health Journal, 49*(4), 419–426. https://doi.org/10.1007/s10597-012-9567-1

Longchoopol, C., Thapinta, D., Ross, R., & Lertwatthanawilat, W. (2018). The Thai group cognitive behavior therapy intervention program for depressive symptoms among older women: A randomized controlled trial. *Pacific Rim International Journal of Nursing Research, 22*(1), 74–85. Retrieved from https://he02.tci-thaijo.org/index.php/PRIJNR/article/view/78778

Luanaigh, C. Ó., & Lawlor, B. A. (2008). Loneliness and the health of older people. *International Journal of Geriatric Psychiatry, 23*(12), 1213–1221. https://doi.org/10.1002/gps.2054

Mangialasche, F., Kivipelto, M., Solomon, A., & Fratiglioni, L. (2012). Dementia prevention: Current epidemiological evidence and future perspective. *Alzheimer's Research & Therapy, 4*(1), 6. https://doi.org/10.1186/Alzrt104

Maier, A., Riedel-Heller, S. G., Pabst, A., & Luppa, M. (2021). Risk factors and protective factors of depression in older people 65+. A systematic review. *PloS one, 16*(5), e0251326. https://doi.org/10.1371/journal.pone.0251326

Noradechanunt, C., Worsley, A., & Groeller, H. (2017). Thai Yoga improves physical function and well-being in older adults: A randomised controlled trial. *Journal of Science and Medicine in Sport, 20*(5), 494–501. https://doi.org/10.1016/j.jsams.2016.10.007

Norton, S., Matthews, F. E., Barnes, D. E., Yaffe, K., & Brayne, C. (2014). Potential for primary prevention of Alzheimer's disease: An analysis of population-based data. *The Lancet Neurology, 13*(8), 788–794. https://doi.org/10.1016/S1474-4422(14)70136-X

O'Connor, M., Piet, J., & Hougaard, E. (2014). The effects of mindfulness-based cognitive therapy on depressive symptoms in older people bereaved people with loss-related distress: A controlled pilot study. *Mindfulness, 5*(4), 400–409. https://doi.org/10.1007/s12671-013-0194-x

Patel, V., Flisher, A. J., Nikapota, A., & Malhotra, S. (2008). Promoting child and adolescent mental health in low and middle income countries. *Journal of Child Psychology and Psychiatry, 49*(3), 313–334. https://doi.org/10.1111/j.1469-7610.2007.01824.x

Petersen, I., Barry, M., Lund, C., & Bhana, A. (2014). Mental health promotion and the prevention of mental disorders (245-275). In V. Patel, H. Minas, A. Cohen, & M. J. Prince (Eds.), *Global mental health: Principles and practice*. Oxford University Press.

Phansuea, P., Tangwongchai, S., Rattananupong, T., Lohsoonthorn, V., & Lertmaharit, S. (2020). Qigong programme among community-dwelling older adults at risk of depression: A randomised controlled study. *Cogent Medicine, 7*(1), 1711655. https://doi.org/10.1080/2331205X.2020.1711655

Pot, A. M., Bohlmeijer, E. T., Onrust, S., Melenhorst, A.-S., Veerbeek, M., & De Vries, W. (2010). The impact of life review on depression in older adults: A randomized controlled trial. *International Psychogeriatrics, 22*(4), 572–581. https://doi.org/10.1017/S104161020999175X

Power, C., Greene, E., & Lawlor, B. A. (2017). Depression in late life: Etiology, presentation, and management. In H. Chiu & K. Shulman (Eds.), *Mental health and illness of the elderly*. Springer.

Ramanathan, M., Bhavanani, A. B., & Trakroo, M. (2017). Effect of a 12-week yoga therapy program on mental health status in older people women inmates of a hospice. *International journal of yoga, 10*(1), 24–28. https://doi.org/10.4103/0973-6131.186156

Read, J., Sharpe, L., Burton, A. L., Arean, P. A., Raue, P. J., McDonald, S., Titov, N., Gandy, M., & Dear, B. F. (2020). A randomized controlled trial of internet-delivered cognitive behaviour therapy to prevent the development of depressive disorders in older adults with multimorbidity. *Journal of Affective Disorders, 264*, 464–473. https://doi.org/10.1016/j.jad.2019.11.077

Resnick, B., Luisi, D., & Vogel, A. (2008). Testing the Senior Exercise Self-efficacy Project (SESEP) for use with urban dwelling minority older adults. *Public Health Nursing, 25*(3), 221–234. https://doi.org/10.1111/j.1525-1446.2008.00699.x

Reynolds, C. F., III, Cuijpers, P., Patel, V., Cohen, A., Dias, A., Chowdhary, N., et al. (2012). Early intervention to reduce the global health and economic burden of major depression in older adults. *Annual Review of Public Health, 33*, 123–135. https://doi.org/10.1146/annurev-publhealth-031811-124544

Santini, Z. I., Koyanagi, A., Tyrovolas, S., Mason, C., & Haro, J. M. (2015). The association between social relationships and depression: A systematic review. *Journal of Affective Disorders, 175*, 53–65. https://doi.org/10.1016/j.jad.2014.12.049

Sherman, L. (2012). Tai chi increases testosterone and improves prostate symptoms. *The Journal of Chinese Medicine, 98*, 73–74. https://doi.org/10.1155/2012/624692

Sonnenberg, C., Deeg, D., Van Tilburg, T., Vink, D., Stek, M., & Beekman, A. (2013). Gender differences in the relation between depression and social support in later life. *International Psychogeriatrics, 25*(1), 61–70. https://doi.org/10.1017/S1041610212001202

Spitzer, R. L., & Wakefield, J. C. (1999). DSM-IV diagnostic criterion for clinical significance: Does it help solve the false positives problem? *American Journal of Psychiatry, 156*(12), 1856–1864.

Stahl, S. T., Smagula, S. F., Dew, M. A., Schulz, R., Albert, S. M., & Reynolds, C. F. (2020). Digital monitoring of sleep, meals, and physical activity for reducing depression in older spousally-bereaved adults: A pilot randomized controlled trial. *The American Journal of Geriatric Psychiatry, 28*(10), 1102–1106. https://doi.org/10.1016/j.jagp.2020.02.013

Titov, N., Dear, B. F., Ali, S., Zou, J. B., Lorian, C. N., Johnston, L., Terides, M. D., Kayrouz, R., Klein, B., Gandy, M., & Fogliati, V. J. (2015). Clinical and cost-effectiveness of therapist-guided internet-delivered cognitive behavior therapy for older adults with symptoms of depression: A randomized controlled trial. *Behavior Therapy, 46*(2), 193–205. https://doi.org/10.1016/j.beth.2014.09.008

Torres de Galvis, Y., & Montoya, I. D. (1997). *Segundo Estudio Nacional de Salud Mental y Consumo de Sustancias Psicoactivas, Colombia 1997*. Ministerio de Salud Pública.

Toth, S., Petrenko, C., Gravener-Davis, J., & Handley, E. (2016). Advances in prevention science: A developmental psychopathology perspective. In D. Cicchetti (Ed.), *Developmental psychopathology* (Vol. 4, pp. 815–873). Wiley and Sons. https://doi.org/10.1002/9781119125556.devpsy416

Tsang, H. W. H., Tsang, W. W. N., Jones, A. Y. M., Fung, K. M. T., Chan, A. H. L., Chan, E. P., & Au, D. W. H. (2013). Psycho-physical and neurophysiological effects of qigong on depressed elders with chronic illness. *Aging & Mental Health, 17*(3), 336–348. https://doi.org/10.1080/13607863.2012.732035

Uemura, K., Yamada, M., & Okamoto, H. (2021). The effectiveness of an active learning program in promoting a healthy lifestyle among older adults with low health literacy: A randomized controlled trial. *Gerontology, 67*(1), 25–35. https://doi.org/10.1159/000511357

Underwood, M., Lamb, S. E., Eldridge, S., Sheehan, B., Slowther, A.-M., Spencer, A., Thorogood, M., Atherton, N., Bremner, S. A., Devine, A., Diaz-Ordaz, K., Ellard, D. R., Potter, R., Spanjers, K., & Taylor, S. J. C. (2013). Exercise for depression in older people residents of care homes: A cluster-randomised controlled trial. *Lancet, 382*(9886), 41–49. https://doi.org/10.1016/S0140-6736(13)60649-2

van der Aa, H. P. A., van Rens, G. H. M. B., Bosmans, J. E., Comijs, H. C., & van Nispen, R. M. A. (2017). Economic evaluation of stepped-care versus usual care for depression and anxiety in older adults with vision impairment: Randomized controlled trial. *BMC Psychiatry, 17*(1), 280. https://doi.org/10.1186/s12888-017-1437-5

van Zoonen, K., Buntrock, C., Ebert, D. D., Smit, F., Reynolds, C. F., III, Beekman, A. T., & Cuijpers, P. (2014). Preventing the onset of major depressive disorder: A meta-analytic review of psychological interventions. *International Journal of Epidemiology, 43*(2), 318–329. https://doi.org/10.1093/ije/dyt175

van't Veer-Tazelaar, P. J., van Marwijk, H. W., van Oppen, P., van der Horst, H. E., Smit, F., Cuijpers, P., & Beekman, A. T. (2011). Prevention of late-life anxiety and depression has sustained effects over 24 months: A pragmatic randomized trial. *American Journal of Geriatric Psychiatry, 19*(3), 230–239. https://doi.org/10.1097/JGP.0b013e3181faee4d

van't Veer-Tazelaar, P., Smit, F., van Hout, H., van Oppen, P., van der Horst, H., Beekman, A., & van Marwijk, H. (2010). Cost effectiveness of a stepped care intervention to prevent depression and anxiety in late life: Randomised trial. *British Journal of Psychiatry, 196*, 319–325. https://doi.org/10.1192/bjp.bp.109.069617

Wang, S. Y., & Kim, G. (2020). The relationship between physical-mental comorbidity and subjective well-being among older adults. *Clinical Gerontologist, 43*(4), 455–464. https://doi.org/10.1080/07317115.2019.1580810

Winocur, G., Palmer, H., Dawson, D., Binns, M. A., Bridges, K., & Stuss, D. T. (2007). Cognitive rehabilitation in the older people: An evaluation of psychosocial factors. *Journal of the International Neuropsychological Society, 13*(1), 153–165. https://doi.org/10.1017/S135561770707018X

Yang, K., & Victor, C. R. (2011). Age and loneliness in 25 European nations. *Ageing and Society, 31*(08), 1368–1388. https://doi.org/10.1017/S0144686X1000139X

Zhang, J.-X., Liu, X.-H., Xie, X.-H., Zhao, D., Shan, M.-S., Zhang, X.-L., Kong, X.-M., & Cui, H. (2015). Mindfulness-based stress reduction for chronic insomnia in adults older than 75 years: A randomized, controlled, single-blind clinical trial. *Explore, 11*(3), 180–185. https://doi.org/10.1016/j.explore.2015.02.005

Zhao, J., Yin, H., Wang, X., Zhang, G., Jia, Y., Shang, B., Zhao, J., Wang, C., & Chen, L. (2020). Effect of humour intervention programme on depression, anxiety, subjective well-being, cognitive function and sleep quality in Chinese nursing home residents. *Journal of Advanced Nursing, 76*(10), 2709–2718. https://doi.org/10.1111/jan.14472

Chapter 10
Depressive Disorders Among Family Caregivers of People Living with Dementia

Claudia Miranda-Castillo, Thamara Tapia-Muñoz, Déborah Oliveira, and Sebastián Sáez

10.1 Dementia

The global number of older people (aged ≥60 years) is expected to more than double by 2050 and more than triple by 2100, increasing from 962 million in 2017 to 2.1 billion in 2050, and 3.1 billion in 2100 (United Nations, 2020). Although dementia does not affect only older people, it is one of the leading causes of care dependency and disability among older people, being one of the top ten causes of years of healthy life lost due to disability (YLDs) (World Health Organization, 2021). The WHO estimates that 55.2 million people are living with dementia worldwide, and this number is forecasted to rise to 78 million by 2030 and 139 million by 2050 (World Health Organization, 2021). In 2019, the estimated global cost of dementia was US$1.3 trillion and is projected to increase to US$1.7 trillion by

C. Miranda-Castillo (✉)
Facultad de Enfermería, Universidad Andres Bello, Santiago, Chile

Millennium Institute for Research in Depression and Personality (MIDAP), Santiago, Chile

Millennium Institute for Care Research (MICARE), Santiago, Chile
e-mail: claudia.miranda@unab.cl

T. Tapia-Muñoz
Millennium Institute for Care Research (MICARE), Santiago, Chile

Department of Behavioural Science and Health, University College London, London, UK

Millennium Nucleus on Sociomedicine (SocioMed), Santiago, Chile

D. Oliveira
Medical School, Department of Psychiatry, Universidade Federal de São Paulo (UNIFESP), São Paulo, Brazil

S. Sáez
Millennium Institute for Care Research (MICARE), Santiago, Chile

V. Martínez, C. Miranda-Castillo (eds.), *Prevention and Early Treatment of Depression Through the Life Course*, Depression and Personality,
https://doi.org/10.1007/978-3-031-13029-8_10

2030. However, if projections are corrected for increases in care costs, global dementia costs can reach US$2.8 trillion by 2030 (World Health Organization, 2021).

Dementia is a neuropsychiatric syndrome characterized by progressive and chronic cognitive impairment, behavioral and psychological symptoms, and decreased functional capacity. It is a multifaceted condition caused by a myriad of brain disorders, such as Alzheimer's disease, vascular diseases in the brain, and Lewy body dementia, among others. Approximately 40% of all cases of dementia are thought to be caused by modifiable risk factors, such as diabetes, obesity, hypertension, tobacco smoking, alcohol abuse, brain injury, hearing impairment, and excessive exposure to air pollution (Livingston et al., 2020b). Known non-modifiable causes of dementia include advanced age, female sex, and genetic causes. The number of people with dementia is significantly higher in lower-income countries, with nearly 70% living in such settings, and dementia is twice as likely to affect women (World Health Organization, 2021). In the United Kingdom, for example, 61% of all people living with dementia are women, and dementia is the leading cause of death in all women (Alzheimer's UK, 2018).

The symptoms and other disease manifestations affecting each person living with dementia will vary and depend on, for example, the type of the disease affecting the brain, the parts of the brain affected by the disease, and the point of the disease trajectory at which the person is. Some pharmacological and non-pharmacological interventions can help control the neuropsychiatric manifestations that affect the quality of life of both the person living with dementia and their family caregivers (Watt et al., 2019). However, dementia has no cure and no treatment can effectively modify the disease progression.

10.2 Care and Support for People Living with Dementia

Throughout the years, dementia progressively leads to a deterioration in the person's ability to independently perform activities of daily living, which leads to an increase in the need for care and support from others. In more advanced stages of dementia, the person will need care and support to perform basic activities, such as cooking and feeding, as well as personal hygiene.

Most people living with dementia live at home, particularly in low- and middle-income countries (96%) (World Health Organization, 2021), and receive the care and support they need from family members and friends. Family caregivers (often also called "care partners," "informal caregivers," or "unpaid caregivers") perform this role without receiving any payment and with little support and training from services and governments. Globally, 70–80% of all family caregivers are women (World Health Organization, 2021), who bear not only the physical and mental health impact of care provision but also most of the care-related costs (Wimo et al., 2018).

The majority of the family caregivers of people living with dementia are spouses or adult and middle-aged daughters. Spouses are often older people themselves and have their own health needs, whereas adult and middle-aged daughters are likely to have to compete for other caring needs (i.e., childcare), household chores, and work responsibilities (Conde-Sala et al., 2010; Greenwood & Smith, 2016; Oliveira et al., 2019; Rigby et al., 2019). Several studies show that providing unpaid care can impact the mental and physical health of caregivers differently depending on their age, gender, and relationship to the person cared for, suggesting that interventions might need to be tailored to each group to have optimal effects (Walter & Pinquart, 2020).

10.3 Depression in Family Caregivers of People Living with Dementia

It is widely known that family caregivers of people living with dementia experience a negative impact on their physical and emotional health. Possible explanations for this effect have been formulated around two main perspectives. The first relates to stress. It has been reported that the experience of stress in caregivers can lead to high risks of illness (Haley et al., 2010; Martire & Schulz, 2012) and death (Perkins et al., 2013). The second explanatory perspective considers emotional, economic, and family-related costs that dementia caregivers have to face, which have been linked to mental health problems such as burden, anxiety, and depression (Cheng, 2017; De Fazio et al., 2015; Madaleno et al., 2019; Pinquart & Sörensen, 2003). According to a recent review, the latter is one of the most studied issues in dementia caregivers (Queluz et al., 2020).

Depression differs according to symptomatology and timing. The World Health Organization's diagnostic manual, ICD-11, classifies different types of depressive disorders as single episode depressive disorder, recurrent depressive disorder, dysthymic disorder, mixed depressive and anxiety disorder, going from single episodes to chronic disorders (World Health Organization, 2018). Depending on the methodology and instrument used to measure depression, there is a 30–60% prevalence in dementia caregivers (Madaleno et al., 2019; Sallim et al., 2015; Tzuang & Gallagher-Thompson, 2015). Furthermore, there have been reports indicating that there is a higher prevalence of depression and/or depressive symptomatology in caregivers of people living with dementia compared to individuals caring for people with chronic or psychiatric disorders (D'Aoust et al., 2015; Schoenmakers et al., 2010) and anxiety (Cooper et al., 2007; Joling et al., 2010).

Characteristics of caregivers themselves, which have been related to depressive symptoms, are being younger (O'Rourke et al., 2010), having a close relationship with the person with dementia (Fauth et al., 2012; Ornstein et al., 2014), high levels of burden (Epstein-Lubow et al., 2008), low levels of self-efficacy, few leisure activities (Romero-Moreno et al., 2012), low levels of mastery in dealing with caregiving (Mausbach et al., 2007), poor perception of caregiving as a challenge and lack of control over the situation (O'Rourke et al., 2010), perception of poor physical health, and previous presence of depressive symptoms (Joling et al., 2015).

In addition, more dysfunctional, disengaging, or less emotional coping is more robustly associated with depressive and anxious symptoms (García-Alberca et al., 2012; Li et al., 2014). A review by Watson et al. (2019) identified a set of factors that are consistently associated with the presence of depressive symptoms in dementia caregivers, namely, being a female and adult-child caregiver, coping strategies employed, activity restrictions, the severity of problematic behaviors associated with dementia, as well as the nature and quality of relationships that caregivers establish with care recipients (Watson et al., 2019).

Contextual factors that have been related to higher depressive symptomatology in family caregivers include low socioeconomic status, lower satisfaction with social support received (Clay et al., 2008), higher educational level (O'Rourke et al., 2010), and unemployment (Ornstein et al., 2014).

Evidence also suggests that family caregivers of people living with dementia are a high-risk group for suicide. In this regard, O'Dwyer et al. (2016), in a cross-sectional study of over 500 caregivers, found that 16% of caregivers had contemplated suicide more than once in the previous year. In addition, low satisfaction with social support received and the use of dysfunctional coping strategies had an indirect effect on suicidal ideation through depression. Meanwhile, Joling et al. (2018) assessed 192 family caregivers who did not have a clinical diagnosis of depression or anxiety at baseline for 2 years. Thirty-nine percent of them presented depressive symptomatology, and of the latter, 11.8% (4.7% of the total sample) reported suicidal thoughts at different times in the caregiving trajectory. This last group, compared to the rest of the sample, had more severe depressive and anxious symptoms and a lower sense of competence and mastery, felt less happy, and had more health problems, less family support, and more feelings of loneliness.

There is little evidence related to trajectories of depressive disorders among dementia caregivers. A study by Joling et al. (2012) reported that, after 18 months, 24.8% of 725 at-risk caregivers developed depression, with 58% of them showing high levels of depressive symptoms at all points of assessment. In addition, several cohort studies have shown that increases in caregiver depressive symptoms over time are related to factors associated with the person with dementia, the caregivers themselves, and the context. The severity of behavioral and psychological symptoms, as well as more time since the diagnosis of dementia, has been associated with higher levels of caregivers' depression over time (Cheng, 2017; O'Rourke et al., 2010).

A relevant dimension to understanding depressive symptomatology in caregivers of people living with dementia is gender. It is known that women are more likely to carry out the duties of caregiving. In addition, there is current evidence suggesting that female caregivers of people living with dementia are at higher risk for depression and have worse mental health outcomes overall (Verma & Anand, 2012; Watson et al., 2019; Xiong et al., 2020).

Although different perspectives have been proposed to address gender differences relative to mental health in caregivers, such explanations are linked to traditional gender role expectations. Stress and coping theory have shown the main evidence relative to differences between male and female caregivers. It has been reported that female dementia caregivers experience higher impacts from caregiving, as well as a larger effect on their depressive symptoms and somatic activity, which, in turn, has been explained by their inefficient use of coping styles (Pillemer et al., 2018). However, so far, evidence about the role of coping strategies by gender is limited and sometimes contradictory (Sharma et al., 2016). Additionally, literature also shows that women who provide care for their spouses are at higher risk of presenting depressive symptoms, which are more likely to appear near the end of the caregiving trajectory (Kaufman et al., 2018; Schulz & Sherwood, 2008).

Given this background, Sharma et al. (2016) proposed that the impact of gender may be mediated by other variables such as sociodemographic characteristics of patients and caregivers, as well as the sociocultural context. For example, specifically focusing on Latin America and the Caribbean, with their unique particularities in confronting dementia compared to the European scenario (Baez & Ibáñez, 2016), it can be noted that there are structural/systemic problems that contribute to the difficulties that dementia caregivers face in terms of prevention and promotion of mental health. Among such obstacles, the following have been mentioned: a scarcity of mental health facilities, cultural barriers and socioeconomic vulnerabilities, and shortage of formal long-term care (Ibáñez et al., 2021; Parra et al., 2018). All of this has placed most of the burden on informal care (Thrush & Hyder, 2014) and consequently led, in this group, to a higher vulnerability to experiencing depressive symptoms.

10.4 Management of Depressive Symptoms Among Dementia Caregivers

An early diagnosis improves the prognosis and effective management of mental health disorders. The WHO Mental Health Gap Action Program (mhGAP) recommends a combination of both antidepressant drugs and psychosocial interventions to address moderate to severe disorders (World Health Organization, 2011). Depression among caregivers of people living with dementia is managed with the same treatments available in primary and specialist care (NICE guideline, 2018). There are, however, specific interventions for dementia caregivers that have shown to be cost-effective with long-term effects in reducing depressive symptoms (Livingston et al., 2020a).

10.4.1 Psychoeducational Programs

Psychoeducational interventions have shown the most positive results in reducing depression symptoms among caregivers (Chien et al., 2011; Lee et al., 2020; Liu et al., 2017; Piersol et al., 2017). A recent systematic review compared the efficacy of remotely delivered interventions offering information (determined by the professional with the participant having a passive role), training (practical skills to manage the burden of care with an active role of caregivers) and support (participants discuss and share feelings, problems, or issues related to caring with peers or professionals), or a mixture of these. When compared to usual treatment, waiting list, or attention control, any of the above interventions have little or no effect on depressive symptoms (SMD = −0.05; 95% CI = −0.22 to 0.12). However, compared to a control group with only information, remotely delivered interventions involving training, support, or both had a small effect on caregivers' depressive symptoms (SMD = −0.25; 95% CI = −0.43 to −0.06; $I_2 = 53\%$) (González-Fraile et al., 2021).

10.4.2 Cognitive Behavioral Therapy

Cognitive behavioral therapy (CBT) has had the largest amount of evidence and has shown significant effects to reduce depressive symptoms among caregivers (Lee et al., 2020). CBT aims to empower people and promote self-agency, by working on automatic and dysfunctional thoughts (Hopkinson et al., 2019). In the case of caregivers, the principal outcomes are to change dysfunctional thoughts about caregiving and behavioral activation that enhances self-care strategies including leisure activities (Losada et al., 2011).

CBT has shown effectiveness in reducing depressive symptoms among caregivers of people living with dementia (Cheng et al., 2019). In a meta-analysis carried out by Hopkinson et al. (2019) including 25 randomized controlled trials (RCTs) published between 1996 and 2016, moderate quality of evidence was found for the effectiveness of CBT to reduce depression among caregivers. The authors reported statistically significant improvements of depression symptoms immediately after completing the intervention (standardized mean differences (SMD) = −0.34; 95% CI = −0.47–0.21; $p < 0.001$) and after up to 3 months of follow-up (SMD = −0.99; 95% CI = −1.35–0.64; $p < 0.001$). The authors also reported that brief versions (up to eight sessions) and longer versions (more than eight sessions) significantly improved caregivers' depressive symptoms.

Similarly, Sun et al. (2022) conducted a meta-analysis that aimed to compare CBT formats. They included 37 RCTs published between 2000 and 2021, obtaining standardized mean differences (SMD) and conducting a rank analysis based on P-scores to compare different formats to control groups. Higher P-score indicated a higher probability of a specific format being the best intervention. They found no significant differences between the formats of CBT. However, compared to control groups (no intervention or treatment as usual), CBT delivered over the Internet (SMD = −1.45; CI = −2.31, −0.28), telephone (SMD = −1.28; CI = −1.78, −0.53), and individual (SMD = −1.19; CI = −2.29, −0.31) reduced depressive symptoms and had the higher probabilities of being the best treatment for caregivers ($P_{\text{Internet}} = 0.811$; $P_{\text{telephone}} = 0.803$; $P_{\text{individual}} = 0.771$; $P_{\text{group}} = 0.440$; $P_{\text{combine}} = 0.334$; $P_{\text{control}} = 0.107$).

Finally, low-intensity CBT, which includes the delivery of the intervention in a short format or by a nonspecialized therapist, has shown effectiveness in reducing depressive symptoms among caregivers. Even though the effect size is smaller than the one found for traditional CBT, this format might be useful for countries with fewer resources for highly trained therapists (Kaddour et al., 2019).

10.4.3 Mindfulness-Based Interventions

Mindfulness interventions are based on meditative exercises, like meditation or yoga, to connect people with the present while helping them be aware of their experiences (thoughts, feelings, body sensations) and accept them. Mindfulness-based interventions (MBIs) are combinations between psychological therapies and mindfulness practices (Zhang et al., 2021). The most recognized ones are mindfulness-based cognitive therapy (MBCT) and mindfulness-based stress reduction (MBSR) (Han, 2021). Acceptance and commitment therapy (ACT) is also considered an MBI, but it will be reviewed separately in the following section.

MBIs have shown positive results to help caregivers with depression (Cheng & Zhang, 2020). Liu et al. (2017) reviewed seven RCTs focused on MBIs for dementia caregivers. The authors reported small heterogeneity across studies ($I_2 = 7\%$) and, compared with control groups, mindfulness training significantly decreased caregivers' depressive symptoms (SMD = −0.58; 95% CI = −0.79 to −0.37). Moreover, Cheng et al. (2020) analyzed 131 studies (RCTs and quasi RCTs) published between 2006 and 2018, including nine MBI studies. They converted the SMD to Hedges to correct for small samples bias. The authors found that MBIs were effective in reducing depressive symptoms ($g = 0.58$; $k = 7$; $N = 258$). Similarly, Han (2021) carried out a meta-analysis of 15 RCTs published between 1966 and 2021. From them, 11 were exclusively for caregivers with dementia and 4 had caregivers of other chronic conditions. The study analyzed the effectiveness of MBIs including MBCT, MBSR, ACT, and other forms of mindfulness. The authors reported that the effect of MBIs on reducing depressive symptoms was related to the type of control groups. At immediate posttest, a large effect was found when compared to passive control groups (SMD = 1.21; 95% CI = 0.67, 1.75), and a medium effect was found when compared to active control groups (SMD = 0.60; 95% CI = 0.39, 0.80).

10.4.4 Acceptance and Commitment Therapy

ACT is part of the contextualistic approaches of CBT, but it does not completely fit into traditional categories because of its flexibility in integrating mindfulness (Hayes, 2004). It addresses topics like feelings, values, or spirituality within specific contexts using techniques to overcome avoidant behaviors and thoughts while keeping the person in the present instead of focusing on the past or future experiences (Hayes, 2004).

According to ACT theory fundaments, psychological problems are rooted in six processes: (1) experiential avoidance, (2) cognitive fusion or controlling behavior through rigid verbal use, (3) loss of contact with values, (4) inaction produced by unalignment between behavior and values, (5) loss of contact with the present moment, and (6) conceptualized self, judging one's thoughts and emotions (Hayes, 2004; Hayes et al., 2006; Pachana & Laidlaw, 2014). Therefore, ACT's clinical aim is to reach behavioral flexibility to adapt and accept difficult scenarios. It focuses on helping people to solve problems by validating and accepting their experiences (feelings, thoughts, and behaviors) and connecting them with their values in life (Márquez-González et al., 2014). Rigidly believing the content of our thoughts, feelings, and body sensations, disconnected from our immediate experiences with the environment, creates avoidant behaviors and dysfunctional coping mechanisms and ultimately an unalignment between values and meaning of life. Therefore, ACT works with the client's use of language to redefine the problem and potential solutions (Hayes, 2004).

ACT has shown a moderate size effect and quality of evidence to reduce depression among the general population (Bai et al., 2020) and family caregivers of children, people with cancer or in palliative care, and people living with dementia (Han et al., 2020).

In the case of dementia caregivers, ACT aims to change the ideas or verbal rules related to caregiving (Pachana & Laidlaw, 2014). ACT has gained notice to support dementia caregivers because of the challenges of caring for a relative with multiple needs and progressive levels of dependency (Losada et al., 2015). Most dementia caregivers think about their relatives as completely dependent; therefore, they focus their lives to become the perfect caregiver. They usually reject help and avoid engaging in leisure activities or using their time to take care of themselves, including seeking health support. They also experience confronted feelings for their relatives (love, pain, frustration, tiredness, anger) and, consequently, feelings of guilt (Márquez-González et al., 2014). So far, ACT effectiveness for dementia caregivers' depression has been evaluated in two RCTs. Losada et al. (2015) carried out an RCT with 135 dementia family caregivers in Madrid, Spain. They designed a specific ACT intervention for caregivers that was compared to a minimal treatment condition. The intervention improved depressive symptoms immediately after the intervention (time by treatment effect estimate = 10.47; $p < 0.001$), but these differences did not remain at 6-month follow-up (time by treatment effect estimate = 3.48; $p = 0.196$). The authors also compared ACT with CBT for depressive symptoms. They did not find significant differences from baseline to posttreatment or from baseline to follow-up. Similarly, Márquez-González et al. (2020) conducted an RCT with 92 dementia caregivers. They were allocated to functional analysis-guided modular intervention (FAMI), ACT, CBT, or control group (CG) with 2 hours of psychoeducation workshop. The authors found that there was a higher decrease in depressive symptoms among the three treatment conditions compared to CG ($p < 0.005$), and this improvement was maintained in time (6-month follow-up).

There were no significant differences between FAMI, ACT, and CBT to treat caregivers' depression ($F_{(4, 78)} = 0.250$; $p = 0.909$). These promising results should, however, be further explored because of their attrition rate and sample sizes.

10.4.5 Other Non-pharmacological Interventions

Due to their easy access during the daytime and their adaptability, telephone- and computer-delivered interventions have been developed to support caregivers of people living with dementia. Telephone counseling and face-to-face technology-based counseling are effective interventions to address mental health issues among dementia caregivers (Teahan et al., 2020; Waller et al., 2017; Zhu et al., 2021). However, the effectiveness of both technological systems, used separately or combined, to reduce depressive symptoms, has had inconsistent results, and the quality of the studies has been rated as low or moderate. Thus, their impact still needs to be verified (Teahan et al., 2020; Waller et al., 2017; Zhu et al., 2021).

Physical exercise interventions have been widely recommended because of the number of RCTs that had reported statistically significant effects on reducing depressive symptoms and other mental health issues. However, the internal validity of their evidence makes it difficult to determine the quality of those results (Cuthbert et al., 2017).

Finally, multicomponent interventions have been developed to support family caregivers. Recently, Cheng and Zhang (2020) did not find advantages of multicomponent interventions over single interventions. However, the Strategies for Relatives (START) program, a multicomponent intervention for dementia caregivers, showed to be cost-effective for reducing depressive symptoms with an effect lasting from after the intervention up to 5 years. START is a manualized intervention delivered by graduate psychologists with no clinical training, which is key in health systems with a low rate of clinical specialists (Knapp et al., 2013; Livingston et al., 2013; Livingston et al., 2020b).

10.5 Conclusion

The relationship between caregivers' mental health and the quality of life and prognosis of people living with dementia has led to the inclusion of caregivers in dementia policies and national care plans (Livingston et al., 2020a). Comprehensive management of dementia usually encompasses psychoeducation, training, and counseling in coordination with mental health-care interventions. Linking caregivers with support networks is essential for helping them, and it has been considered among different dementia national plans in Europe and countries in other regions (Tokovska et al., 2021). In addition, exchanging experiences with people living with dementia and other relatives has improved caregivers' mental health, including the reduction of depressive symptoms (Carter et al., 2020). Evidence confirms the use of non-pharmacological interventions to manage caregivers' depressive symptoms (González-Fraile et al., 2021), especially CBT, and mindfulness-based programs (Cheng et al., 2019; Han, 2021; Hopkinson et al., 2019; Kaddour et al., 2019; Liu et al., 2017; Sun et al., 2022). ACT has shown promising results; however, more research is needed to find out whether its effects are long-lasting and cost-effective (Losada et al., 2015; Márquez-González et al., 2020). Other interventions have been analyzed including social peer support groups, exercise, and counseling or a combination of all. Evidence does not support dyadic or multicomponent interventions over single-component interventions (Cheng & Zhang, 2020).

Acknowledgments This work was supported by ANID – Millennium Science Initiative Program – ICS13_005 and ICS2019_024. In addition, CM-C received funding from ANID – FONDECYT – 1191726, and TT-M from ANID – Doctorado Internacional/2020-72210393.

References

Alzheimer's UK. (2018). *Women and dementia: A marginalised majority*. https://www.alzheimersresearchuk.org/about-us/our-influence/policy-%0Awork/reports/women-dementia/

Baez, S., & Ibáñez, A. (2016). Dementia in Latin America: An emergent silent tsunami. *Frontiers in Aging Neuroscience, 8*, 253. https://doi.org/10.3389/fnagi.2016.00253

Bai, Z., Luo, S., Zhang, L., Wu, S., & Chi, I. (2020). Acceptance and commitment therapy (ACT) to reduce depression: A systematic review and meta-analysis. *Journal of Affective Disorders, 260*, 728–737. https://doi.org/10.1016/j.jad.2019.09.040

Carter, G., Monaghan, C., & Santin, O. (2020). What is known from the existing literature about peer support interventions for carers of individuals living with dementia: A scoping review. *Health & Social Care in the Community, 28*(4), 1134–1151. https://doi.org/10.1111/hsc.12944

Cheng, S.-T. (2017). Dementia caregiver burden: A research update and critical analysis. *Current Psychiatry Reports, 19*(9), 64. https://doi.org/10.1007/s11920-017-0818-2

Cheng, S.-T., Au, A., Losada, A., Thompson, L. W., & Gallagher-Thompson, D. (2019). Psychological interventions for dementia caregivers: What we have achieved, what we have learned. *Current Psychiatry Reports, 21*(7), 59. https://doi.org/10.1007/s11920-019-1045-9

Cheng, S.-T., Li, K.-K., Losada, A., Zhang, F., Au, A., Thompson, L. W., & Gallagher-Thompson, D. (2020). The effectiveness of nonpharmacological interventions for informal dementia caregivers: An updated systematic review and meta-analysis. *Psychology and Aging, 35*(1), 55–77. https://doi.org/10.1037/pag0000401

Cheng, S.-T., & Zhang, F. (2020). A comprehensive meta-review of systematic reviews and meta-analyses on nonpharmacological interventions for informal dementia caregivers. *BMC Geriatrics, 20*(1), 137. https://doi.org/10.1186/s12877-020-01547-2

Chien, L.-Y., Chu, H., Guo, J.-L., Liao, Y.-M., Chang, L.-I., Chen, C.-H., & Chou, K.-R. (2011). Caregiver support groups in patients with dementia: A meta-analysis. *International Journal of Geriatric Psychiatry, 26*(10), 1089–1098. https://doi.org/10.1002/gps.2660

Clay, O. J., Roth, D. L., Wadley, V. G., & Haley, W. E. (2008). Changes in social support and their impact on psychosocial outcome over a 5-year period for African American and White dementia caregivers. *International Journal of Geriatric Psychiatry, 23*(8), 857–862. https://doi.org/10.1002/gps.1996

Conde-Sala, J. L., Garre-Olmo, J., Turró-Garriga, O., Vilalta-Franch, J., & López-Pousa, S. (2010). Differential features of burden between spouse and adult-child caregivers of patients with

Alzheimer's disease: An exploratory comparative design. *International Journal of Nursing Studies, 47*(10), 1262–1273. https://doi.org/10.1016/j.ijnurstu.2010.03.001

Cooper, C., Balamurali, T. B. S., & Livingston, G. (2007). A systematic review of the prevalence and covariates of anxiety in caregivers of people with dementia. *International Psychogeriatrics, 19*(2), 175–195. https://doi.org/10.1017/S1041610206004297

Cuthbert, C. A., King-Shier, K., Ruether, D., Tapp, D. M., & Culos-Reed, S. N. (2017). What is the state of the science on physical activity interventions for family caregivers? A systematic review and RE-AIM evaluation. *Journal of Physical Activity & Health, 14*(7), 578–595. https://doi.org/10.1123/jpah.2016-0280

D'Aoust, R. F., Brewster, G., & Rowe, M. A. (2015). Depression in informal caregivers of persons with dementia. *International Journal of Older People Nursing, 10*(1), 14–26. https://doi.org/10.1111/opn.12043

De Fazio, P., Ciambrone, P., Cerminara, G., Barbuto, E., Bruni, A., Gentile, P., Talarico, A., Lacava, R., Gareri, P., & Segura-García, C. (2015). Depressive symptoms in caregivers of patients with dementia: Demographic variables and burden. *Clinical Interventions in Aging, 10*, 1085–1090. https://doi.org/10.2147/CIA.S74439

Epstein-Lubow, G., Davis, J. D., Miller, I. W., & Tremont, G. (2008). Persisting burden predicts depressive symptoms in dementia caregivers. *Journal of Geriatric Psychiatry and Neurology, 21*(3), 198–203. https://doi.org/10.1177/0891988708320972

Fauth, E., Hess, K., Piercy, K., Norton, M., Corcoran, C., Rabins, P., Lyketsos, C., & Tschanz, J. (2012). Caregivers' relationship closeness with the person with dementia predicts both positive and negative outcomes for caregivers' physical health and psychological well-being. *Aging & Mental Health, 16*(6), 699–711. https://doi.org/10.1080/13607863.2012.678482

García-Alberca, J. M., Cruz, B., Lara, J. P., Garrido, V., Lara, A., & Gris, E. (2012). Anxiety and depression are associated with coping strategies in caregivers of Alzheimer's disease patients: Results from the MÁLAGA-AD study. *International Psychogeriatrics, 24*(8), 1325–1334. https://doi.org/10.1017/S1041610211002948

González-Fraile, E., Ballesteros, J., Rueda, J.-R., Santos-Zorrozúa, B., Solà, I., & McCleery, J. (2021). Remotely delivered information, training and support for informal caregivers of people with dementia. *The Cochrane Database of Systematic Reviews, 1*(1), CD006440. https://doi.org/10.1002/14651858.CD006440.pub3

Greenwood, N., & Smith, R. (2016). The oldest carers: A narrative review and synthesis of the experiences of carers aged over 75 years. *Maturitas, 94*, 161–172. https://doi.org/10.1016/j.maturitas.2016.10.001

Hayes, S. C. (2004). Acceptance and commitment therapy, relational frame theory, and the third wave of behavioral and cognitive therapies. *Behavior Therapy, 35*, 639–665. https://doi.org/10.1016/S0005-7894(04)80013-3

Hayes, S. C., Luoma, J. B., Bond, F. W., Masuda, A., & Lillis, J. (2006). Acceptance and commitment therapy: model, processes and outcomes. *Behaviour Research and Therapy, 44*(1), 1–25. https://doi.org/10.1016/j.brat.2005.06.006

Haley, W. E., Roth, D. L., Howard, G., & Safford, M. M. (2010). Caregiving strain and estimated risk for stroke and coronary heart disease among spouse caregivers: Differential effects by race and sex. *Stroke, 41*(2), 331–336. https://doi.org/10.1161/STROKEAHA.109.568279

Han, A. (2021). Effects of mindfulness-based interventions on depressive symptoms, anxiety, stress, and quality of life in family caregivers of persons living with dementia: A systematic review and meta-analysis. *Research on Aging, 44*(7-8), 494–509. https://doi.org/10.1177/01640275211043486

Han, A., Yuen, H. K., & Jenkins, J. (2020). Acceptance and commitment therapy for family caregivers: A systematic review and meta-analysis. *Journal of Health Psychology, 26*(1), 82–102. https://doi.org/10.1177/1359105320941217

Hopkinson, M. D., Reavell, J., Lane, D. A., & Mallikarjun, P. (2019). Cognitive behavioral therapy for depression, anxiety, and stress in caregivers of dementia patients: A systematic review and meta-analysis. *The Gerontologist, 59*(4), e343–e362. https://doi.org/10.1093/geront/gnx217

Ibáñez, A., Pina-Escudero, S. D., Possin, K. L., Quiroz, Y. T., Peres, F. A., Slachevsky, A., Sosa, A. L., Brucki, S. M. D., & Miller, B. L. (2021). Dementia caregiving across Latin America and the Caribbean and brain health diplomacy. *The Lancet Healthy Longevity, 2*(4), e222–e231. https://doi.org/10.1016/S2666-7568(21)00031-3

Joling, K. J., O'Dwyer, S. T., Hertogh, C. M. P. M., & van Hout, H. P. J. (2018). The occurrence and persistence of thoughts of suicide, self-harm and death in family caregivers of people with dementia: A longitudinal data analysis over 2 years. *International Journal of Geriatric Psychiatry, 33*(2), 263–270. https://doi.org/10.1002/gps.4708

Joling, K. J., Smit, F., van Marwijk, H. W. J., van der Horst, H. E., Scheltens, P., Schulz, R., & van Hout, H. P. J. (2012). Identifying target groups for the prevention of depression among caregivers of dementia patients. *International Psychogeriatrics, 24*(2), 298–306. https://doi.org/10.1017/S1041610211001633

Joling, K. J., van Hout, H. P. J., Schellevis, F. G., van der Horst, H. E., Scheltens, P., Knol, D. L., & van Marwijk, H. W. J. (2010). Incidence of depression and anxiety in the spouses of patients with dementia: A naturalistic cohort study of recorded morbidity with a 6-year follow-up. *The American Journal of Geriatric Psychiatry: Official Journal of the American Association for Geriatric Psychiatry, 18*(2), 146–153. https://doi.org/10.1097/JGP.0b013e3181bf9f0f

Joling, K. J., van Marwijk, H. W. J., Veldhuijzen, A. E., van der Horst, H. E., Scheltens, P., Smit, F., & van Hout, H. P. J. (2015). The two-year incidence of depression and anxiety disorders in spousal caregivers of persons with dementia: Who is at the greatest risk? *The American Journal of Geriatric Psychiatry: Official Journal of the American Association for Geriatric Psychiatry, 23*(3), 293–303. https://doi.org/10.1016/j.jagp.2014.05.005

Kaddour, L., Kishita, N., & Schaller, A. (2019). A meta-analysis of low-intensity cognitive behavioral therapy-based interventions for dementia caregivers. *International Psychogeriatrics, 31*(7), 961–976. https://doi.org/10.1017/S1041610218001436

Kaufman, J. E., Lee, Y., Vaughon, W., Unuigbe, A., & Gallo, W. T. (2018). Depression associated with transitions into and out of spousal caregiving. *The International Journal of Aging and Human Development, 88*(2), 127–149. https://doi.org/10.1177/0091415018754310

Knapp, M., King, D., Romeo, R., Schehl, B., Barber, J., Griffin, M., Rapaport, P., Livingston, D., Mummery, C., Walker, Z., Hoe, J., Sampson, E. L., Cooper, C., & Livingston, G. (2013). Cost effectiveness of a manual based coping strategy programme in promoting the mental health of family carers of people with dementia (the START (STrAtegies for RelaTives) study): A pragmatic randomised controlled trial. *British Medical Journal, 347*, f6342. https://doi.org/10.1136/bmj.f6342

Lee, M., Ryoo, J. H., Chung, M., Anderson, J. G., Rose, K., & Williams, I. C. (2020). Effective interventions for depressive symptoms among caregivers of people with dementia: A systematic review and meta-analysis. *Dementia (London, England), 19*(7), 2368–2398. https://doi.org/10.1177/1471301218822640

Li, R., Cooper, C., & Livingston, G. (2014). Relationship of coping style to mood and anxiety disorders in dementia carers. *Current Opinion in Psychiatry, 27*(1), 52–56. https://journals.lww.com/co-psychiatry/Fulltext/2014/01000/Relationship_of_coping_style_to_mood_and_anxiety.10.aspx

Liu, Z., Chen, Q.-L., & Sun, Y.-Y. (2017). Mindfulness training for psychological stress in family caregivers of persons with dementia: A systematic review and meta-analysis of randomized controlled trials. *Clinical Interventions in Aging, 12*, 1521–1529. https://doi.org/10.2147/CIA.S146213

Livingston, G., Barber, J., Rapaport, P., Knapp, M., Griffin, M., King, D., Livingston, D., Mummery, C., Walker, Z., Hoe, J., Sampson, E. L., & Cooper, C. (2013). Clinical effectiveness of a manual based coping strategy programme (START, STrAtegies for RelaTives) in promoting the mental health of carers of family members with dementia: Pragmatic randomised controlled trial. *British Medical Journal (Clinical Research Ed.), 347*, f6276. https://doi.org/10.1136/bmj.f6276

Livingston, G., Huntley, J., Sommerlad, A., Ames, D., Ballard, C., Banerjee, S., Brayne, C., Burns, A., Cohen-Mansfield, J., Cooper, C., Costafreda, S. G., Dias, A., Fox, N., Gitlin, L. N., Howard, R., Kales, H. C., Kivimäki, M., Larson, E. B., Ogunniyi, A., et al. (2020a). Dementia prevention, intervention, and care: 2020 report of the Lancet Commission. *Lancet (London, England), 396*(10248), 413–446. https://doi.org/10.1016/S0140-6736(20)30367-6

Livingston, G., Manela, M., O'Keeffe, A., Rapaport, P., Cooper, C., Knapp, M., King, D., Romeo, R., Walker, Z., Hoe, J., Mummery, C., & Barber, J. (2020b). Clinical effectiveness of the START (STrAtegies for RelaTives) psychological intervention for family carers and the effects on the cost of care for people with dementia: 6-year follow-up of a randomised controlled trial. *The British Journal of Psychiatry, 216*(1), 35–42. https://doi.org/10.1192/bjp.2019.160

Losada, A., Márquez-González, M., & Romero-Moreno, R. (2011). Mechanisms of action of a psychological intervention for dementia caregivers: Effects of behavioral activation and modification of dysfunctional thoughts. *International Journal of Geriatric Psychiatry, 26*(11), 1119–1127. https://doi.org/10.1002/gps.2648

Losada, A., Márquez-González, M., Romero-Moreno, R., Mausbach, B. T., López, J., Fernández-Fernández, V., & Nogales-González, C. (2015). Cognitive-behavioral therapy (CBT) versus acceptance and commitment therapy (ACT) for dementia family caregivers with significant depressive symptoms: Results of a randomized clinical trial. *Journal of Consulting and Clinical Psychology, 83*(4), 760–772. https://doi.org/10.1037/ccp0000028

Madaleno, T. R., Moriguti, J. C., Ferriolli, E., De Carlo, M. M. R. P., & Lima, N. K. C. (2019). Mood, lifestyle and cardiovascular risk factors among older caregivers of patients with Alzheimer's disease dementia: A case-control study. *Aging Clinical and Experimental Research, 31*(11), 1609–1614. https://doi.org/10.1007/s40520-019-01212-8

Márquez-González, M., Losada, A., & Romero-Moreno, R. (2014). Acceptance and commitment therapy with dementia care-givers. In N. Pachana & K. Laidlaw (Eds.), *The Oxford handbook of clinical geropsychology*. Oxford University Press.

Márquez-González, M., Romero-Moreno, R., Cabrera, I., Olmos, R., Pérez-Miguel, A., & Losada, A. (2020). Tailored versus manualized interventions for dementia caregivers: The functional analysis-guided modular intervention. *Psychology and Aging, 35*(1), 41–54. https://doi.org/10.1037/pag0000412

Martire, L. M., & Schulz, R. (2012). Caregiving and care receiving in later life: Health effects and promising interventions. In *Handbook of health psychology* (2nd ed., pp. 293–307). Psychology Press.

Mausbach, B. T., Patterson, T. L., Von Känel, R., Mills, P. J., Dimsdale, J. E., Ancoli-Israel, S., & Grant, I. (2007). The attenuating effect of personal mastery on the relations between stress and Alzheimer caregiver health: A five-year longitudinal analysis. *Aging & Mental Health, 11*(6), 637–644. https://doi.org/10.1080/13607860701787043

NICE Guideline. (2018). *Dementia: Assessment, management and support for people living with dementia and their carers*. https://www.nice.org.uk/guidance/ng97/resources/dementia-assessment-management-and-support-for-people-living-with-dementia-and-their-carers-pdf-1837760199109

O'Dwyer, S. T., Moyle, W., Zimmer-Gembeck, M., & De Leo, D. (2016). Suicidal ideation in family carers of people with dementia. *Aging & Mental Health, 20*(2), 222–230. https://doi.org/10.1080/13607863.2015.1063109

O'Rourke, N., Kupferschmidt, A. L., Claxton, A., Smith, J. Z., Chappell, N., & Beattie, B. L. (2010). Psychological resilience predicts depressive symptoms among spouses of persons with Alzheimer disease over time. *Aging & Mental Health, 14*(8), 984–993. https://doi.org/10.1080/13607863.2010.501063

Oliveira, D., Vass, C., & Aubeeluck, A. (2019). Quality of life on the views of older family carers of people with dementia. *Dementia (London, England), 18*(3), 990–1009. https://doi.org/10.1177/1471301217700741

Ornstein, K., Gaugler, J. E., Zahodne, L., & Stern, Y. (2014). The heterogeneous course of depressive symptoms for the dementia caregiver. *International Journal of Aging & Human Development, 78*(2), 133–148. https://doi.org/10.2190/AG.78.2.c

Pachana, N., & Laidlaw, K. (Eds.). (2014). *The Oxford handbook of clinical geropsychology*. Oxford University Press. https://doi.org/10.1093/oxfordhb/9780199663170.001.0001

Parra, M. A., Baez, S., Allegri, R., Nitrini, R., Lopera, F., Slachevsky, A., Custodio, N., Lira, D., Piguet, O., Kumfor, F., Huepe, D., Cogram, P., Bak, T., Manes, F., & Ibanez, A. (2018). Dementia in Latin America: Assessing the present and envisioning the future. *Neurology, 90*(5), 222–231. https://doi.org/10.1212/WNL.0000000000004897

Perkins, M., Howard, V. J., Wadley, V. G., Crowe, M., Safford, M. M., Haley, W. E., Howard, G., & Roth, D. L. (2013). Caregiving strain and all-cause mortality: Evidence from the REGARDS study. *The Journals of Gerontology. Series B, Psychological Sciences and Social Sciences, 68*(4), 504–512. https://doi.org/10.1093/geronb/gbs084

Piersol, C. V., Canton, K., Connor, S. E., Giller, I., Lipman, S., & Sager, S. (2017). Effectiveness of interventions for caregivers of people with Alzheimer's disease and related major neurocognitive disorders: A systematic review. *The American Journal of Occupational Therapy: Official Publication of the American Occupational Therapy Association, 71*(5), 7105180020p1–7105180020p10. https://doi.org/10.5014/ajot.2017.027581

Pillemer, S., Davis, J., & Tremont, G. (2018). Gender effects on components of burden and depression among dementia caregivers. *Aging & Mental Health, 22*(9), 1156–1161. https://doi.org/10.1080/13607863.2017.1337718

Pinquart, M., & Sörensen, S. (2003). Differences between caregivers and noncaregivers in psychological health and physical health: A meta-analysis. *Psychology and Aging, 18*(2), 250–267. https://doi.org/10.1037/0882-7974.18.2.250

Queluz, F. N. F. R., Kervin, E., Wozney, L., Fancey, P., McGrath, P. J., & Keefe, J. (2020). Understanding the needs of caregivers of persons with dementia: A scoping review. *International Psychogeriatrics, 32*(1), 35–52. https://doi.org/10.1017/S1041610219000243

Rigby, T., Ashwill, R. T., Johnson, D. K., & Galvin, J. E. (2019). Differences in the experience of caregiving between spouse and adult child caregivers in dementia with Lewy bodies. *Innovation in Aging, 3*(3), igz027. https://doi.org/10.1093/geroni/igz027

Romero-Moreno, R., Márquez-González, M., Mausbach, B. T., & Losada, A. (2012). Variables modulating depression in dementia caregivers: A longitudinal study. *International Psychogeriatrics, 24*(8), 1316–1324. https://doi.org/10.1017/S1041610211002237

Sallim, A. B., Sayampanathan, A. A., Cuttilan, A., & Ho, R. (2015). Prevalence of mental health disorders among caregivers of patients with Alzheimer disease. *Journal of the American Medical Directors Association, 16*(12), 1034–1041. https://doi.org/10.1016/j.jamda.2015.09.007

Schoenmakers, B., Buntinx, F., & Delepeleire, J. (2010). Factors determining the impact of care-giving on caregivers of elderly patients with dementia. A systematic literature review. *Maturitas, 66*(2), 191–200. https://doi.org/10.1016/j.maturitas.2010.02.009

Schulz, R., & Sherwood, P. R. (2008). Physical and mental health effects of family caregiving. *The American Journal of Nursing, 108*(9 Suppl), 23–27. https://doi.org/10.1097/01.NAJ.0000336406.45248.4c

Sharma, N., Chakrabarti, S., & Grover, S. (2016). Gender differences in caregiving among family – caregivers of people with mental illnesses. *World Journal of Psychiatry, 6*(1), 7–17. https://doi.org/10.5498/wjp.v6.i1.7

Sun, Y., Ji, M., Leng, M., & Wang, Z. (2022). Which cognitive behavioral therapy delivery formats work for depressive symptoms in dementia caregivers?—A systematic review and network meta-analysis of randomized controlled trials. *Journal of Affective Disorders, 308*, 181–187. https://doi.org/10.1016/j.jad.2022.04.055

Teahan, Á., Lafferty, A., McAuliffe, E., Phelan, A., O'Sullivan, L., O'Shea, D., Nicholson, E., & Fealy, G. (2020). Psychosocial interventions for family carers of people with dementia: A systematic review and meta-analysis. *Journal of Aging and Health, 32*(9), 1198–1213. https://doi.org/10.1177/0898264319899793

Thrush, A., & Hyder, A. A. (2014). The neglected burden of caregiving in low- and middle-income countries. *Disability and Health Journal, 7*(3), 262–272. https://doi.org/10.1016/j.dhjo.2014.01.003

Tokovska, M., Nour, M. M., Sørensen, A., & Småland Goth, U. (2021). Informal caregivers and psychosocial support: Analysis of European Dementia Policy documents. *Journal of Public Health Research, 11*(1), 2416. https://doi.org/10.4081/jphr.2021.2416

Tzuang, M., & Gallagher-Thompson, D. (2015). Caring for care-givers of a person with dementia. In N. Pachana & K. Laidlaw (Eds.), *The Oxford handbook of clinical geropsychology* (pp. 797–836). Oxford University Press.

United Nations. (2020). *World population ageing 2019: Highlights*. https://www.un.org/en/development/desa/population/publications/pdf/ageing/WorldPopulationAgeing2019-Highlights.pdf

Verma, R., & Anand, K. S. (2012). Gender differences in anxiety and depression among the caregivers of patients with dementia. *Advances in Alzheimer's Disease, 1*(3), 17–21. https://doi.org/10.4236/aad.2012.13003

Waller, A., Dilworth, S., Mansfield, E., & Sanson-Fisher, R. (2017). Computer and telephone delivered interventions to support caregivers of people with dementia: A systematic review of research output and quality. *BMC Geriatrics, 17*(1), 265. https://doi.org/10.1186/s12877-017-0654-6

Walter, E., & Pinquart, M. (2020). How effective are dementia caregiver interventions? An updated comprehensive meta-analysis. *The Gerontologist, 60*(8), 609–619. https://doi.org/10.1093/geront/gnz118

Watson, B., Tatangelo, G., & McCabe, M. (2019). Depression and anxiety among partner and offspring carers of people with dementia: A systematic review. *The Gerontologist, 59*(5), e597–e610. https://doi.org/10.1093/geront/gny049

Watt, J. A., Goodarzi, Z., Veroniki, A. A., Nincic, V., Khan, P. A., Ghassemi, M., Thompson, Y., Tricco, A. C., & Straus, S. E. (2019). Comparative efficacy of interventions for aggressive and agitated behaviors in dementia: A systematic review and network meta-analysis. *Annals of Internal Medicine, 171*(9), 633–642. https://doi.org/10.7326/M19-0993

Wimo, A., Prince, M., & Gauthier, S. (2018). *Global estimates of informal care*. https://www.alz.co.uk/adi/pdf/global-estimates-of-informal-care.pdf

World Health Organization. (2011). *mhGAP Intervention Guide for mental, neurological and substance use disorders in non-specialized health settings*.

World Health Organization. (2018). *ICD11 – The International Classification of Diseases* (11th rev.). https://www.who.int/classifications/icd/en/

World Health Organization. (2021). *Global status report on the public health response to dementia*. https://apps.who.int/iris/handle/10665/344701

Xiong, C., Biscardi, M., Astell, A., Nalder, E., Cameron, J. I., Mihailidis, A., & Colantonio, A. (2020). Sex and gender differences in caregiving burden experienced by family caregivers of persons with dementia: A systematic review. *PLoS One, 15*(4), e0231848. https://doi.org/10.1371/journal.pone.0231848

Zhang, D., Lee, E. K. P., Mak, E. C. W., Ho, C. Y., & Wong, S. Y. S. (2021). Mindfulness-based interventions: An overall review. *British Medical Bulletin, 138*(1), 41–57. https://doi.org/10.1093/bmb/ldab005

Zhu, A., Cao, W., Zhou, Y., Xie, A., Cheng, Y., & Chu, S.-F. (2021). Tele-health intervention for carers of dementia patients-a systematic review and meta-analysis of randomized controlled trials. In *Frontiers in aging neuroscience* (Vol. 13, p. 612404). https://doi.org/10.3389/fnagi.2021.612404

Index

V. Martínez, C. Miranda-Castillo (eds.), *Prevention and Early Treatment of Depression Through the Life Course*, Depression and Personality,
https://doi.org/10.1007/978-3-031-13029-8

Ingram Content Group UK Ltd.
Milton Keynes UK
UKHW020643170323
418722UK00003B/63

9 783031 130281